CASE REVIEW

Genitourinary Imaging

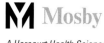

Mosby

A Harcourt Health Sciences Company

St. Louis   London   Philadelphia   Sydney   Toronto

Glenn A. Tung, MD
Associate Professor
Department of Diagnostic Imaging
Brown University School of Medicine
Providence, Rhode Island

Ronald J. Zagoria, MD
Professor of Radiology
Wake Forest University School of Medicine
Winston-Salem, North Carolina

William W. Mayo-Smith, MD
Associate Professor
Department of Diagnostic Imaging
Brown University School of Medicine
Providence, Rhode Island

WITH 413 ILLUSTRATIONS

CASE REVIEW

Genitourinary Imaging

CASE REVIEW SERIES

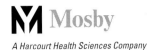

Acquisitions Editor: Stephanie Smith Donley
Project Manager: Carol Sullivan Weis
Project Specialist: Christine Carroll Schwepker
Designer: Mark Oberkrom

Mosby, Inc.
A Harcourt Health Sciences Company
11830 Westline Industrial Drive
St. Louis, Missouri 63146

Printed in the United States of America

Library of Congress Cataloging in Publication Data

Tung, Glenn A.
   Gastrointestinal imaging: case review / Glenn A. Tung, Ronald J. Zagoria,
William W. Mayo-Smith.
       p. ; cm. — (Case review series)
Cross-referenced to: Genitourinary radiology / Ronald J. Zagoria, Glenn A. Tung. c1997.
   Includes bibliographical references and index.
   ISBN 0-323-00657-4
     1. Genitourinary organs—Imaging—Case studies. I. Zagoria, Ronald J. II. Mayo-
Smith, William W. III. Zagoria, Ronald J. Genitourinary radiology. IV. Title. V. Series.
     [DNLM: 1. Urogenital Diseases—diagnosis—Examination Questions. 2. Diagnostic
Imaging—Examination Questions. WJ 18.2 T926g 2000]
RC874.T76 2000
616.6'0754'076—dc21

        00-028387

00 01 02 03 04 TG/MVY 9 8 7 6 5 4 3 2 1

To my parents, C.C. and Lillian,
To my dear wife, Nadine, and our sons,
Matthew and Eric,
Thank you for your love and encouragement.

To my colleagues, Jeffrey M. Brody,
John J. Cronan, and Jeffrey M. Rogg,
You have taught me as much through your
friendship as through your intellect.
GAT

To my wife and sons,
The joys of my life.
RJZ

To Margaret and Bill, who cultivate intellectual
curiosity,
To Leslie, who has supported me throughout,
And to the cool hat trick of James, Andrew, and
Christopher, who keep it all in perspective.
WWM-S

My experience in teaching medical students, residents, fellows, practicing radiologists, and clinicians has been that they love the case conference format more than any other approach. I hope that the reason for this is not a reflection on my lecturing ability, but rather that people stay awake, alert, and on their toes more when they are in the hot seat (or may be the next person to assume the hot seat). In the dozens of continuing medical education courses I have directed, the case review sessions are almost always the most popular parts of the courses.

The idea of this Case Review series grew out of a need for books designed as exam preparation tools for the resident, fellow, or practicing radiologist about to take the boards or the certificate of additional qualification (CAQ) exams. Anxiety runs extremely high concerning the content of these exams, administered as unknown cases. Residents, fellows, and practicing radiologists are very hungry for formats that mimic this exam setting and that cover the types of cases they will encounter and have to accurately describe. In addition, books of this ilk serve as excellent practical reviews of a field and can help a practicing board-certified radiologist keep his or her skills sharpened. Thus heads banged together, and Mosby and I arrived at the format of the volume herein, which is applied consistently to each volume in the series. We believe that these volumes will strengthen the ability of the reader to interpret studies. By formatting the individual cases so that they can "stand alone," these case review books can be read in a leisurely fashion, a case at a time, on the whim of the reader.

The content of each volume is organized into three sections based on difficulty of interpretation and/or the rarity of the lesion presented. There are the Opening Round cases, which graduating radiology residents should have relatively little difficulty mastering. The Fair Game section consists of cases that require more study, but most people should get into the ballpark with their differential diagnoses. Finally, there is the Challenge section. Most fellows or fellowship-trained practicing radiologists will be able to mention entities in the differential diagnoses of these challenging cases, but one shouldn't expect to consistently "hit home runs" a la Mark McGwire. The Challenge cases are really designed to whet one's appetite for further reading on these entities and to test one's wits. Within each of these sections, the selection of cases is entirely random, as one would expect at the boards (in your office or in Louisville).

For many cases in this series, a specific diagnosis may not be what is expected—the quality of the differential diagnosis and the inclusion of appropriate options are most important. Teaching how to distinguish between the diagnostic options (taught in the question and answer and comment sections) will be the goal of the authors of each Case Review volume.

The best way to go through these books is to look at the images, guess the diagnosis, answer the questions, and then turn the page for the answers. If there are two cases on a page, do them two at a time. No peeking!

Mosby (through the strong work of Liz Corra) and I have recruited most of the authors of THE REQUISITES series (editor, James Thrall, MD) to create Case Review books for their subspecialties. To meet the needs of certain subspecialties and to keep each of the volumes to a consistent, practical size, some specialties will have more than one volume (e.g., ultrasound, interventional and vascular radiology, and neuroradiology). Nonetheless, the pleasing tone of THE REQUISITES series and its emphasis on condensing the fields of radiology into its foundations will be inculcated into the Case Review volumes. In many situations, THE REQUISITES authors have enlisted new coauthors to breathe a novel approach and excitement into the cases submitted. I think the fact that so many of THE REQUISITES authors are "on board" for this new series is a testament to their dedication to teaching. I hope that the success of THE REQUISITES is duplicated with the new Case Review series. Just as THE REQUISITES series provides coverage of the essentials in each subspecialty and successfully meets that overwhelming need in the market, I hope that the Case Review series successfully meets the overwhelming need in the market for practical, focused case reviews.

David M. Yousem, MD

The goal of the Case Review series is to supplement and reinforce the concepts and teachings that are put in a more didactic form in THE REQUISITES series. It was recognized that whereas some students learn best in a noninteractive "study-book" mode, others need the anxiety or excitement of being quizzed, being put on the hot seat. The format that was selected for the Case Review series (i.e., showing a limited number of images needed to construct a differential diagnosis and asking a few clinical and imaging questions) was designed to simulate the boards experience. The only difference is that the Case Review books provide the correct answer and immediate feedback. Cases are scaled from relatively easy to very hard to test the limit of the reader's knowledge. In addition, a brief authors' commentary, a link back to THE REQUISITES volume, and an up-to-date reference to the literature are provided. Most importantly the images in the cases are of the highest pictorial quality and relevance.

Glenn Tung, Ron Zagoria, and Bill Mayo-Smith are well known to students of radiology, having already produced the critically acclaimed *Genitourinary Radiology: THE REQUISITES.* These authors know the most effective means to teach residents, update private practitioners, and tweak the academic superstars with interesting cases in their field. They have certainly fulfilled the mission of the Case Review series by providing a balanced array of cases from different modalities, pathologies, and difficulty. From a ball to a bean and the lesions in between, the reader is treated to a tour de force of genitourinary radiology via the Case Review approach. The result is "must" reading.

I welcome the Genitourinary Imaging volume by Drs. Tung, Zagoria, and Mayo-Smith to the previously published Gastrointestinal Imaging (by Peter Feczko and Robert Halpert), Brain Imaging (by Laurie Loevner), and Head and Neck Imaging (by David Yousem) contributions to the Case Review series.

David M. Yousem, MD

When David Yousem, the Case Review series editor, approached Ron and me to write a companion book to *Genitourinary Radiology: THE REQUISITES* textbook, I wish I could tell you that we agreed to the project immediately. The truth is that Ron bought into the concept immediately and my first reaction was "I'll need a good psychiatrist to get through another book." My second thought was "I'll need Bill Mayo-Smith to get through another book." Bill was much more helpful than the psychiatrist (although he's not much of a poet [see below]), and voilà, here is the book.

In all honesty, Ron, Bill, and I like the format of this book. It is modeled after both the oral board examination in radiology (for which both Ron and Bill have served as testers) and the teaching conferences that we give to our residents. The case series format is straightforward. On each right-hand page, one or two cases are illustrated by one or two figures each and followed by four related questions. On the back page are the answers to those questions, key references to the recent literature, a cross-reference to *Genitourinary Radiology: THE REQUISITES*, and a one- or two-paragraph comment section. In many ways this book is an excellent companion to our first book because the types of cases were selected from the subject matter of Chapters 2 through 10 of THE REQUISITES textbook. The organization of the 200 cases into three groups based on difficulty is a standard that Dave Yousem insisted on and adds to the challenge of the book. We hope that *Genitourinary Imaging: Case Review* helps you to learn about this interesting and challenging subspecialty of radiology.

Oh, by the way, Bill adds the following words of wisdom:

Lectures can be boring,
Most textbooks are long,
We hope cases are the answer,
To keep your knowledge strong.

See what I mean?

Glenn A. Tung, MD

I gratefully acknowledge Drs. Ronald J. Zagoria, Jeffrey M. Brody, and Damian Dupuy for contributing many of their most interesting teaching cases to this book. In addition, many residents and fellows in the Department of Diagnostic Imaging at the Brown University School of Medicine made substantive contributions to this book. My sincere thanks are extended to Drs. Sun-ho Ahn, Jane A. Auger, Patricia B. Delzell, Mark A. Geist, Allan I. Hoffman, Khursheed Imam, Asim A. Khwaja, Michael Merport, John A. Pezzullo, and Catherine Petchprapa for contributing cases and text. I would also like to acknowledge Dr. Judy Song for her help in organizing my teaching case material. Finally, I want thank my colleagues in the Department of Diagnostic Imaging for their support of academic efforts and for their dedication to teaching our residents, fellows, and medical students.

GAT

Writing a book, I have found, is no small task and requires the efforts of many people. Thanks to the residents at Brown, who keep me honest. In particular, I want to thank Drs. Sun-ho Ahn, Jane Auger, Mark Geist, Himanshu Gupta, Allan Hoffman, Khursheed Imam, Asim Khwaja, Michael Merport, John Pezzullo, and Catherine Petchprapa, each of whom contributed specific cases. If you like a case, credit our residents; if you do not, blame the authors! Special thanks to John Cronan and Mark Ridlen, who lead by example and have always been supportive of academics. I am grateful to the staff radiologists at Brown University, who gave us time to write this book, and to Drs. Joseph Callahan and Walter Gajewski, who provided a useful patient management perspective and edited some of the cases. And finally, my thanks to Debbie Desjardins and Angel Crouse, who typed the original manuscript and corrected all my misspellings.

WWM-S

CONTENTS

Opening Round Cases

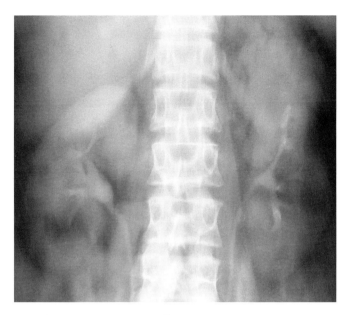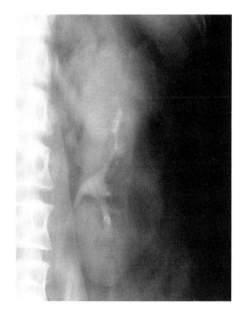

1. What is the most cost-effective technique that can be used to further evaluate an abnormality such as the one seen in the left kidney?
2. Is the mass in the left kidney exophytic or infiltrative?
3. Are renal cell carcinomas (RCCs) of more, less, or equal echogenicity to the kidney?
4. What imaging technique is most accurate for staging RCC?

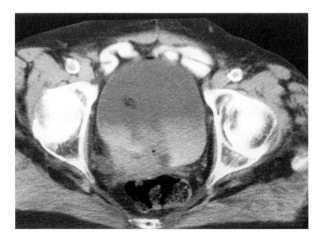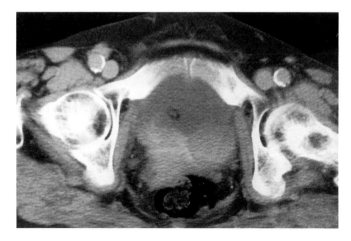

1. What is the most prevalent carcinogen for carcinoma of the urinary bladder?
2. What are some "markers" for transitional cell carcinoma that can be identified in urine samples?
3. What is the traditional classification of bladder cancers with respect to depth of invasion?
4. What is the most important prognostic factor with respect to recurrence and the development of metastatic disease?

CASE 1

Renal Cell Carcinoma

1. Renal sonography.

2. Exophytic.

3. All of the aforementioned, with approximately one third of RCCs in each category.

4. CT with contrast infusion and MRI are of equally high accuracy when performed properly.

Reference

Zagoria RJ, Wolfman NT, Karstaedt N, et al: CT features of renal cell carcinoma with emphasis on relation to tumor size, *Invest Radiol* 25:261-266, 1990.

Cross-Reference

Genitourinary Radiology: THE REQUISITES, pp 89-100.

Comment

This patient has a large exophytic mass extending from the upper pole of the left kidney. This mass would be classified as a ball-shaped lesion. Because simple cysts are the most common cause of ball-shaped lesions in the kidney, further evaluation of renal masses is performed most cost effectively using sonography. Of renal masses, 80% can be characterized with sonography alone, requiring no additional imaging evaluation. In this case the mass appears to be solid, and an argument could be made to proceed directly with CT or MRI. However, because of superimposed structures, enhancement of a renal mass can sometimes be difficult to determine on urography. Therefore sonography is a reasonable next step in the evaluation. Furthermore, for the characterization and staging of a renal mass, CT should not be performed immediately after urography because it is ideal to obtain scans before and after the infusion of contrast material.

Renal cell carcinoma is the most common primary renal malignancy. It is generally seen in the elderly, with a slight male predominance. There is a markedly increased risk of RCC in patients with von Hippel-Lindau disease and in those on long-term dialysis. RCC occurs in both kidneys in approximately 2% of patients. Unlike urothelial tumors, which progress in an infiltration pattern, RCC tends to grow by expansion, leading to an exophytic, ball-shaped mass. As evidenced on sonography, approximately one third of RCCs are hyperechoic, one third isoechoic, and one third hypoechoic compared with the kidney. Most are heterogeneous in echotexture. Small RCCs tend to be hyperechoic and should not be mistaken for angiomyolipomas. CT and MRI, when performed properly, can achieve an accuracy approaching 100% for preoperative staging of RCC.

Notes

CASE 2

Epidemiology and Prognosis of Bladder Cancer

1. In the United States, it is cigarette tobacco.

2. Bladder tumor antigen (BTA), nuclear matrix protein (NMP) 22, and telomerase.

3. Superficial tumors are confined to the mucosa or lamina propria and are traditionally distinguished from invasive bladder cancers.

4. Depth of invasion.

Reference

Droller MM: Bladder cancer: state of the art care, *CA Cancer J Clin* 48:269-284, 1998.

Cross-Reference

Genitourinary Radiology: THE REQUISITES, pp 197-204.

Comment

Bladder cancer was one of the earliest cancers in which carcinogens were found to play a significant role. Cigarette smoking increases the risk of developing transitional cell bladder cancer by 2 to 4 times. The hope is that the development of tumor markers in the urine might obviate the need for surveillance cystoscopy. Potential tumor markers include BTA (a substance released from the extracellular matrix in the presence of bladder cancer), NMP 22 (derived from the nuclear matrix protein mitotic apparatus), telomerase (a ribonucleoprotein enzyme responsible for producing telomeres, DNA sequences that protect chromosomes during DNA replication), and fibrin or fibrin degradation products.

The superficial cancers are papillary tumors confined to the mucosa (T_a), papillary and nodular tumors that infiltrate the lamina propria (T_1), and nonexophytic, in situ lesions that replace or undermine the normal bladder mucosa. Stage T_a tumors have only a 3% chance of progressing and usually are of low or moderate grade, whereas tumors that have penetrated the lamina propria progress in about 25% of cases and are high grade in 40% of cases. Invasive tumors are generally more nodular neoplasms that infiltrate the muscularis propria or the serosa (T_2 to T_3). Tumors that penetrate the muscularis only superficially may be associated with a lower incidence of metastases than are more deeply invasive tumors, but this is a difficult clinical distinction and one that is more often made after evaluation of the cystectomy specimen. Of the tumors that invade deeply into the muscularis propria, 50% are associated with occult metastatic disease at presentation and usually advance to gross metastases within 2 years of diagnosis.

Notes

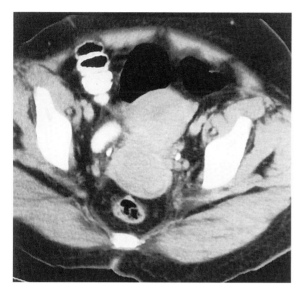 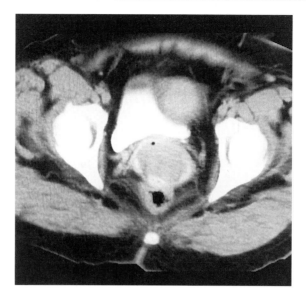

1. What is the most likely type and stage of this tumor?
2. What are the current International Federation of Gynecology and Obstetrics (FIGO) guidelines for staging this tumor?
3. Has the incidence of this disease increased or decreased over the past 30 years?
4. What are the risk factors associated with this disease?

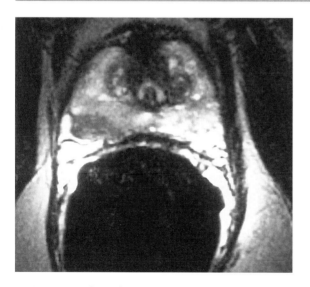 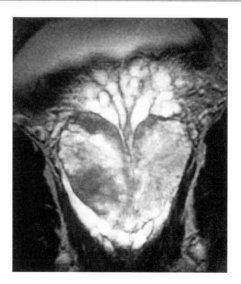

1. True or False: The majority of prostate adenocarcinomas arise from the peripheral zone.
2. Nodules of benign prostate hyperplasia arise from which zone of the prostate?
3. What is the clinicopathologic significance of the neurovascular bundle?
4. The ejaculatory ducts are located in which zone of the prostate?

Cervical Carcinoma

1. Stage IIa.

2. Clinical staging of cervical carcinoma requires bimanual pelvic examination, chest radiography, barium enema, excretory urography, cystoscopy, and sigmoidoscopy.

3. The incidence of invasive carcinoma is decreasing as a result of increased patient awareness and routine Papanicolaou smear screening. However, the overall incidence of cervical dysplasia is increasing presumably as a result of the increased incidence of sexually transmitted diseases.

4. Low socioeconomic status, multiple sexual partners, immunosuppression, and human papillomavirus infection.

Reference
Hricak H, Yu KK: Radiology in invasive cervical cancer, *Am J Roentgenol* 167:1101-1107, 1996.

Cross-Reference
Genitourinary Radiology: THE REQUISITES, pp 295-301.

Comment
Cervical carcinoma is the third most common gynecologic malignancy, after endometrial and ovarian carcinomas. Clinically, the patient with cervical cancer may have abnormal vaginal discharge or vaginal bleeding, but usually there are no symptoms. The diagnosis is confirmed most often by a cervical biopsy or by Papanicolaou testing. In situ disease (stage 0) requires no imaging. Biopsy-confirmed invasive disease requires staging. The goal of imaging is to accurately stage disease and direct therapy. Stage I cervical cancer is confined to the cervix. In stage II disease the cancer extends beyond the cervix, and in stage III disease the tumor spreads to the pelvic sidewall or causes ureteral obstruction. Stage IV cervical cancer invades the bladder or rectum directly or extends beyond the true pelvis.

Patients with a superficial cervical carcinoma can undergo a transvaginal cone excision (in which the tumor is excised and the uterus is left in place). Patients with tumor that has not invaded the parametria (stage Ib) usually undergo radical hysterectomy and pelvic lymph node dissection. Patients who have parametrial invasion (stage IIb and higher) are treated with radiation therapy in combination with radiation-sensitizing chemotherapy. The take-home point about cervical cancer staging recalls Shakespeare, "To be or not to be, that is the question . . . ." With respect to treatment options, stage IIb is an important staging threshold. Critical imaging observations in the staging of cervical carcinoma include parametrial invasion, pelvic lymphadenopathy, and hydroureter and extrapelvic metastatic disease. The presence of any of these findings connotes advanced disease and precludes surgery. Hydronephrosis is an important diagnosis that upstages the classification to stage IIIb.

Notes

Zonal Anatomy of the Prostate on MRI

1. True.

2. The transitional zone.

3. It is a common site where adenocarcinoma transgresses the prostatic capsule.

4. The central zone.

Reference
McNeal JE: Normal anatomy of the prostate and changes in benign prostatic hypertrophy and carcinoma, *Semin Ultrasound CT MR* 9:329-334, 1988.

Cross-Reference
Genitourinary Radiology: THE REQUISITES, pp 21, 32, 306, 307.

Comment
On these turbo spin-echo T2W images the cancer is a hypointense area in the right side of the peripheral zone at the midgland level. At surgery, there was microscopic spread of adenocarcinoma through the capsule and into the right neurovascular bundle.

Prostate anatomy was redefined more than a decade ago through the meticulous analysis of the microscopic structure of the acinar and ductal patterns of the glandular prostate. Discrete glandular "zones" of the prostate were defined and have impacted our understanding of prostate adenocarcinoma and benign prostatic hyperplasia (BPH). The central zone consists of an acinar-ductal system that empties into the verumontanum, close to the orifices of the ejaculatory duct. Its branches ramify proximally to the base of the prostate gland (i.e., closer to the bladder neck) and surround the ejaculatory ducts. The other major glandular zone, the peripheral zone, has no contact with the verumontanum but is more extensive; it extends from the prostatic apex inferiorly to the base of the gland superiorly. Together, the ducts of the peripheral and central zones compose roughly 95% of the glandular tissue of the prostate. Acinar mucin traps water and is what gives the peripheral and central zones their high signal intensity on long TR/TE MRI. The preprostatic segment of the urethra is proximal to the verumontanum and is surrounded by a smaller glandular system called the *transitional zone.* This zone contributes negligibly to prostate function.

Benign prostatic hyperplasia has been found to be a disease exclusively of the preprostatic region; nodules arise from either the transition zone or the submucosal tissues of the periurethral gland. The central zone is relatively immune from disease, but the peripheral zone is the site of chronic inflammatory processes, atypical hyperplasias, and most prostatic carcinomas. Rarer transition zone cancers arise in BPH nodules.

Notes

CASE 5

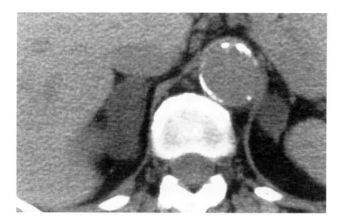

1. What is the most likely diagnosis?
2. What is the physiologic basis for the imaging findings?
3. What is the role of MRI in evaluating these findings?
4. What is the significance of mass size and density?

CASE 6

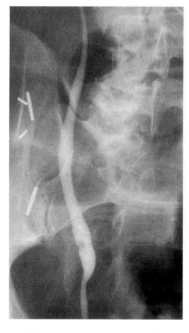 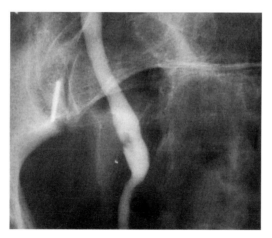

1. What are the major differential diagnoses for this filling defect?
2. When a ureteral transitional cell carcinoma (TCC) is detected, what is the risk of a synchronous or metachronous TCC elsewhere in the urinary tract?
3. Most radiolucent stones are composed of what substance?
4. What imaging characteristics of this mass suggest that it is a mucosal lesion?

Evaluation of Adrenal Masses: Size versus Density

1. Bilateral adrenal adenomas.

2. Intracellular lipid is present in adrenal adenomas but not in metastases, carcinomas, or pheochromocytomas.

3. Chemical shift MRI is sensitive and specific for differentiating an adenoma from a metastasis when CT is equivocal.

4. Historically, increased adrenal size is associated with increased risk of malignancy because of the late clinical presentation of primary carcinoma and metastases. This factor is probably less relevant since the increased use of cross-sectional imaging, which identifies incidental masses. In this case the low density is more important than the adrenal size.

Reference

McNicholas MMJ, Lee MJ, Mayo-Smith WW, Hahn PF, Boland GW, Mueller PR: An imaging algorithm for differential diagnosis of adrenal adenomas and metastases, *Am J Roentgenol* 165:1453-1459, 1995.

Cross-Reference

Genitourinary Radiology: THE REQUISITES, pp 346-351.

Comment

Adrenal adenoma is one of the more common incidentally discovered masses; these benign tumors are discovered in 1% to 8% of autopsy cases and in 1% of patients undergoing abdominal CT examination. Adenomas are typically less than 3 cm in diameter and can be bilateral. The differential diagnosis for bilateral adrenal masses includes bilateral adenomas, metastases, hemorrhage (bilateral in 10% of neonates and 20% of adults), granulomatous adrenalitis, and pheochromocytomas (10% are bilateral).

This case demonstrates the typical findings of bilateral adrenal adenomas (i.e., bilateral, well-circumscribed, low density masses without other evidence of metastases). The low density (less than 18 HU) is caused by cytoplasmic lipid, which also explains signal loss on opposed-phase chemical shift MRI. Adenomas enhance vigorously with the administration of intravenous contrast material, and the contrast material washes out of the gland on delayed imaging. This washout is greater in adenomas than in metastases. A threshold value of more than 50% contrast washout on 15-minute delayed CT has been used to differentiate adenomas from metastases. For equivocal findings, either MRI or follow-up CT can be performed. If immediate pathologic diagnosis is required, adrenal biopsy using CT or ultrasound guidance is safe and accurate.

Notes

Transitional Cell Carcinoma

1. TCC, radiolucent stone, blood clot, infection debris, and air bubble.

2. 40%.

3. Uric acid.

4. It has acute margins with the wall of the ureter, and there is slight indentation of the ureter wall adjacent to the lesion.

Reference

Wong-You-Cheong JJ, Wagner BJ, Davis CJ, Jr: Transitional cell carcinoma of the urinary tract: radiologic-pathologic correlation, *Radiographics* 18:123-142, 1998.

Cross-Reference

Genitourinary Radiology: THE REQUISITES, pp 184-188.

Comment

The most common causes of radiolucent filling defects seen in the urinary tract are radiolucent stones, followed by TCC, blood clots, infectious debris, air bubbles, sloughed papillae, indentation by an extrinsic mass, other urothelial neoplasms, and submucosal inflammation. The majority of these lesions in most patients are the result of radiolucent stones and ureteral tumors, mainly TCC. Closely scrutinizing the details of these lesions can often help in the diagnosis. Acute angles where the filling defect abuts the urothelium suggest an intraluminal or a mucosal process. Retraction of the ureteral wall, as seen in this case, indicates that this is a mucosal lesion and probably a TCC. TCCs, such as that shown in this case, least commonly develop in the ureter. Of TCCs, 90% develop in the bladder, with approximately 9% arising in the pyelocalyceal system. When a TCC develops in one of the more unusual sites, there is a markedly increased risk of synchronous or metachronous TCC developing elsewhere along the urothelial lining. Smokers, patients exposed to benzene compounds or some oncologic chemotherapy agents, patients with Balkan nephropathy, and analgesic abusers are at increased risk of developing TCC.

Notes

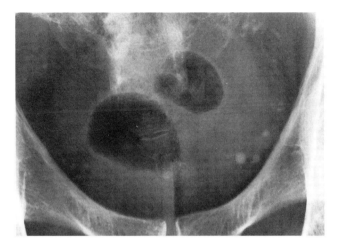 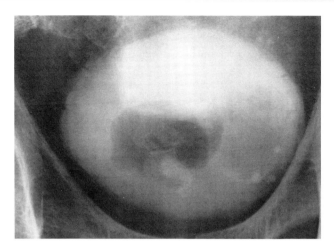

1. What is the purpose of the scout radiograph?
2. What is the finding on the urogram?
3. What is the differential diagnosis for this finding, and what can be done at the time of examination to differentiate these possibilities?
4. What maneuvers can be performed to optimize visualization of the distal ureters during an intravenous urogram?

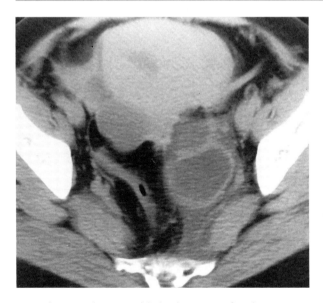 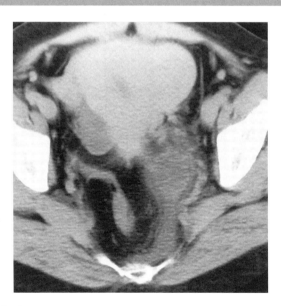

1. What are the most likely diagnoses for these imaging findings?
2. What should be done next?
3. It has been determined that an infection is most likely. True or False: Percutaneous drainage is the treatment of choice.
4. What are the complications of this disease?

Bladder Tumor on Intravenous Urography

1. To differentiate calcifications from contrast-opacified genitourinary structures before administration of contrast media and to differentiate air in the rectum from radiolucent filling defects. The scout radiograph also helps the clinician assess bowel preparation and the presence of confounding radiopacities (e.g., retained barium).

2. A lobulated filling defect along the levolateral wall of the bladder.

3. Neoplasm, calculus, blood clot, or fungus ball. The last three are mobile filling defects, so imaging after a change in position may be helpful.

4. The abdomen can be compressed and the patient can be moved into the prone position.

Reference

Kowalchuk RM, Banner MP, et al: Efficacy of prone positioning during intravenous urography in patients with hematuria or urothelial tumor but no obstruction, *Acad Radiol* 5:415-422, 1998.

Cross-Reference

Genitourinary Radiology: THE REQUISITES, pp 197-204, 219-226.

Comment

Intravenous urography is frequently used to evaluate the urinary tract in patients with gross or microscopic hematuria. The major clinical concern is detection of stone disease and urothelial cancer (i.e., transitional cell carcinoma [TCC]). Many patients with urinary tract calculi have a history of episodic, groin-radiating back pain. Noncontrast CT has become the modality of choice for evaluation of these patients. In older patients with painless hematuria, malignancy is of greater concern. Intravenous urography is a relatively noninvasive technique for screening the collecting system for sources of malignancy. However, excretory urography is not sensitive enough to detect small bladder neoplasms, but larger lesions, such as the one shown in this case, should be detected readily.

Intravenous urography also can be used to evaluate the upper urinary tract for synchronous lesions or smaller TCCs when the bladder is normal. Patients who do not have a mass on intravenous urography but have persistent hematuria should usually undergo cystoscopy and retrograde pyelography to directly image the bladder and upper urinary tract, respectively. When the distal ureters cannot be visualized on routine views, urography performed while the patient is in the prone position can improve visualization of the distal ureters, as evidenced by 100 of 510 patients (20%) in the study referenced above. This maneuver is easy to perform and may obviate the need for retrograde pyelography.

Notes

Tuboovarian Abscess

1. Pelvic inflammatory disease (PID) and ovarian neoplasm.

2. The radiologist should talk to the referring physician about the clinical history and physical examination findings.

3. False. Antimicrobial therapy is the first line of therapy. Percutaneous aspiration is useful to decrease the volume of the ovarian abscess and to determine the causative organisms in patients who do not respond to antibiotic therapy.

4. Fallopian tube scarring and paratubal adhesions, recurrent PID, infertility, and chronic pelvic pain.

Reference

Caspi B, Zalel Y, et al: Sonographically guided aspiration: an alternative therapy for tubo-ovarian abscess (see comments), *Ultrasound Obstet Gynecol* 7(6):439-442, 1996.

Cross-Reference

Genitourinary Radiology: THE REQUISITES, pp 264-267.

Comment

Pelvic inflammatory disease is a term used to describe ascending infection and inflammation of the endometrium, fallopian tubes, and ovaries. PID refers to a disease continuum that may progress from cervicitis, to endometritis, to salpingitis, to pelvic peritonitis, and then finally to generalized peritonitis, perihepatitis, or pelvic abscess. Tuboovarian abscess (TOA) refers to a more advanced form of the disease in which there are microabscesses involving the tubes and ovaries. Approximately 1% of patients treated for acute PID progress to development of a TOA, as in this case.

Imaging plays a role in cases in which the clinical diagnosis is unclear. Ultrasound is the first-line imaging modality for evaluation of pelvic pain in young women. Ultrasound of TOAs typically demonstrates an enlarged ovary in or adjacent to a heterogeneous mass. A heterogeneous mass is detected in more than 90% of patients with proven TOAs. On CT a TOA may appear as a complex mass with heterogeneous enhancement and thickened internal septations. The inflammation causes stranding of the adnexal fat. TOAs have a similar imaging appearance to ovarian carcinoma, but the clinical presentation is quite different. Patients who have a TOA are acutely ill, with fever and marked tenderness on examination, whereas patients with ovarian carcinoma have fewer clinical symptoms.

Most cases of TOA are treated first with intravenous antibiotics (e.g., doxycycline and cefoxitin or cefotetan or clindamycin plus gentamicin). If treatment with intravenous antibiotics fails, percutaneous aspiration may be performed. Aspiration of the TOA is usually sufficient, and placement of a drainage catheter is usually unnecessary.

Notes

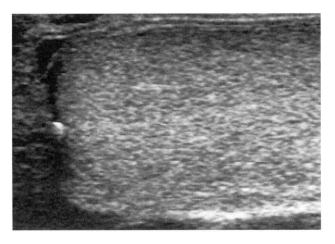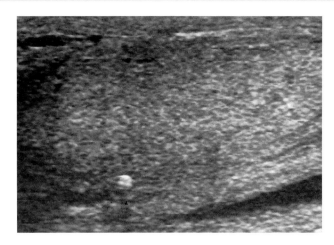

1. What is the most likely diagnosis?
2. Is this lesion intratesticular or extratesticular? What is the significance of this distinction?
3. Is this a benign or a premalignant condition?
4. What is one common associated condition?

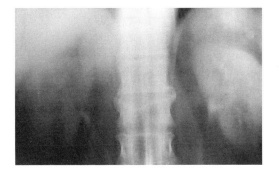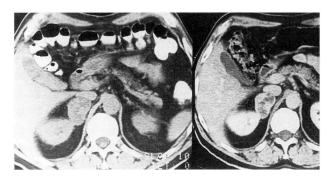

1. What is the differential diagnosis for this lesion?
2. On nonenhanced CT, what measured attenuation value helps to distinguish a nonmalignant lesion from a malignant adrenal mass?
3. If an incidental adrenal mass is discovered on enhanced CT, what is the strategy for evaluation, short of biopsy?
4. What are the essential clinical questions that should guide management of this lesion?

Scrotal Pearl

1. Scrotal calculus, or scrotal pearl.

2. Extratesticular. It is unlikely to be malignant.

3. Benign.

4. Hydrocele.

Reference

Linkowski GD, Avvelone A, Gooding GAW: Scrotal calculi: sonographic detection, *Radiology* 156:484, 1985.

Cross-Reference

Genitourinary Radiology: THE REQUISITES, p 316.

Comment

Scrotal calculi, also called *scrotal pearls* or *fibrinoid loose bodies,* are benign and mobile concretions found between the membranes of the tunica vaginalis. Pathologically there is a central nidus of hydroxyapatite surrounded by fibrinoid material. The calculi can be single or multiple and may be larger than 4 mm in diameter (as large as 10 mm). Scrotal calculi may be the result of a nonspecific inflammatory process of the tunica vaginalis or torsion of a testicular appendage. Nonspecific scrotal inflammation may cause granulation tissue to form from exfoliated vaginal endothelial cells. With time, a fibrinoid nidus develops and gradually calcifies. Alternatively the scrotal pearl may form as a result of calcification of a torsed and infarcted appendix testis or epididymis. In either case, secondary hydroceles are commonly associated with scrotal pearls.

A large calcification in the tunica vaginalis must be distinguished from a peripheral intratesticular calcification. Testicular microliths are usually multiple and smaller than 3 mm in diameter. Larger parenchymal calcifications may be associated with old testicular trauma or a testicular neoplasm. For instance, large focal calcifications have been reported in cases of "burned out" primary testicular neoplasms and large cell calcifying Sertoli cell tumors of the testis. The latter is a rare tumor that has been associated with gynecomastia, sexual precocity, and Carney's complex (cardiac myxoma, pigmented skin lesions, cutaneous myomas, myxoid mammary fibroadenomas, primary pigmented nodule adrenocortical disease, and pituitary adenoma).

Notes

Evaluation of an Incidental Adrenal Mass on CT

1. Adenoma, metastasis, pheochromocytoma, and myelolipoma.

2. 18 Hounsfield units (HU).

3. Measure its attenuation coefficient on contrast-enhanced CT; if it exceeds a threshold value of 25 HU on "early" delayed scanning (approximately 15 minutes after contrast administration), consider measuring the coefficient value after 1-hour delayed CT, noncontrast CT at another time, or chemical shift MRI.

4. Is there biochemical evidence of adrenal hyperfunction? Is there a clinical history of primary tumor metastasizing to the adrenal gland?

References

Boland GW, Hahn PF, Pena C, Mueller PF: Adrenal masses: characterization with delayed contrast-enhanced CT, *Radiology* 202(3):693-696, 1997.

Korobkin M, Brodeur FJ, Yutzy GG, et al: Differentiation of adrenal adenomas from nonadenomas using CT attenuation values, *Am J Roentgenol* 166:531-536, 1996.

Cross-Reference

Genitourinary Radiology: THE REQUISITES, pp 346-349.

Comment

Adenomas tend to be round or oval, have a well-defined margin, and are usually less than 3 cm in diameter. This case is atypical in that, on noncontrast CT, adenomas typically have a uniform low attenuation. Because of the large amount of intracytoplasmic lipid, measured attenuation values are efficacious for characterizing adenomas. In a study of 135 adrenal masses, Korobkin and colleagues reported that all lesions with an attenuation value of less than 18 HU on nonenhanced CT were adenomas.

However, adrenal adenomas are more often discovered as incidental lesions on enhanced CT. Recent clinical research has explored the value of attenuation coefficient measurements in this setting. On enhanced CT performed 12 to 18 minutes after contrast infusion, Boland and colleagues reported that an attenuation threshold of 24 HU resulted in the differentiation of adenomas (usually <25 HU) from metastases (usually >25 HU), with a sensitivity and specificity of 96%. When the CT examination is repeated after more than 1 hour, relatively rapid washout of contrast material occurs for adenomas, and attenuation measurements for nonenhanced CT can be used to characterize the adrenal mass.

Notes

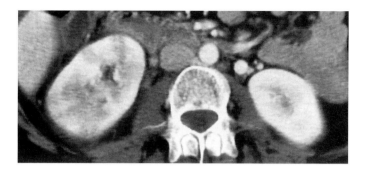
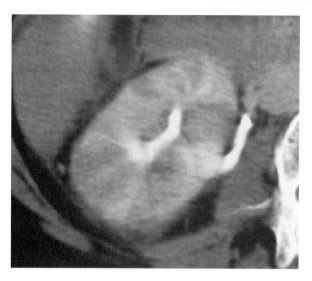

1. What is the diagnosis in this febrile patient?
2. What causes the areas of decreased enhancement in the right kidney?
3. In the setting of blunt trauma, what type of renal injury can have an identical radiographic appearance?
4. True or False: When hydronephrosis is present with this type of renal abnormality, it is the result of ureteral obstruction.

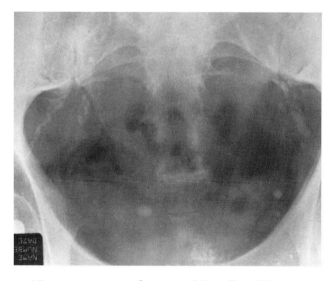
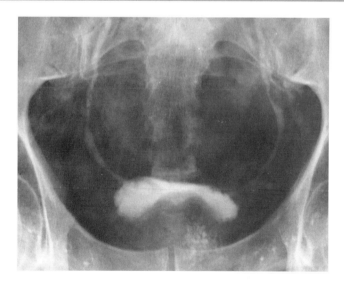

1. Name two causes of an immobile, off-midline stone in the bladder.
2. What is a pseudoureterocele?
3. What triad of findings on intravenous urography suggests the diagnosis of ureterocele on a duplex ureter?
4. Name three complications of intravesical ureteroceles.

Acute Pyelonephritis

1. Acute pyelonephritis.

2. Interstitial edema of the kidney leads to urinary stasis in some of the tubules in the medulla. These tubules do not opacify to the degree of normal or near-normal areas of kidney filled with opacified urine.

3. Renal contusion.

4. False. Some bacteria that cause acute pyelonephritis release an endotoxin, which leads to smooth muscle paralysis and nonobstructive hydronephrosis.

Reference

Gash JR, Zagoria RJ, Dyer RB: Imaging features of infiltrating renal lesions, *Crit Rev Diagn Imaging* 33:293-310, 1992.

Cross-Reference

Genitourinary Radiology: THE REQUISITES, pp 116-118, 173-176.

Comment

Acute pyelonephritis is almost always the result of infection ascending from the bladder via reflux of infected urine or lymphatic communication with bladder infection. It usually is a unilateral process. Radiographically, acute pyelonephritis may be focal or diffuse, as in this case. On intravenous urography, most commonly the findings are normal, as evidenced by 70% of patients with pyelonephritis. However, CT is much more sensitive for the detection of abnormalities caused by pyelonephritis. Typical CT findings include unilateral nephromegaly, striated nephrogram, and patchy, wedge-shaped areas of low attenuation in the otherwise enhanced kidney. The bacteria often secrete an endotoxin, which can cause hydronephrosis as a result of diminished peristalsis and flaccidity of the smooth muscle of the ureter. This finding should not be confused with ureteral obstruction.

Imaging is not usually required to diagnose pyelonephritis because it is easily diagnosed on a clinical basis. However, symptoms of pyelonephritis can be confused with those of other entities, such as urolithiasis or cholecystitis, possibly necessitating cross-sectional imaging studies. On occasion, imaging findings of pyelonephritis may precede detectable bacteriuria and fever by several days. Acute pyelonephritis is usually successfully treated with appropriate antibiotic therapy. Possible complicating features include emphysematous pyelonephritis, abscess formation, and xanthogranulomatous pyelonephritis, all of which may require additional treatment.

Notes

Calculus in an Orthotopic Ureterocele

1. Displacement of a bladder stone by a mass or an enlarged prostate, bladder diverticulum, or ureterocele.

2. A dilation of the intramural ureter secondary to contiguous bladder disease.

3. An upper pole renal mass, a radiolucent filling defect in the bladder, and ipsilateral or bilateral hydronephrosis.

4. Recurrent urinary tract infection, stone or milk of calcium formation, bladder outlet obstruction, and hydronephrosis.

Reference

Thornbury JR, Silver TM, Vinson RK: Ureteroceles vs. pseudo-ureteroceles in adults: urographic diagnosis, *Radiology* 122: 81-84, 1977.

Cross-Reference

Genitourinary Radiology: THE REQUISITES, pp 158, 159.

Comments

A ureterocele is a focal dilation of the distal end of the ureter and may be intravesical (simple) or ectopic. When the ureterocele and its orifice are both within the bladder, it is termed *intravesical.* The orifice of an intravesical ureterocele opens in the normal location but is stenotic. However, there is usually only slight dilation of the distal ureter above the ureterocele. Intravesical ureteroceles can be associated with single or duplex ureters. In contrast to those discovered in children, ureteroceles in adults usually form in single ureters that insert orthotopically, thus the term *adult ureterocele.* In most cases adult ureteroceles are incidentally discovered, but they may occur with (1) obstructive signs and symptoms, especially when large; (2) recurrent urinary tract infections; or (3) stones or milk of calcium formation.

Because renal function is typically normal, the intravesical ureterocele is distended with urine on intravenous urography, is shaped like a spring onion or cobra head, and protrudes into the lumen of the bladder. The wall of the ureterocele is visible as a lucent line or halo between the contrast-opacified urine in the ureterocele and the bladder lumen. In this case an impacted stone is isodense compared with the contrast-opacified urine in the ureterocele. On voiding cystourethrography the ureterocele often appears as a filling defect, but it can also intussuscept into the distal ureter and mimic a bladder diverticulum.

In contrast to the thin radiolucent halo associated with a ureterocele, a pseudoureterocele has an irregularly thick and nodular wall. The reported causes of pseudoureterocele include obstruction of the ureteral orifice caused by carcinoma of the bladder or cervix, a benign bladder tumor, radiation cystitis, a stone confined to the intravesical portion of the ureter, or transurethral prostatic resection.

Notes

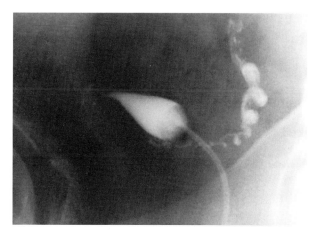 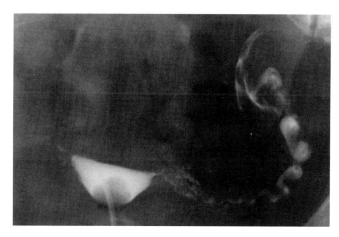

1. What is the differential diagnosis? How often is tubal patency demonstrated?
2. What are the major clinical complications associated with this disease?
3. Given a referral for primary infertility, state at least two reasons for not doing a hysterosalpingogram.
4. What are the major differences between the types of contrast media used for hysterosalpingograms?

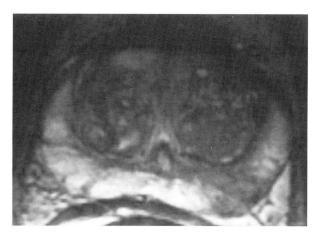 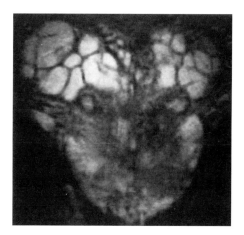

1. What is the differential diagnosis for a focal area of hypointense signal in the peripheral zone on a T2W image of the prostate?
2. True or False: For MRI of the prostate in which an endorectal surface coil is used, contrast-enhanced MRI is usually unnecessary.
3. True or False: MRI is as sensitive for the detection of central zone cancers as it is for peripheral zone adenocarcinoma.
4. True or False: Some peripheral zone cancers are of high signal intensity on T2W images.

CASE 13

Salpingitis Isthmica Nodosa

1. Salpingitis isthmica nodosa, tuberculosis of the fallopian tube, and tubal adenomyosis. "Free spill" of contrast is seen in about one fourth of all cases.

2. Infertility and ectopic uterine gestation.

3. Active menstrual bleeding, acute pelvic inflammatory disease, within 4 days of D & C, and pregnancy.

4. Image detail and peritoneal absorption.

Reference

Creasy JL, Clark RL, Cuttino JT, Groff TR: Salpingitis isthmica nodosa: radiologic and clinical correlates, *Radiology* 154:597-600, 1985.

Cross-Reference

Genotourinary Radiology: THE REQUISITES, pp 13-16, 45, 277, 278.

Comment

The term *salpingitis isthmica nodosa* (SIN) was coined by German pathologist Hans Chiari in 1887 to describe the predominant location, pathologic appearance, and presumed cause of a disease typified by epithelial inclusions within the walls of the fallopian tube. The classic findings of SIN on hysterosalpingogram (HSG) include numerous, small diverticular outpouchings in the ampullary part of one or both fallopian tubes. SIN can involve the entire tube, although usually only the proximal two thirds of the fallopian tube is involved. Tubal patency is observed in about 25% of cases. The cause of SIN has been debated, but a medical history of genital infection is frequently obtained, and the development of SIN after exposure to gonococci has been reported.

The clinical importance of this condition is its association with both infertility and extrauterine gestation. In the report referenced earlier, the prevalence of SIN was 4% in a group of women referred for HSG because of infertility. These authors also report a high rate of ectopic pregnancy (9.4%)

Tuberculous salpingitis and tubal adenomyosis are in the differential diagnosis of findings attributed to SIN. Tubal narrowing, occlusion, and fistula formation have also been observed in some cases of tuberculous salpingitis.

The authors recommend water-soluble contrast mediums for HSG because they provide better mucosal detail than the oil-based contrast agents and are more readily taken up by the peritoneal epithelium. Oil-soluble contrast material gained popularity after initial reports of an association between use of this material and successful impregnation after HSG. However, these oily contrast agents are not absorbed as well and have been linked to the development of fibrosis or granulomatosis.

Notes

CASE 14

MRI of the Prostate: Rules and Pitfalls

1. Adenocarcinoma, hyperplasia (fibrous, fibromuscular, muscular, and atypical adenomatous types), prostatitis, and hemorrhage after biopsy.

2. True. In most cases enhanced MRI is of no added benefit.

3. False.

4. True. Mucinous or signet ring adenocarcinoma.

Reference

Schiebler ML, Schnall MD, Pollack HM, et al: Current role of MR imaging in the staging of adenocarcinoma of the prostate, *Radiology* 189:339-352, 1993.

Cross-Reference

Genitourinary Radiology: THE REQUISITES, pp 32, 323.

Comment

First, some comments about a few standard techniques and sequences for endorectal MRI (erMRI) of the prostate. This study is most often performed with the intent of staging prostate cancer. Intravenous glucagon 1 mg should be administered to reduce artifact resulting from bowel peristalsis. After a digital rectal examination is performed, the endorectal coil is positioned directly behind the prostate gland, and the coil balloon is inflated with about 100 ml of air. Transverse axial fast or turbo spin echo, T2W images with thin (3-mm) slices form the cornerstone of prostate erMRI; supplemental fast spin echo T2W images in the coronal (as in this case) or sagittal plane may be performed as needed to confirm the diagnosis based on evaluation of the transaxial images. A transaxial T1W sequence through the prostate gland is also performed before the endorectal coil is removed. Finally, transaxial T1W images of the pelvis and lower abdomen are performed to evaluate for pelvic-retroperitoneal lymphadenopathy and metastases to the bone marrow. The routine use of contrast material is not necessary.

On fast spin echo T2W images the majority of prostate adenocarcinomas appear as focal areas of decreased signal in the normally hyperintense peripheral zone. Mucinous adenocarcinoma, which occurs in about 5% of cases, may be of high signal intensity on T2W images and is the major exception to this rule. Hemorrhage from a recent biopsy also may result in a hypointense focus in the peripheral zone. Hemorrhage after biopsy usually appears as a focal area of increased signal on the T1W image and corresponds in location to the hypointense area on the T2W image. Tumor surrounded by hemorrhage resulting from a recent biopsy should be suspected if, on the T1W image, only a rim of hyperintensity is visible around the suspicious focus. Alternatively, to avoid confusion, the clinician may delay the staging study until 3 or 4 weeks after prostate biopsy.

Notes

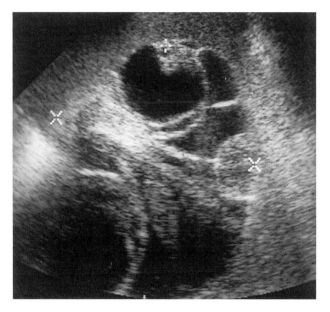
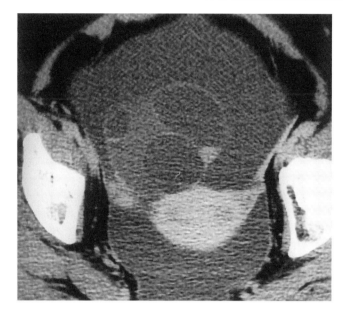

1. What is the most likely diagnosis? What findings on the ultrasound image support this diagnosis?
2. What role do serum markers play in screening for this disease?
3. Name a few risk factors for this disease.
4. What treatment is recommended for patients who have a strong familial history of this disease?

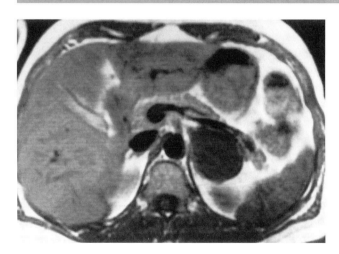
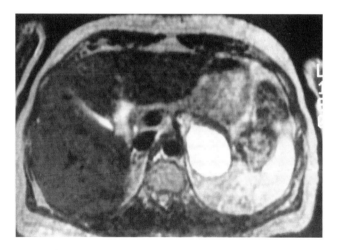

1. Does a predominantly cystic adrenal mass exclude the diagnosis of adrenal neoplasm?
2. What is the most common type of true adrenal cyst?
3. Is mural calcification a common feature of adrenal cysts?
4. True or False: Mural enhancement is not a feature of a simple, uncomplicated cyst and suggests a pseudocyst or cystic neoplasm.

Epithelial Ovarian Carcinoma

1. Ovarian carcinoma. Ovarian mass, with multiple septations (several of which are abnormally thick) and solid peripheral nodules, and ascites.

2. Measuring CA-125 levels alone is not an effective screening test for ovarian cancer.

3. Some risk factors, including early menarche, nulliparity, infertility, and late menopause, support the "incessant ovulation" theory of ovarian cancer; family history is also a risk factor.

4. Oral contraceptive use to decrease ovulation. Prophylactic oophorectomy may be recommended for high-risk patients with an extremely strong familial history of the disease.

Reference

Mayo-Smith WW, Lee MJ: MR imaging of the female pelvis, *Clin Radiol* 5:667-676, 1995.

Cross-Reference

Genitourinary Radiology: THE REQUISITES, pp 278-289.

Comment

Because there is no effective screening test, the NIH Consensus Conference has recommended against screening for ovarian cancer in members of the general population with no known risk factors for the disease. The tumor marker CA-125 is more than 65 U/mL in half of women with stage I or II disease. CA-125 levels also can be elevated in patients with benign diseases, such as uterine leiomyoma, endometriosis, and pelvic inflammatory disease, or during early pregnancy. Only 1% of healthy women have serum CA-125 levels higher than 35 U/mL. The primary value of CA-125 is in monitoring for tumor recurrence in those with an elevated level at the time of diagnosis.

Ultrasound is the initial imaging modality of choice for a suspected ovarian mass. If the ovarian mass is not a small, simple cyst, sonographic criteria that should raise the suspicion of ovarian malignancy include increased ovarian size (diameter >7.5 cm); presence of a solid component, mural nodules, internal papillary projections, or thickened septations; lymphadenopathy; and ascites. Enhancement of the nodular component of an ovarian mass on CT, as in this case, or on MRI suggests malignancy. Enhanced CT and MRI can be used to detect pelvic and retroperitoneal adenopathy and to evaluate the lung and liver for metastatic disease but are not sensitive enough to detect the small peritoneal implants that are present in patients with stage III disease.

Notes

Adrenal Cyst

1. No.

2. Endothelial cyst. Lymphangioma is much more common than hemangioma.

3. Yes. In one series 54% of 37 cysts showed calcification on CT scans.

4. False.

Reference

Rozenblit A, Morehouse HT, Amis ES Jr: Cystic adrenal lesions: CT features, *Radiology* 201:541-548, 1996.

Cross-Reference

Genitourinary Radiology: THE REQUISITES, pp 358, 359.

Comment

True cysts of the adrenal gland account for about 6% of incidentally discovered adrenal masses. At the time of discovery, adrenal cysts may be up to 20 cm in diameter. Some patients complain of back or flank pain when very large cysts compress surrounding organs; symptoms also may develop when hemorrhage or infection complicates an adrenal cyst.

Rozenblit, Morehouse, and Amis propose that nonhyperfunctional cystic adrenal masses be classified into (1) uncomplicated cysts that can be managed with observation, (2) complicated cystic masses that should be surgically removed, and (3) indeterminate cysts that may benefit from diagnostic (and occasionally therapeutic) cyst aspiration. An uncomplicated cyst is homogeneous, and the attenuation value of its content ranges from −20 to +20 HU; fine, thin mural enhancement may represent normal adrenal tissue draped over the cyst. Cysts can be unilocular or multilocular, may have mural or septal linear calcification, and may have walls that are 3 mm or less in thickness. Complicated cystic lesions have one or more of the following characteristics: thick (>5 mm) or nodular wall, inhomogeneous cyst contents, cyst attenuation value exceeding 30 HU, and stippled central or thick rim calcification. Because cystic neoplasm cannot be excluded, the complicated adrenal cyst should be surgically resected. Indeterminate cysts do not have the features of complicated cysts, are larger than 5 cm, have walls more than 3 mm in thickness, and have measured attenuation values in excess of simple water (up to 30 HU). Evaluation of cyst fluid, obtained by fine needle aspiration, may confirm the benign nature and adrenal origin of these indeterminate cysts by revealing high concentrations of cortisol or weak adrenal androgens or visible cholesterol crystals.

Notes

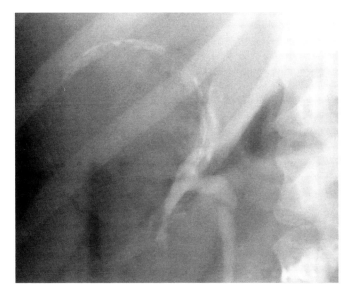

1. What is the most likely diagnosis for the calcified renal mass shown?
2. What percentage of lesions such as the one shown here are malignant?
3. Regardless of the calcification pattern, what diagnosis encompasses the majority of calcified renal masses?
4. What imaging test should be recommended for further evaluation of this abnormality?

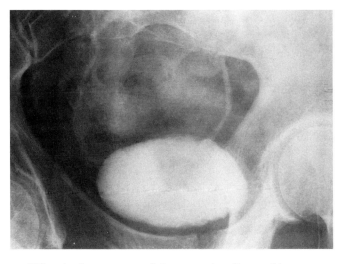 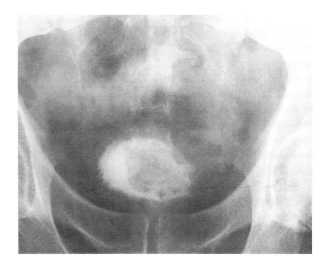

1. What is the purpose of the second radiograph?
2. Does a large amount of residual contrast material demonstrated on the postvoid radiograph indicate bladder dysfunction?
3. What is the differential diagnosis of this finding?
4. What other tests might be performed for further evaluation?

Calcified Renal Mass

1. Complicated renal cyst.

2. 20%.

3. Renal cell carcinoma.

4. CT or MRI.

Reference

Daniel WW Jr, Hartman GW, Witten DM, et al: Calcified renal masses: a review of ten years experience at the Mayo Clinic, *Radiology* 103:503-508, 1972.

Cross-Reference

Genitourinary Radiology: THE REQUISITES, pp 82-84, 88.

Comment

The patient shown has a spherical, ball-shaped mass arising from the middle portion of the right kidney. This mass displaces the calyces with compression and splaying. There is a calcified rim around the upper half of this mass.

Of calcified renal masses, 60% are renal cell carcinoma. Overall, renal cell carcinomas calcify in approximately 20% to 30% of cases. Renal cysts calcify in 1% to 2% of cases. The diagnosis for this patient is renal cell carcinoma; however, the rim of calcification that is visible is more commonly seen with complicated cysts than with renal cell carcinoma. Of those masses in which the calcification is purely rimlike, as in this case, 80% are cysts that have been complicated with hemorrhage or infection. Significantly, 20% of those lesions are renal cell carcinomas, as shown here. The bottom line is that a calcified renal mass requires further evaluation because the risk of malignancy is high. Further imaging evaluation should be recommended for diagnosis and staging, if necessary. Although renal sonography is the standard test for evaluating noncalcified renal masses, CT before and after contrast material infusion is the standard technique for further characterization and possible staging of calcified renal masses. With CT or MRI, which are of comparable efficacy, the internal architecture of the mass can be better evaluated. If delicate, peripheral calcification is the only complex feature in an otherwise simple cyst, further evaluation is probably unnecessary. Alternatively, numerous septations, enhancement, or solid internal components would qualify this mass as a surgical renal mass, most likely a malignancy.

Notes

Transitional Cell Carcinoma of the Bladder

1. The postvoid film is used to evaluate the bladder mucosa and also provides a crude measurement of bladder function.

2. Not necessarily. A large amount of contrast material in the bladder on a postvoid radiograph also may be due to a long delay between the initial radiograph and the postvoid film.

3. The finding is a focal filling defect in the bladder. The differential diagnosis is neoplasm, large calculus, blood clot, or less likely, focal cystitis, ureterocele, or fungus ball.

4. Cystoscopy, CT, ultrasound, or MRI.

Reference

Hillman BJ, Silvert M, et al: Recognition of bladder tumors by excretory urography, *Radiology* 138(2):319-323, 1981.

Cross-Reference

Genitourinary Radiology: THE REQUISITES, pp 6, 193-205.

Comment

Bladder carcinoma accounts for 4% of all malignancies and has a peak incidence in the fifth to sixth decades of life. There is a 3:1 male predominance. Of malignant bladder neoplasms, 95% are carcinomas (88% are transitional cell carcinoma, 5% are squamous cell carcinoma, and 2% are adenocarcinoma). Seventy-five percent are superficial-papillary lesions and 25% are invasive. Synchronous lesions occur in the upper urinary tract in approximately 2% of patients, and metachronous lesions occur in 7% of patients.

Intravenous urography has limited sensitivity for the detection of bladder neoplasms; small lesions are overlooked in up to 40% of patients with known bladder tumors. Early filling views and postvoid images of the bladder may be useful because the radiodense distended bladder may obscure subtle masses. CT and MRI are the imaging modalities of choice for staging known bladder neoplasms because they are most sensitive for detecting extramural extension and nodal metastases.

Notes

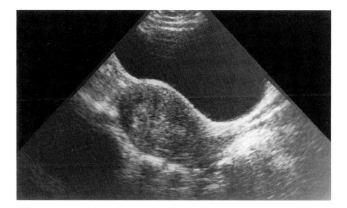 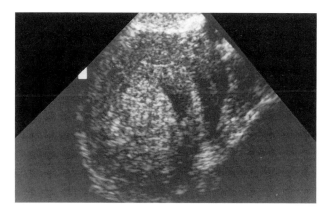

1. Of the following, which are accepted risk factors for endometrial carcinoma: being 20 lb or more overweight, having no children, beginning menopause late, having diabetes, maintaining unopposed estrogen replacement therapy, undergoing tamoxifen therapy, and using oral contraceptives.

2. True or False: An endometrial thickness of 4 mm or less, even in women with bleeding, is associated with endometrial atrophy.

3. True or False: For a postmenopausal woman with vaginal bleeding and an endometrial thickness of 8 mm, endometrial biopsy should be performed.

4. True or False: In postmenopausal women taking sequential hormones, a single endometrial thickness measurement exceeding 8 mm should trigger an endometrial biopsy.

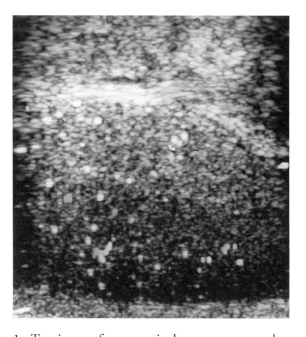 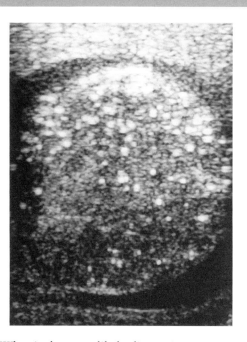

1. Two images from a testicular sonogram are shown. What is the most likely diagnosis?

2. What is the clinical significance of this lesion?

3. Name three associated clinical conditions.

4. True or False: Burned-out primary testicular cancer is pathologically indistinguishable from this lesion.

CASE 19

Endometrial Measurements on Ultrasound in Postmenopausal Women

1. All are risk factors.

2. True.

3. True.

4. False.

References

Levine D, Gosink BB, Johnson LA: Change in endometrial thickness in postmenopausal women undergoing hormone replacement therapy, *Radiology* 197:603-608, 1995.

Rose PG: Medical progress: endometrial carcinoma, *N Engl J Med* 335(9):640-649, 1996.

Cross-Reference

Genitourinary Radiology: THE REQUISITES, pp 17-20, 289.

Comment

Of women with endometrial carcinoma, 75% are postmenopausal and 50% have risk factors for this disease. Most of these risk factors have one factor in common—excessive estrogen exposure. Excessive estrogen exposure causes continuous endometrial stimulation, which can lead to hyperplasia.

Estrogen replacement therapy (ERT) prevents bone loss and alleviates menopausal symptoms. Unopposed exogenous estrogens were popular in the 1970s, but their use resulted in an eightfold increase in the incidence of endometrial cancer. Combined estrogen-progesterone preparations have reduced the risk of endometrial cancer, but there is still an increased risk associated with combined regimens that include less than the recommended 12 days of progesterone monthly.

In the study by Levine and colleagues, sonographic measurements of endometrial thickness were compared between postmenopausal women taking three different ERT regimens (unopposed estrogen, continuous combined estrogen and progestogen, and sequential estrogen and progesterone) and a group of control patients on no hormone replacement. A little over half of the women taking unopposed estrogens had endometrial thickness of 8 mm or more. Given the great risk of endometrial carcinoma in this group of women, biopsy should be recommended when endometrial thickness equals or exceeds 8 mm. Slightly more than half of the women taking sequential estrogen and progesterone hormones had endometrial thickness of 8 mm or more, and change in endometrial thickness was as great as 13 mm during the monthly cycle. Levine and colleagues recommend biopsy only if endometrial thickness is at least 8 mm on a follow-up scan performed early (before day 13) or late (after day 23) in the cycle. Because endometrial width decreases during these periods of the cycle, a measurement of 8 mm or more is more likely to indicate endometrial disease.

Notes

CASE 20

Testicular Microlithiasis

1. Testicular microlithiasis.

2. An association with primary testicular neoplasm has been reported.

3. In addition to primary testicular neoplasm, undescended testes, testicular atrophy, and infertility have been associated.

4. False.

Reference

Backus ML, Mack LA, Middleton WD, King BF, Winter TC III, True LD: Testicular microlithiasis: imaging appearances and pathologic correlation, *Radiology* 192:781-785, 1994.

Cross-Reference

Genitourinary Radiology: THE REQUISITES, p 316.

Comment

Testicular microlithiasis (TM) is a benign but possibly premalignant condition typified by the presence of multiple (from 5 to more than 60), small punctate intratesticular calcifications. In the majority of patients, these calcifications are 1 mm in diameter or smaller, although in some patients, calcifications can be as large as 3 mm. The condition usually affects both testicles but may be asymmetric. Pathologically, TM consists of psammoma bodies (a dense core of calcium surrounded by laminations of collagen) in seminiferous tubules. These calcifications may be the result of a failure of the Sertoli cell to phagocytose degenerating cells. In contrast, burned-out primary testicular cancers consist of a fibrous scar with acellular collagenous tissue that stains with hematoxylin (hematoxyphilic bodies).

Testicular microlithiasis has been associated with a number of other diseases, including cryptorchid testes, testicular atrophy, and infertility; rarer associations with Klinefelter's syndrome, male pseudohermaphroditism, Down syndrome, pulmonary alveolar microlithiasis, and intratubular germ cell neoplasia have also been reported. An association between ultrasound-detectable TM and germ cell tumors was noted in 40% of the 42 patients in the study referenced above. In the reported cases the associated tumor appeared as a discrete testicular mass on ultrasound, separate from the TM. In another case report a yolk sac tumor was discovered on the fourth annual follow-up sonogram of a 17-year-old boy with TM. Semiannual or annual testicular sonography has been recommended for patients with TM between the ages of 20 and 50 years; however, this screening recommendation is controversial.

Notes

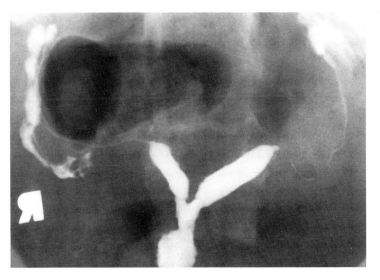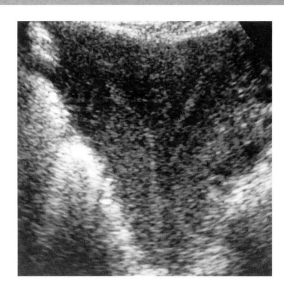

1. What is the most likely diagnosis in this case?
2. This represents a malformation of what embryonic genital duct system?
3. In men, what causes regression of this duct system?
4. What are the diagnostic criteria for this malformation on hysterosalpingography?

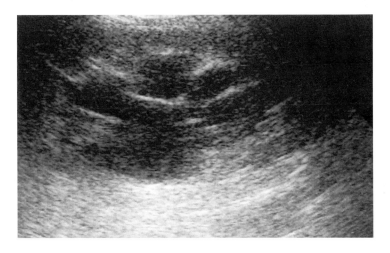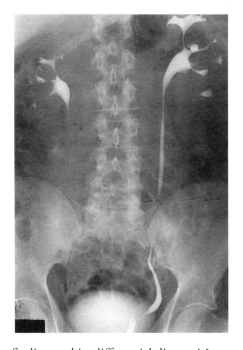

1. A sagittal sonogram of the left kidney is shown. What is the major finding and its differential diagnosis?
2. What examination is shown in the second image?
3. What is the correct diagnosis?
4. What other test (or tests) could be performed to confirm this diagnosis?

Septate Uterus on Ultrasound and Hysterosalpingography

1. Septate uterus.

2. Müllerian or paramesonephric.

3. Müllerian inhibiting factor (produced by the testes).

4. Intercornuate distance less than 4 cm and intercornual angle less than or equal to 75 degrees.

Reference

Reuter KL, Daly DC, Cohen SM: Septate versus bicornuate uteri: errors in imaging diagnosis, *Radiology* 172:749-752, 1989.

Cross-Reference

Genitourinary Radiology: THE REQUISITES, pp 253-257.

Comment

Through fusion, the müllerian or paramesonephric ducts form the upper vagina, uterus, and fallopian tubes in the female embryo. A müllerian inhibiting or suppression factor is secreted by the embryonic testes and suppresses the development of the paramesonephric ducts. Thus phenotypic women with testicular feminization syndrome (androgen insensitivity caused by abnormal testosterone receptors) do not have an internal female genital tract because the normal but often undescended testes produce müllerian regression factor and androgens. In contrast, phenotypic women with gonadal dysgenesis (failure of testicular differentiation) usually have female internal genital ducts because the abnormal gonads do not retain the ability to secrete this factor.

This case illustrates a septate uterus on transvaginal sonography and hysterosalpingography (HSG). Septate uterus represents the most common anomaly of müllerian duct fusion and is classified as a Class V anomaly in the American Fertility Society system. Various degrees of failure of absorption of the midline septum can be observed in this anomaly. Complete failure gives rise to a complete septate uterus; the septum can extend from the fundus to the endocervical canal. Partial absorption failure results in a septum that is confined to the endometrial cavity (subseptate uterus). Spontaneous abortion may occur in as many as 90% of patients with septate uteri because a fertilized ovum quickly outgrows the blood supply of the poorly vascularized septum. Some of the diagnostic features of a septate uterus on transvaginal ultrasound and HSG include a convex, flat, or minimally concave uterine fundal contour; intercornual distance less than or equal to 4 cm; and intercornual angle less than or equal to 75 degrees.

Notes

Peripelvic Cysts

1. Multiple anechoic and echo-poor areas in the renal sinus. The differential diagnosis is pelvocaliectasis from obstruction or reflux and multiple peripelvic cysts.

2. Retrograde pyelogram.

3. Multiple, peripelvic renal cysts.

4. Intravenous urography and enhanced CT scan.

Reference

In der Maur GAP, Puylaert JBCM: Peripelvic renal cysts, hydronephrosis and sinus lipomatosis, *J Med Imag* 3:22-26, 1989.

Cross-Reference

Genitourinary Radiology: THE REQUISITES, pp 9-11, 153-155.

Comment

Not all hypoechoic structures in the renal sinus represent hydronephrosis. The ultrasound shows multiple echo-poor areas in the renal sinus. These areas could represent caliectasis resulting from ureteral obstruction or possibly from a ureteropelvic junction obstruction. The collecting system also may appear dilated when there is severe vesicoureteral reflux. However, with this degree of pelvocaliectasis resulting from reflux, a smaller kidney and cortical thinning over the upper and lower renal poles might be expected. The third consideration in this patient is multiple peripelvic cysts.

Peripelvic cysts are common and are often multiple. Typically, peripelvic cysts insinuate themselves in the sinus fat. They are believed to be secondary to lymphatic obstruction. In contrast, parapelvic cysts originate from the renal parenchyma and extend into the renal sinus. They are usually larger than peripelvic cysts and are not as often multiple. Peripelvic cysts often distort the renal calyces and may stretch or attenuate the infundibuli, which is illustrated well on the retrograde pyelogram.

In this case a retrograde pyelogram was performed. A cystoscope was used to place a catheter in the distal ureter. Contrast material was then instilled by syringe or by drip infusion. This procedure requires cystoscopy and is routinely performed in the operating room with the patient under sedation. In contrast to the intravenous urogram, on a retrograde pyelogram the renal parenchyma is not opacified. Retrograde pyelography is commonly performed (1) to evaluate the ureters and intrarenal collecting system when they have not been completely imaged on intravenous urography, (2) to evaluate a filling defect that is visible on either excretory urography or CT, and (3) to evaluate the patient for whom no explanation for hematuria has been found on other imaging studies.

Notes

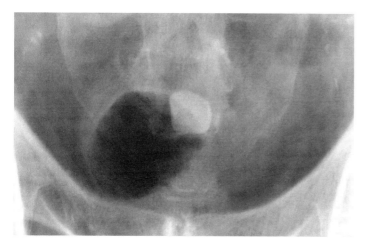 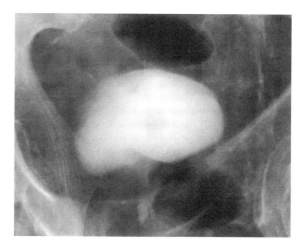

1. Name three risk factors for the development of bladder stones. Which one of these factors is probably the most prevalent?

2. Urinary infection with which bacterium is most often associated with bladder stones?

3. What are "hanging" bladder stones?

4. On a conventional radiograph of a supine patient, what is the significance of a bladder stone that is not in the midline?

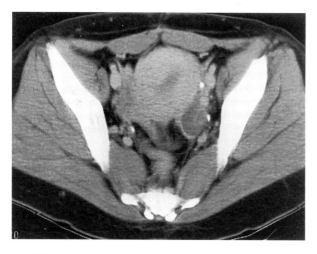 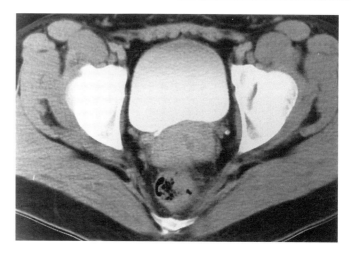

1. What are the abnormal findings on these two CT images?

2. The development of cervical cancer has been linked with which infectious agent?

3. True or False: Pelvic lymph node metastasis has been associated with a significant decrease in the 5-year survival in patients with early stage disease.

4. True or False: The recurrence of cervical cancer is usually in the lung or bone.

CASE 23

Bladder Calculus

1. Urinary stasis, urinary tract infection, foreign body, intestinal mucosa in the urinary tract. Bladder outlet obstruction is probably the most common risk factor.

2. *Proteus* species.

3. Stones that form on nonabsorbable suture material can be suspended from the bladder wall.

4. The stone may be in a diverticulum or ureterocele or may be displaced by a bladder mass or an enlarged prostate.

Reference

Trevino R, Goldstein AMB, Vartanian NL, et al: Vesical bladder stones formed around nonabsorbable sutures and possible explanation for their delayed appearance, *J Urol* 122:849-853, 1979.

Cross-Reference

Genitourinary Radiology: THE REQUISITES, pp 215-217.

Comment

There are three main causes of vesical stone disease: (1) urinary stasis or presence of a foreign body, (2) primary endemic stone disease, and (3) migrant calculi from the kidney. In children and adults the most important risk factor is urinary stasis caused by bladder outlet obstruction. For instance, most migrant calculi from the kidney are passed through the urethra unless the bladder outlet is relatively small, as in children, or is obstructed. Notice that the prostate gland is moderately enlarged in this case.

Foreign bodies, such as a long-term indwelling catheter, nonabsorbable suture material, pubic hairs, or fracture fragments, may form the nidus for stone formation and growth. Nonabsorbable suture material over time may migrate through the bladder wall, penetrate the mucosa, and act as a nidus. Stones formed in this manner may not change in position. In contrast, other bladder calculi are mobile. Mobility is an important distinguishing feature of bladder stones because neoplastic, inflammatory, and metabolic calcifications of the bladder wall are immobile.

A few points should be noted regarding the imaging of bladder calculi. First, low kilovoltage technique (60 to 70 kVp) increases the contrast on a conventional radiograph and aids the detection of faintly opaque stones. On the excretory urogram, most calcified bladder stones produce filling defects in the contrast-filled bladder. As with ureteral stones, all bladder stones are radiopaque on CT. Bladder stones can be treated by cystoscopic removal, litholapaxy, chemolysis, or (when large) suprapubic cystolithotomy.

Notes

CASE 24

Cancer of the Uterine Cervix

1. Enlarged cervix and hydrometra.

2. Human papillomavirus.

3. True.

4. False.

Reference

Cannistra SA, Niloff JM: Cancer of the uterine cervix, *N Engl J Med* 336(16):1030-1038, 1996.

Cross-Reference

Genitourinary Radiology: THE REQUISITES, pp 295-300.

Comment

Cervical cancer usually occurs in postmenopausal women, and the mean age at diagnosis is 54 years. Cervical intraepithelial dysplasia, a common precursor lesion, consists of dysplastic changes and varying degrees of disordered maturation confined to the cervical epithelium. The human papillomavirus genome has been linked to the DNA composition of both intraepithelial lesions and cervical cancer.

The staging of cervical cancer is a critical component in managing the disease. Patients with microinvasive tumors have cancer that invades less than 5 mm into the cervical stroma. Some preliminary work suggests that enhanced MRI may be helpful in identifying this minimally invasive disease, which is typically treated with simple hysterectomy (removal of the uterine corpus and cervix, without resection of the parametria, uterosacral ligaments, or any part of the vagina). The majority of patients with cervical cancer have stage Ib or IIa disease (i.e., grossly visible tumor that may involve the upper two thirds of the vagina but not the parametrium). For these patients, radical hysterectomy and radiotherapy are equivalent treatments; the 5-year survival rate is 85%. Pelvic lymph node metastasis in patients with stage Ib or IIa disease decreases the 5-year survival rate to 45%.

Patients with extensive locoregional disease involving the parametrium (stage IIb), the lower third of the vagina (stage IIIa), the pelvic sidewall (stage IIIb), or the bladder or the rectum (stage IVa) often relapse when treated with surgery. Cervical cancer often recurs locally but may metastasize to distant sites, such as the lungs and bone (stage IVb).

Notes

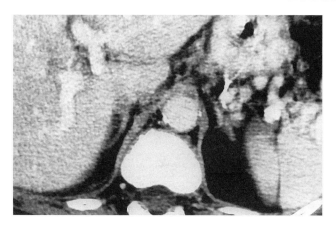 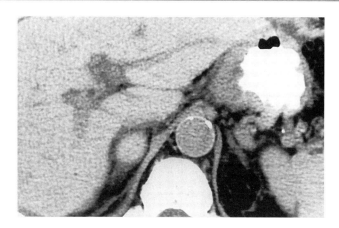

1. What abnormality is visible in the image on the left?
2. What is the finding on the image on the right (which was obtained from a CT scan performed 1 week after the image on the left was taken)?
3. How often is this lesion bilateral?
4. Which modality is most specific for this diagnosis—ultrasound, CT, or MRI?

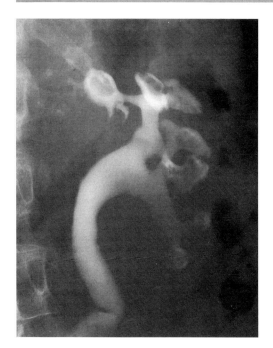

1. Are the filling defects seen in this case located within the calyx or the medulla of the kidney?
2. What is the most likely diagnosis for these filling defects?
3. What processes may cause unilateral papillary necrosis?
4. What is this radiologic appearance of filling defects surrounded by contrast material called in this location?

CASE 25

Acute Adrenal Hemorrhage on CT

1. Gastric wall thickening consistent with the pathologic diagnosis of gastric adenocarcinoma.

2. Acute adrenal hemorrhage.

3. In up to 20% of cases.

4. MRI.

Reference

Hoeffel C, et al: Spontaneous unilateral adrenal hemorrhage: computerized tomography and magnetic imaging findings in 8 cases, *J Urol* 154:1647-1651, 1995.

Cross-Reference

Genitourinary Radiology: THE REQUISITES, pp 357, 358.

Comment

Adrenal hemorrhage can be a complication of blunt abdominal trauma, sepsis, coagulopathy, anticoagulation therapy, liver transplant surgery, or adrenal venography. Spontaneous adrenal hemorrhage is less common. Some of the clinical situations with which spontaneous hemorrhage is associated are septicemia (Waterhouse-Friderichsen syndrome), severe physiologic stress, hypotension, surgery, and adrenal tumors. Metastatic melanoma can be associated with adrenal hemorrhage. The most common symptoms include abdominal pain, a palpable abdominal mass, hypotension, and anemia. However, the clinical diagnosis is often elusive because adrenal hemorrhage is usually asymptomatic. Up to 20% of the cases are bilateral.

The radiologist should be aware of the appearance of acute adrenal hemorrhage on cross-sectional imaging. On ultrasound, adrenal hemorrhage may appear as a hyperechoic mass. The echogenicity gradually decreases as the hematoma resolves, and the eventual appearance may mimic that of an adrenal cyst. On unenhanced CT the adrenal gland is enlarged and has increased attenuation as a result of acute blood products (as in this case). MRI is the most accurate imaging modality for detecting adrenal hemorrhage because of imaging features that are sensitive and specific for blood products. As a result of the presence of methemoglobin, signal intensity is increased in acute adrenal hemorrhage on T1W images. On T2W images, serpiginous, linear low signal within an area of heterogeneous signal may be visible, depending on the age of the bleed. In older hemorrhages a cystic area of T2-hyperintense fluid surrounded by a dark rim may be present as a result of hemosiderin within macrophages.

Notes

CASE 26

Papillary Necrosis

1. Medulla.

2. Papillary necrosis.

3. Pyelonephritis, ureteral obstruction, tuberculosis, and renal vein thrombosis.

4. Signet ring.

Reference

Davidson AJ, Hartman DS, editors: In *Radiology of the kidney and urinary tract,* ed 2, Philadelphia, 1994, WB Saunders, pp 177-189.

Cross-Reference

Genitourinary Radiology: THE REQUISITES, p 71.

Comment

Papillary necrosis is a cause of gross hematuria and a common cause of chronic renal insufficiency. It usually results from ischemia of the medulla of the kidneys. Common causes of papillary necrosis can be remembered by the mnemonic *POSTCARD,* which abbreviates the following common causes: *p*yelonephritis, *o*bstruction, *s*ickle cell disease, *t*uberculosis, *c*irrhosis/pancreatitis, *a*nalgesic abuse, *r*enal vein thrombosis, and *d*iabetes mellitus. Necrosis of the papillae may be predominantly central, causing a cavity that communicates with the nadir of the calyceal concavity. The result is the "ball on tee" pattern that is seen on contrast studies. Alternatively, papillary necrosis originating at the margins of the papilla initially causes sloughing of the edges of the papilla, resulting in apparent elongation of the fornices (angles) of the calyx and causing a "lobster claw" pattern. Further necrosis leads to complete sloughing of a large segment of the papillary tip. Contrast material can then extend from the calyx and surround this necrotic segment of the medulla. If this tissue remains in place, it causes the signet ring appearance, as seen in this case. All of these radiologic patterns are typical of papillary necrosis. The necrotic papilla may pass into the calyx and advance into the ureter, causing ureteral obstruction and a radiologic appearance similar to that seen with a ureteral stone. Clues that help diagnose a sloughed papilla include a roughly triangular filling defect and evidence of papillary necrosis in the upper tract of the kidney on the involved side.

Notes

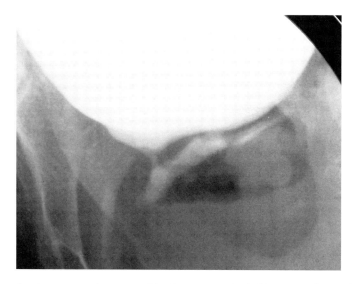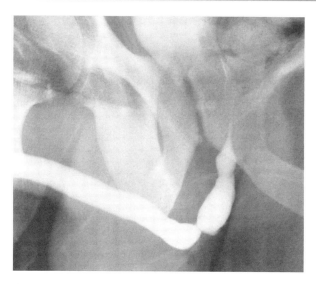

1. A cystourethrogram (the image on the left) was performed in this patient who had contracture of the bladder neck and had just undergone transurethral prostatic resection. What is the abnormal finding, and what might have caused it?

2. What are some of the causes for the lesion shown on the retrograde urethrogram (the image on the right), which was performed on another patient?

3. What causes "watering can" perineum?

4. Should squamous cell carcinoma of the bulbar urethra be included in the differential diagnosis for the lesion shown on the retrograde urethrogram?

Iatrogenic Urethral Injuries

1. "False passage" caused by repeated attempts to pass a transurethral catheter.

2. Focal urethral stricture can be caused by infection, noninfectious urethritis, iatrogenic injury, or traumatic injury.

3. Chronic tuberculosis of the perineum may result in urethral obstruction, fistula formation, and periurethral abscess.

4. No.

Reference

Shaver WA, Richter PH, Orandi A: Changes in the male urethra produced by instrumentation or transurethral resection of the prostate, *Radiology* 116:623-628, 1975.

Cross-Reference

Genitourinary Radiology: THE REQUISITES, pp 237-239.

Comment

Iatrogenic injury to the urethra may result from open surgery, instrumentation, or catheter placement. Urethral strictures have been reported in 3% to 17% of patients who have had transurethral prostatectomy. The majority of strictures in children are iatrogenic; the patient with the stricture on retrograde urethrogram had repetitive cystoscopy as a child. Any indwelling transurethral catheter predisposes a patient to urethritis and increases the risk of stricture. Iatrogenic stricture is most common at the penoscrotal junction and membranous urethra; the meatus and bladder neck also are common sites. Iatrogenic strictures are usually focal and short but may be multifocal or segmental and long. Other causes of urethral stricture include nongonococcal and gonococcal infection (in the bulbous urethra or just proximal to the meatus), noninfectious inflammation (chemical irritation or Reiter's syndrome), traumatic injury (solitary strictures that develop more quickly than inflammatory strictures), or neoplasm (usually causes a long, irregular stricture with or without a fistula).

False passages may be created after numerous failed attempts to pass a catheter or other instrument. Failed catheter placement can produce a tract posterior to the prostatomembranous or bulbar urethra that may enter the prostate or even penetrate the bladder. An even more ominous injury results when the Foley catheter balloon is placed in the membranous urethra and inflated; this mishap is more likely to occur in the patient with spinal cord injury.

Notes

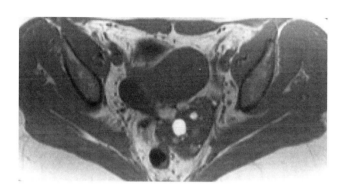
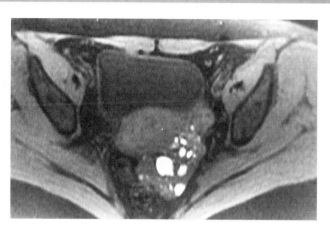
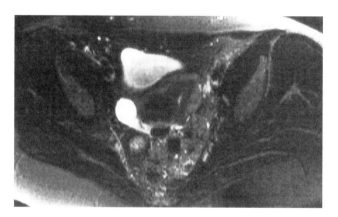

1. What is the differential diagnosis in this case?
2. What are the most common pathologic manifestations of endometriosis?
3. What are the three most common sites for implants from endometriosis?
4. True or False: Serum levels of CA-125 are elevated in women with endometriosis.

MRI of Ovarian Endometriosis

1. Ovarian implants of endometriosis and multiple small hemorrhagic physiologic cysts.

2. Implants, endometrial cysts ("chocolate cysts"), and adhesions.

3. Ovaries, uterine ligaments, and Douglas cul-de-sac.

4. True.

Reference

Seigelman ES, Outwater E, Want T, Mitchell DG: Solid pelvic masses caused by endometriosis: MR imaging features, *Am J Roentgenol* 163:357-361, 1994.

Cross-Reference

Genitourinary Radiology: THE REQUISITES, pp 258-261.

Comment

Endometriosis is defined as the presence of ectopic endometrial glands and stroma in the pelvis or abdomen; it may cause dysmenorrhea, dyspareunia, chronic pelvic pain, or infertility. Approximately one fourth of infertile women of reproductive age have endometriosis. The common manifestations of endometriosis include the endometrial cyst (endometrioma), adhesions resulting from fibrosis, and endometrial implants. In descending order of frequency the most common sites of these implants are the ovaries, uterine ligaments, cul-de-sac of Douglas, serosal surface of the uterus, fallopian tubes, rectosigmoid colon, and bladder dome.

At laparoscopy, endometriosis appears as superficial stains or patches of black or brown on the peritoneal surface of the ovaries, fallopian tubes, uterus or uterosacral ligaments, and bowel. Although most superficial implants ("powder burns") are not identified, high resolution MRI can demonstrate implants in extraperitoneal sites or behind dense adhesions. This case illustrates that small implants may contain foci of hemorrhage and are often hypointense on T2W images; they may be on the surface of the ovary or uterus and may enhance. Frequency-selective fat saturation increases the sensitivity of MRI by increasing the contrast between small endometrial implants and adnexal fat. Dense adhesions may appear as spiculated, hypointense lesions or abnormal stranding in adnexal fat but may be difficult to appreciate. In addition, these adhesions are not specific for endometriosis because they also may develop after pelvic surgery or pelvic inflammatory disease.

Notes

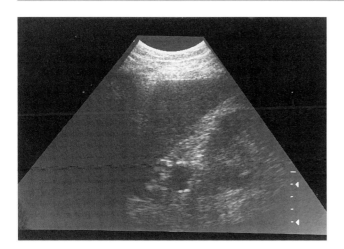

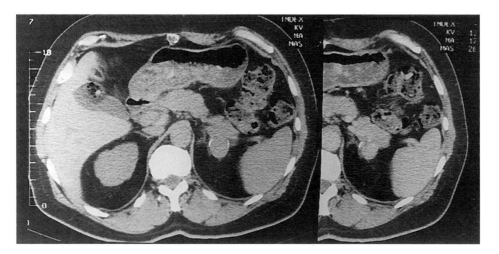

1. A sagittal sonogram of the left kidney and a composite figure of two noncontrast CT images are shown. What is the most likely diagnosis?

2. Name at least three causes for this lesion.

3. True or False: Most adrenal pseudotumors occur on the right side.

4. True or False: Many adrenal pseudotumors are vascular lesions.

Adrenal Pseudotumor

1. Splenic artery aneurysm or pseudoaneurysm.

2. Atherosclerosis with media degeneration, mycosis, inflammation (pancreatitis), trauma, and portal hypertension.

3. False.

4. True.

References

Brady TM, Gross BH, Glazer GM, Williams DM: Adrenal pseudomasses due to varices: angiographic-CT-MRI-pathologic correlations, *Am J Roentgenol* 145:301-304, 1985.

Spitell JA Jr, Fairbairn JF II, Kincaid OW, et al: Aneurysm of the splenic artery, *JAMA* 175:452-456, 1961.

Cross-Reference
Genitourinary Radiology: THE REQUISITES, pp 361-364.

Comment

Normal periadrenal viscera or a vascular lesion may mimic an adrenal mass. Pseudolesions of the adrenal gland are most often detected on intravenous urography, nephrotomography, or ultrasound, and they occur more frequently on the left side. There are several nonvascular causes of a left adrenal pseudotumor, including a splenic lobule, left renal mass, pancreatic body or tail mass, adjacent small bowel, gastric diverticulum, and redundant gastric fundus. Pseudotumor that is caused by bowel may be diagnosed by repeating the radiologic or ultrasound study after oral contrast medium or water, respectively, is administered. Vascular adrenal pseudomasses include a tortuous splenic artery, splenic artery aneurysm or pseudoaneurysm, and periadrenal venous collaterals in portal hypertension. Right adrenal pseudotumors are less common and may be caused by tortuous renal vessels or exophytic renal and hepatic masses.

In this case a splenic artery aneurysm mimicked a left adrenal mass on abdominal sonography. Aneurysms of the splenic artery are the most common cause of visceral artery aneurysms. They occur in women twice as frequently as in men, and 90% of women with splenic pseudoaneurysms have been pregnant at least twice. As many as 75% of those patients who suffer rupture, the most common complication of splenic artery aneurysms, may die; the risk of this complication is higher during pregnancy. Calcification in the aneurysm wall is present in two thirds of cases. Notice the linear focus of mural calcification on both the ultrasound and noncontrast CT examinations. Calcified splenic aneurysms may rupture, but this complication may occur less often with this type of aneurysm than with their noncalcified counterparts.

Notes

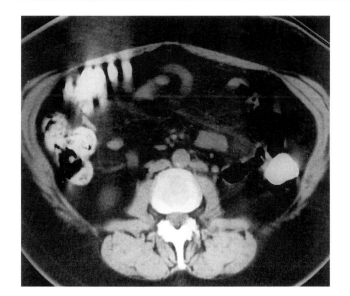
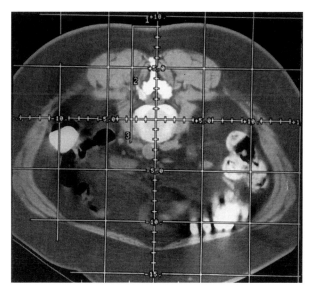

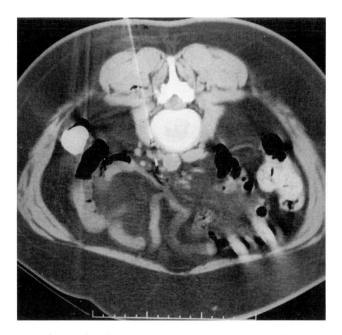

1. What is the abnormal finding in the upper left-hand image?
2. What is the differential diagnosis for this finding?
3. What is the grid shown in the middle of the image on the right?
4. Name two percutaneous techniques for performing biopsy of a retroperitoneal mass.

CASE 30

Percutaneous Biopsy of Retroperitoneal Lymphadenopathy

1. Left paraaortic lymph node.

2. Based on this image alone, a lymph node or duplicated inferior vena cava. Other images showed a single inferior vena cava.

3. An electronic grid used for localization of a biopsy site. Paper grids can also perform this function, although they can be lost or contaminated and are more expensive.

4. Tandem and coaxial.

Reference

Silverman SG, Deuson TE, Kane N, et al: Percutaneous abdominal biopsy: cost-identification analysis, *Radiology* 206:429-435, 1998.

Cross-Reference

Genitourinary Radiology: THE REQUISITES, pp 75-79.

Comment

Staging CT was performed for this patient with carcinoma of the cervix. The only abnormal finding was a small paraaortic lymph node. Accurate staging of cervical carcinoma is critical because treatment may be altered significantly. If this retroperitoneal lymph node contains tumor, the patient has stage IV disease and is not a candidate for surgery. Instead, she must undergo pelvic and paraaortic radiation therapy and possibly chemotherapy. If this node does not contain malignant cells, the patient should undergo radical hysterectomy and pelvic lymph node dissection. The biopsy in this case was positive for carcinoma.

Image-guided biopsy is a routine procedure at most institutions and has achieved general acceptance in the medical community. The study referenced above compared the cost of percutaneous biopsy with surgical biopsy in 400 patients with a newly discovered abdominal mass. The study reported a cost savings of more than $3000 per patient when percutaneous biopsy was performed as the initial procedure to establish the diagnosis.

The techniques used to perform a biopsy vary depending on the institution and the radiologist. A variety of needle types and sizes can be used. Two techniques are used most commonly. The coaxial technique involves placement of a relatively large needle at the edge of a lesion and sampling tissue through a smaller needle placed coaxially through the larger outer needle. This technique is used frequently for the biopsy of lung masses. In addition, this technique is preferable for difficult-to-access lesions because the outer guiding needle needs to be placed only once. Once the outer needle is in place, no further imaging is required to obtain multiple biopsies. For larger lesions, either a coaxial or tandem technique can be used. The tandem technique uses two needles in tandem, the first for localization and the second for performing the biopsy. Using imaging guidance, the first needle is placed in the lesion. Then the second needle is placed in the same plane but adjacent to the first (i.e., tandem to it), and a biopsy is performed. Multiple biopsies can be obtained from the second needle without additional imaging when the first needle serves as a guide. The tandem technique is preferable for larger masses that are easier to access.

Notes

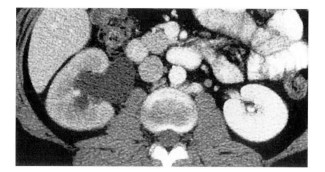
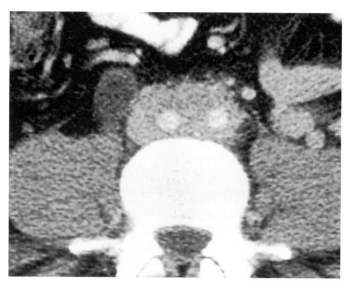

1. What is causing the delayed nephrogram and nephromegaly of the right kidney?

2. What is the likely cause of the soft tissue around the aorta and iliac arteries?

3. What is the fluid-containing structure to the right of the abnormal soft tissue?

4. What is the treatment for this type of hydronephrosis?

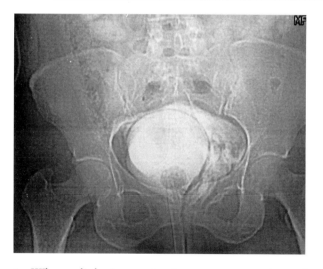
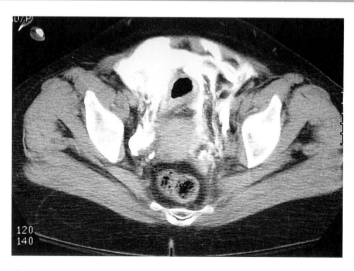

1. What radiologic examinations are commonly used to evaluate traumatic bladder injury?

2. What type of bladder rupture is associated with the collection of extravasated contrast media in the space of Retzius?

3. A "cloudlike" appearance of contrast on conventional cystography is associated with which type of bladder rupture?

4. If the distinction between intraperitoneal and extraperitoneal bladder rupture is still in question after CT cystography, what can be done?

CASE 31

Retroperitoneal Fibrosis

1. Ureteral obstruction.

2. Retroperitoneal fibrosis.

3. Hydroureter.

4. This condition may be managed temporarily with ureteral stents. Definitive therapy usually requires surgical dissection of the ureter, lateralization of the ureter, and ureteral wrapping with omentum or peritoneum to prevent recurrent encasement.

Reference

Amis ES: Retroperitoneal fibrosis, *Am J Roentgenol* 157:321-329, 1991.

Cross-Reference

Genitourinary Radiology: THE REQUISITES, pp 179, 180.

Comment

Retroperitoneal fibrosis (RPF) includes both idiopathic (Ormond's disease) and secondary proliferation of nonneoplastic fibrotic tissues. RPF tends to be centered around the aorta initially, but with progression it encases the inferior vena cava and ureters. RPF is usually centered near the L4-5 level of the spine, but it may arise or extend the entire length of the retroperitoneum, including the renal sinus. Approximately 50% of RPF cases are bilateral. RPF is one of the most common causes of bilateral ureteral obstruction. Obstruction of the ureter is caused by encasement of the ureter by the surrounding RPF. This encasement causes a narrowed, aperistaltic segment of ureter and resulting hydronephrosis. Although only limited success in reversing RPF has been achieved using systemic steroids and chemotherapeutic agents, definitive treatment of the hydronephrosis usually requires surgical intervention, moving the ureter away from the fibrosis and insulating it with protective peritoneum or omentum, thus preventing further progression of the RPF.

Secondary RPF is associated with numerous other entities, including aortic aneurysms, aortic and iliac graft procedures, retroperitoneal hematomas, urinomas, infections, inflammatory bowel disease, sclerosing cholangitis, and fibrosing mediastinitis, and with use of certain drugs, most notably ergot alkaloids.

Lymphoma can present with a similar or identical appearance. Surgical biopsy is often required to obtain adequate tissue to exclude lymphoma. There are no "absolute" imaging characteristics to differentiate RPF from retroperitoneal lymphoma, although extensive soft tissue proliferation behind the aorta strongly suggests lymphoma rather than RPF.

Notes

CASE 32

Radiologic Diagnosis of Bladder Rupture

1. Conventional cystography and CT cystography.

2. Extraperitoneal.

3. Intraperitoneal.

4. Short of surgical exploration, delayed CT scanning or repeat scanning after direct instillation of contrast material into the bladder.

References

Bodner DR, Selzman AA, Spirnak JP: Evaluation and treatment of bladder rupture, *Semin Urol* 13:62-65, 1995.

Sivit CJ, Cutting JP, Eichelberger MR: CT diagnosis and location of rupture of the bladder in children with blunt abdominal trauma: significance of contrast material extravasation in the pelvis, *Am J Roentgenol* 164:1243-1246, 1995.

Cross-Reference

Genitourinary Radiology: THE REQUISITES, pp 224-229.

Comment

The distinction between intraperitoneal and extraperitoneal bladder rupture has important surgical implications. Although conventional cystography is the time-honored method, CT cystography is as accurate and can be performed while the patient is being scanned for evaluation of other abdominopelvic injuries.

The distribution of extravasated contrast material or urine is critical for classifying full-thickness bladder ruptures. In cases of isolated extraperitoneal rupture, like that shown in this case, extravasated fluid or contrast is described as "flame-shaped" and may collect in the perivesical, anterior prevesical (space of Retzius), or retrorectal space. Remember that the prevesical space can extend superiorly to the level of the umbilicus. Extravasated intraperitoneal contrast medium is described as "cloudlike"; contrast or urine may collect in the rectouterine or rectovesical pouch or outline loops of small bowel. If the intraperitoneal leak is large, extravasated contrast may extend to the paracolic gutters or lateral pelvic recesses.

There are several pitfalls associated with CT cystography; it can be difficult to evaluate extravasated urine or contrast material when there is lavage fluid or an extraperitoneal hematoma or when abdominopelvic anatomy is distorted by traumatic injury. In difficult cases, delayed CT scanning (15 to 30 minutes) or repeat scanning after administration of additional intravenous or intravesical contrast material may help.

Notes

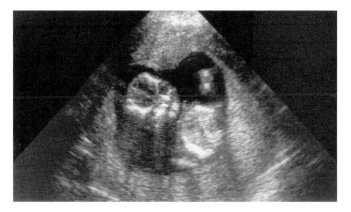 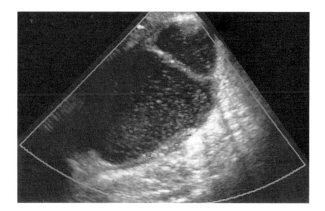

1. After what time in pregnancy (weeks gestational age) are corpus luteum cysts expected to resolve?

2. As a general rule, what is the size threshold (diameter) below which simple ovarian cysts can be managed conservatively when discovered during pregnancy?

3. If removal is indicated, during which trimester is elective excision of an ovarian mass recommended?

4. True or False: The majority of complex ovarian cysts discovered during pregnancy are malignant.

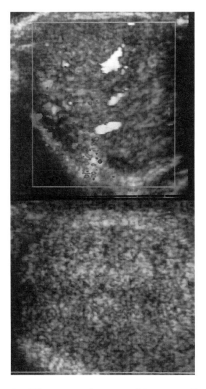 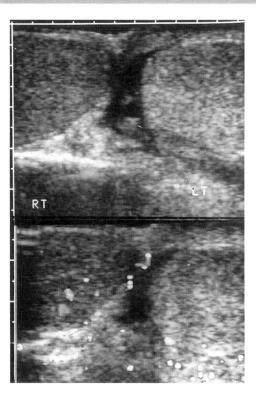

1. These are ultrasound images of an older boy with left hemiscrotal pain and enlargement. The composite image to the left is a sagittal color Doppler image of the right testicle (top) and the left testicle (bottom). The composite image to the right is a coronal gray scale image (top) and a color Doppler image of both testes (bottom). What is the diagnosis?

2. What is the clinical differential diagnosis of spontaneous scrotal pain in the infant or child?

3. Why are false negative diagnoses of torsion diagnosed as epididymitis in older children or adults?

4. For the diagnosis of testicular torsion, is color Doppler imaging more, less, or equally as sensitive as nuclear scintigraphy?

CASE 33

Ovarian Cystadenoma in Pregnancy

1. Approximately 16 weeks gestational age.

2. 5 cm.

3. Second trimester.

4. False. Only about 2% to 5% of adnexal masses removed during pregnancy are malignant.

References

Ghossain MA, Buy JN, Ligneres C, et al: Epithelial tumors of the ovary: comparison of MR and CT findings, *Radiology* 181:863-870, 1991.

Hill LM, Connors-Beatty MA, Norwak A, Tush B: The role of ultrasonography in the detection and management of adnexal masses during the second and third trimesters of pregnancy, *Am J Obstet Gynecol* 179(3):703-707, 1998.

Cross-Reference
Genitourinary Radiology: THE REQUISITES, pp 278-283.

Comment
Cystadenoma is one of the most commonly encountered benign ovarian neoplasms. Serous tumors are often unilocular and commonly contain "simple" fluid. In contrast, mucinous cystadenomas are multilocular and have uniformly thin (less than 3 mm) septations. Fluid within individual loculi may be "complex" because of proteinaceous debris, hemorrhage, or both. Papillary projections are unusual and, if present, should suggest a borderline malignancy or cystadenocarcinoma.

When discovered during pregnancy, ovarian cysts less than 5 cm in diameter tend to resolve between 13 and 30 weeks. It has been recommended that all cysts greater than 10 cm in diameter be removed; controversy exists regarding the appropriate management of cysts between 5 and 10 cm in diameter. Elective excision (before symptoms develop) of an ovarian mass that persists beyond 16 weeks gestation and avoidance of surgery in the first and third trimesters help to decrease the risk of pregnancy termination and preterm labor.

Serous cystadenoma must be differentiated from a functional ovarian cyst, hydrosalpinx, paratubal cyst, peritoneal pseudocyst, and tuboovarian abscess. Functional ovarian cysts are common in women of child-bearing age and may represent follicular cysts, corpus luteum cysts, or corpora albicans cysts. Hydrosalpinx appears as a tortuous, fluid-filled mass containing mucosal infoldings. Paratubal cysts are usually small and are among the most common conditions of the fallopian tubes that can mimic an ovarian cyst. Peritoneal pseudocysts are collections of ascitic fluid trapped within mesothelium-lined cavities. These fluid collections are often associated with endometriosis or prior surgery.

Notes

CASE 34

Testicular Torsion and Infarction

1. The left testicle is heterogeneously hyperechoic and has no flow. The right testicle is normal.

2. Torsion of the spermatic cord, incarcerated hernia, epididymitis, and torsion of the appendix testis.

3. Spontaneous detorsion is often associated with reactive hyperemia of the testis.

4. It is equally as sensitive. Both have reported sensitivities between 85% and 100%.

References

Sanelli PC, Burke BJ, Lee L: Color and spectral Doppler sonography of partial torsion of the spermatic cord, *Am J Roentgenol* 12:49-51, 1999.

Cross-Reference
Genitourinary Radiology: THE REQUISITES, pp 306-309.

Comment
The main vascular supply to the testis is from the testicular artery, which arises from the abdominal aorta. The testicular artery, along with the ipsilateral deferential artery, enters the spermatic cord and divides near the mediastinum of the testis. Branches ramify along the surface of the testis in the tunica vasculosa and then give rise to centripetal branches that enter the testis parenchyma. Through anastomoses between the testicular and deferential arteries, there is a shared vascular supply between the testis and epididymis.

Testicular viability depends on the duration of ischemia and on the number of turns in the twisted spermatic cord. Irreversible ischemic damage can occur within 4 hours after complete torsion ($\geq$450-degree twist), but the testis may remain viable for more than 24 hours when the degree of torsion is low (180- and 360-degree rotations).

Gray scale sonography is of less value in the early stages of testicular torsion and often demonstrates a normal testicle when the torsion has occurred within the last 6 hours. Between 8 and 24 hours after torsion, the testis and epididymis may enlarge and become heterogeneously hypoechoic or hyperechoic, as demonstrated in this case.

Color Doppler imaging is as sensitive as nuclear scintigraphy for the diagnosis of complete torsion in adults and older children, although its sensitivity in small infants is reduced because of limitations in detecting flow in small (less than 1 cm^3) testicles. The *sine qua non* is the demonstration of normal flow in the contralateral normal testicle and absent flow in the ipsilateral symptomatic one. Flow in the epididymis also may be reduced; certainly it should not be increased, which would be expected in epididymitis. False negative diagnoses of torsion have been attributed to intermittent torsion.

Notes

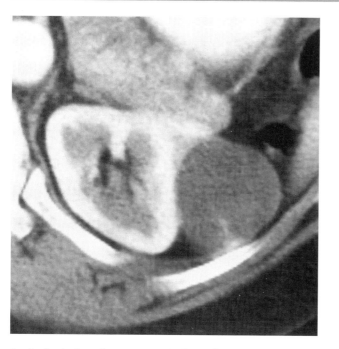 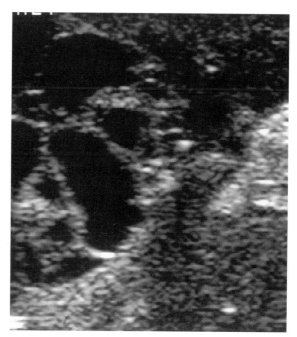

1. Is the lesion shown a surgical renal mass or would it usually be treated conservatively?
2. What are the main differential diagnoses for this type of mass?
3. Using the Bosniak classification, what class is this lesion?
4. What single imaging feature is specific for the diagnosis of multilocular cystic nephroma?

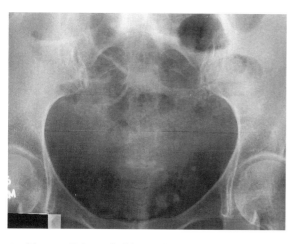 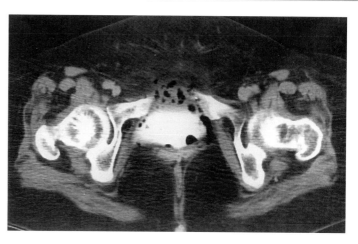

1. True or False: Bladder wall emphysema is equivalent to gangrenous cystitis and therefore should be treated as a life-threatening illness in all cases.
2. Name the two main risk factors for this disease.
3. What is the recommended treatment for this disease?
4. True or False: The most common causative organism is *Clostridium perfringens.*

Cystic Renal Cell Carcinoma

1. Based on the multiple septations and slight thickening of the peripheral margins, this mass should be considered a surgical renal mass. This determination is further confirmed by the sonographic image showing thick septations.

2. Renal cell carcinoma, multilocular cystic nephroma, and renal cyst complicated by infection or hemorrhage.

3. Based on the CT scan this is a Bosniak class III lesion. Cystic lesions with multiple septa and no enhancing solid components are Bosniak class III.

4. Herniation of the mass into the renal pelvis.

Reference
Bosniak MA: Problems in the radiologic diagnosis of renal parenchymal tumors, *Urol Clin North Am* 20:217-230, 1993.

Cross-Reference
Genitourinary Radiology: THE REQUISITES, pp 87-89.

Comment
Any ball-shaped renal mass that is not a simple cyst and does not contain detectable fat should be considered a renal cell carcinoma. Lesions that are predominantly cystic can be further classified using the Bosniak classification system. This system allows for some complex cystic lesions with additional features, such as thin, peripheral calcifications or one or two septa, to be classified as benign cysts. However, Bosniak class III and IV lesions are surgical renal masses, unless there are extenuating circumstances, such as metastatic disease, or features strongly suggestive of an alternative nonsurgical diagnosis, such as an abscess. CT renal masses that appear to be cysts must be scrutinized very carefully. As demonstrated by this case, enhancement can be very subtle; multiple septations are faintly visible within this mass. When there is doubt regarding the diagnosis, sonography can help to further elucidate the internal architecture of a renal mass. Sonography clearly shows the complicated internal architecture of this mass, which was a renal cell carcinoma.

Multilocular cystic nephroma can have an appearance identical to that of renal cell carcinoma. Sometimes multilocular cystic nephromas herniate into the renal sinus. This sign is diagnostic of this entity, but it is not sensitive for this diagnosis. Most multilocular cystic nephromas do not herniate into the renal pelvis.

Notes

Emphysematous Cystitis

1. False.

2. Diabetes mellitus and bladder outlet obstruction.

3. First-line treatment includes antibiotic therapy, adequate bladder drainage, and treatment of hyperglycemia (if present).

4. False.

Reference
Quint EJ, Drach GW, Rappaport WD, Hoffman CJ: Emphysematous cystitis: a review of the spectrum of disease, *J Urol* 147:134-137, 1992.

Cross-Reference
Genitourinary Radiology: THE REQUISITES, p 215.

Comment
Emphysematous cystitis (EC), or cystitis emphysematosa, is a rare infection in which pockets of gas form in the bladder wall. Risk factors include poorly controlled diabetes and urinary stasis (caused by neurogenic bladder or bladder outlet obstruction). Less commonly there is an association with subcutaneous emphysema, hemorrhagic cystitis, and alcoholic liver disease. *Escherichia coli* and *Enterobacter* species are the organisms most commonly isolated, but other bacteria, including *Clostridium perfringens* and *Nocardia* and *Candida* species, also have been linked to EC. Carbon-dioxide gas bubbles form in the bladder wall or lumen when the infecting microbe ferments glucose. Because glucose is consumed in this process, the urine dipstick test may be negative for glucose. The clinical course of this rare cystitis is variable and unpredictable; the course can be benign and reversible, but rare fatalities have been reported. Emphysematous ureteritis, nephritis, and adrenalitis may coexist and cause a more life-threatening infection.

The radiologic appearance of EC may be confused with that of rectal air, pneumatosis cystoides intestinalis, emphysematous vaginitis, and gas gangrene of the uterus. The appearance of linear ring or ovoid clusters of gas in the bladder wall on CT is usually diagnostic. The bladder wall may be thickened or nodular. Bladder luminal gas without mural collections of gas, known as *primary pneumaturia or pneumocystosis,* is not synonymous with EC. Treatment includes appropriate antibiotic therapy and adequate bladder drainage. Elimination of the infecting microorganisms results in gradual absorption of carbon dioxide.

Notes

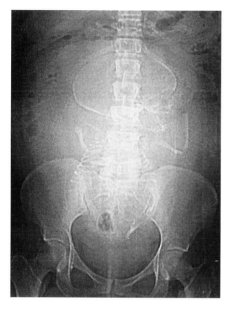
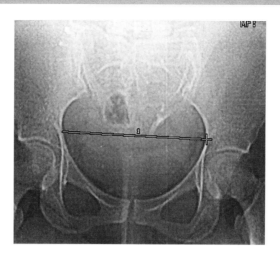

1. Why was this examination performed?
2. What is the indication for the study?
3. What measurements are obtained from the study?
4. From what other imaging techniques can these measurements be obtained?

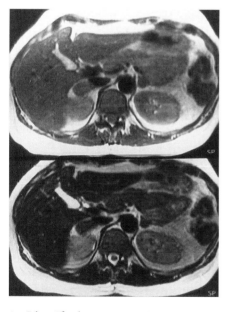
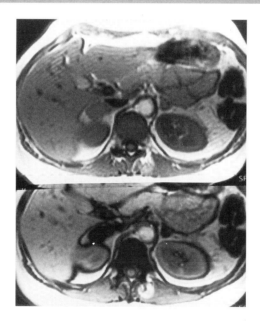

1. Identify these composite MR image pairs.
2. What is the diagnosis in this case?
3. What is the cause for loss of signal in the adrenal mass on the bottom image of the figure to the right?
4. Name two conditions that might result in a change in the appearance of this mass on repeat chemical shift MRI.

Pelvimetry

1. To evaluate maternal pelvis size and determine whether it is large enough to allow vaginal delivery.

2. Breech presentation.

3. Interspinous distance, anteroposterior (AP) pelvic inlet diameter, and transverse pelvic diameter.

4. Conventional and digital radiography and MRI.

References

Thomas SM, Bees NR, et al: Trends in the use of pelvimetry techniques, *Clin Radiol* 53(4):293-295, 1998.

van Loon AJ, Mantigh A, et al: Randomized controlled trial of magnetic resonance pelvimetry in breech presentation at term, *Lancet* 350:1799-1804, 1997.

Cross-Reference

Genitourinary Radiology: THE REQUISITES, pp 48, 49.

Comment

In cases of breech presentation, pelvimetry is used to evaluate maternal pelvis size. The clinical objective is to determine whether vaginal delivery can be safely performed. A relatively small maternal pelvis increases the risk of complications during vaginal delivery and could necessitate an emergency cesarean section.

Pelvimetry was originally performed with conventional radiography, but more recently, low-dose CT, digital fluoroscopy, and MRI have been used. One pelvimetry technique employing CT calls for a single AP scout image, a single lateral scout image, and sometimes a single axial image at the level of the ischial spines (measures the interspinous distance). When the low-dose CT technique is used, the average absorbed radiation dose is approximately half of that absorbed when conventional radiography is used.

Pelvimetry should report the interspinous distance, the AP pelvic inlet diameter, and the transverse pelvic diameter. Measured from an axial image or the AP scout, an interspinous distance of less than 10 cm is considered abnormally small. An AP pelvic inlet diameter is measured from the sacral promontory to the posterior aspect of the symphysis pubis on the lateral scout view; a value of less than 11 cm is considered small. The transverse pelvic diameter is measured between the iliac bones, midway between the inferior sacroiliac joint and the symphysis on the AP scout (as shown in the image on the right). A measurement of less than 12 cm is considered abnormal.

Notes

Characterization of the Adrenal Mass with Chemical Shift MRI

1. The composite figure to the left shows a T1W image (top) and a turbo spin-echo, T2W image (bottom). The composite image to the right shows an in-phase, T1W gradient echo image (top) and an opposed-phase, T1W gradient echo MR image (bottom) of a right adrenal mass.

2. Adenoma of the right adrenal gland.

3. Phase cancellation caused by the presence of both fat and water protons.

4. Metastasis to a gland with an adrenal adenoma (collision tumor) and metyrapone treatment.

Reference

Mitchell DG, Crovello M, Matteucci T, Petersen RO, Miettinen MM: Benign adrenocortical masses: diagnosis with chemical shift MR imaging, *Radiology* 185:345-351, 1992.

Cross-Reference

Genitourinary Radiology: THE REQUISITES, pp 29, 30, 346-349.

Comment

Adrenal cortical cells and tumors derived from these cells contain a large amount of cytoplasmic cholesterol, fatty acids, and neutral fat. Adrenal adenomas can be characterized on both CT and chemical shift MRI because they contain large numbers of "clear" cells (cortical cells with abundant lipids).

On MRI the chemical environment of a proton, and specifically magnetic shielding by nearby electrons, may result in a change or shift in the resonance frequency of that proton. When a slice of tissue is first excited, all of the protons resonate synchronously (in phase) with one another but very soon thereafter, water and fat protons resonate asynchronously (out of phase) with one another because of this chemical shift. The temporal periodicity of this cyclic phase synchrony-asynchrony can be approximated by the quotient of 3.4 ms/T divided by the magnet field strength (in units of Tesla). If the echo time of a gradient echo pulse sequence corresponds with one of the "out-of-phase" times, then the signal intensity of a voxel containing equal populations of both fat and water decreases because of intravoxel phase cancellation. The signal intensity of a voxel is determined by a vectorial average of the amplitude and phase of its constituent protons. However, a voxel containing either mostly fat or mostly water protons will not have significant phase dispersion and therefore will not lose signal on the opposed-phase image. In most cases visual assessment of signal loss is as accurate as quantitative measurements (e.g., lesion-to-spleen signal intensity ratios).

Notes

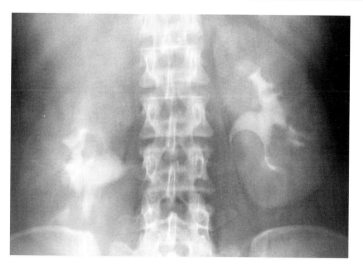
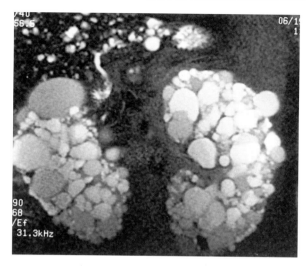

1. What causes the numerous lucencies seen on this patient's intravenous urogram (the image on the right)?

2. What is the most likely underlying diagnosis in these two patients with the same disease?

3. Why are some of the masses of lower signal intensity on the coronal T2W MRI?

4. What is the risk of renal cell carcinoma development in this group of patients?

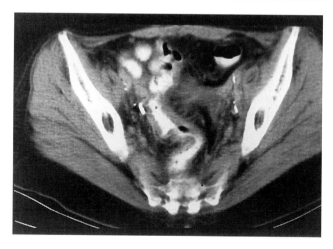
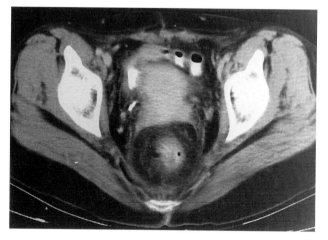

1. This patient received radiation therapy for stage IIB cervical carcinoma. What is the most likely diagnosis?

2. What thickness of the distended rectal wall is considered abnormal?

3. True or False: The frequency of radiotherapy-associated complications is much higher in patients with cervical cancer than in those with endometrial cancer.

4. True or False: Injury to the ascending colon as a result of radiation therapy for cervical cancer is common.

CASE 39

Autosomal Dominant Polycystic Kidney Disease

1. Numerous renal cysts.

2. Autosomal dominant polycystic kidney disease.

3. These represent cysts complicated by infection or hemorrhage, resulting in higher protein content in the fluid.

4. The same as in the general population.

Reference

Hartman DS: An overview of renal cystic disease. In Hartman DS, editor: *Renal cystic disease,* Philadelphia, 1989, Saunders.

Cross-Reference

Genitourinary Radiology: THE REQUISITES, pp 108-110.

Comment

Autosomal dominant polycystic kidney disease (ADPKD) is a hereditary disorder that is inherited in an autosomal dominant pattern. It usually becomes symptomatic in the third or fourth decade of life, with evidence of renal disease. This disease may come to light as a result of hematuria, hypertension, or renal insufficiency. Up to 15% of patients develop intracranial aneurysms that may lead to spontaneous subarachnoid hemorrhage and later discovery of the underlying renal disease. Although there is no increased risk of malignancy development in these patients, the disease, which has a high degree of penetrance, nearly always progresses to complete renal failure and the need for long-term dialysis. As the patient ages, more and more renal cysts develop, leading to complete replacement of the parenchyma by cystic masses, as seen on this MRI. In addition to intracranial aneurysms, these patients often develop cysts in other organs. Hepatic cysts, as seen on the MRI, occur in up to 75% of ADPKD patients. Cysts in other abdominal and pelvic viscera also are relatively common. The numerous lucent lesions corresponding to cysts are described as the "Swiss cheese" nephrogram. This finding is rarely seen today because most patients with this disease are diagnosed by sonography.

Notes

CASE 40

Colitis after Radiation Treatment of Cervical Carcinoma

1. Proctocolitis secondary to radiation treatment.

2. 4 mm or more.

3. True.

4. False.

Reference

Blomlie V, Rofstad EK, Trope C, Lien HH: Critical soft tissues of the female pelvis: serial MR imaging before, during, and after radiation therapy, *Radiology* 203:391-397, 1997.

Cross-Reference

Genitourinary Radiology: THE REQUISITES, pp 301, 302.

Comment

For patients with cervical cancer that involves the parametrial tissues, lower third of the vagina, or pelvic sidewall, radiation therapy is the treatment of choice. Radiation injury to the rectosigmoid colon or to the lower urinary tract may be confused with recurrent disease. Adverse effects occur significantly more often in patients who have cervical cancer compared with those who have endometrial cancer because of higher rectal doses from intracavitary radiation sources. Injury to the rectal wall usually occurs before injury to the bladder; the mean time is 20 to 24 months after the completion of radiation therapy.

Although rectovaginal fistula is the most significant complication, radiation enterocolitis occurs more often, yet still affects fewer than 5% of patients. Patients may complain of abdominal or rectal cramping, diarrhea, or rectal bleeding. Radiation enteritis is less common that proctosigmoiditis, but the patient whose small intestine is fixed in the pelvis by surgical adhesions or who has other pelvic pathologic conditions is at increased risk. Several findings on CT may suggest the diagnosis of radiation proctosigmoiditis. Colon wall thickness of 4 mm or more is considered abnormal and is the most common sign of radiation colitis. Like ischemic colitis, which shares the common pathophysiologic finding of an occlusive arteriopathy, radiation colitis has been associated with pneumatosis. Rarely, there is perirectal fibrofatty proliferation.

The referenced article makes several interesting observations about radiation injury to the lower urinary tract. Pelvic hydroureter may occur because of parametrial cellulitis, trigonal ulceration, or periureteral fibrosis but is transient in about half of cases. Gas in the urinary bladder is a harbinger of vesical fistula, but after cystoscopy, it may remain in the irradiated bladder for more than 1 week because of poor bladder emptying. In the normal bladder, gas after cystoscopy resolves within four micturitions.

Notes

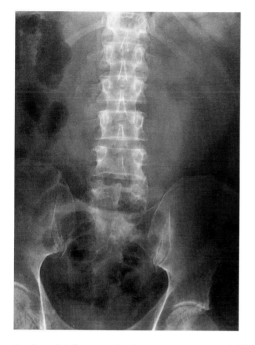 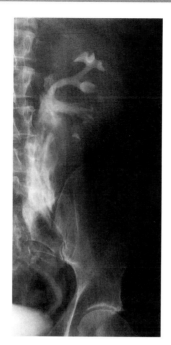

1. In which space is the contrast material located at the L4-5 region of the spine?
2. What is the underlying cause of this contrast material extravasation?
3. At what site does the extravasation usually originate?
4. What is the cause of hydronephrosis?

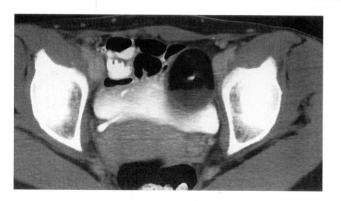 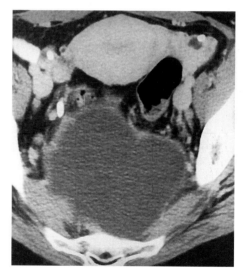

1. These pelvic CT images are from two different patients. What is the diagnosis in both cases?
2. Name the four general pathologic types of ovarian neoplasms.
3. Notice the bilateral ovarian disease in one of these cases. What is the significance of this finding?
4. What is the current treatment for this lesion?

CASE 41

Ureteral Obstruction with Perirenal Contrast Material Extravasation

1. In the perirenal space.

2. Ureteral obstruction.

3. The fornix of a calyx.

4. An impacted stone at the ureterovesical junction.

Reference

Chapman JP, Gonzalez J, Diokno AC: Significance of urinary extravasation during renal colic, *Urology* 6:541-545, 1987.

Cross-Reference

Genitourinary Radiology: THE REQUISITES, pp 79, 131.

Comment

This patient has a 5 mm–diameter stone obstructing the ureter at the left ureterovesical junction. The resulting hydroureteronephrosis has led to spontaneous rupture of a calyceal fornix and contrast material extravasation. Some contrast material is visible in the renal sinus (a part of the perirenal space), superimposed on the lower pole calyces, with most of the contrast material tracking within the perirenal space around the ureter.

Spontaneous forniceal rupture secondary to ureteral obstruction is not a rare phenomenon. However, it must be recognized as the totally benign entity that it is. It should not be confused with significant pathologic problems. This rupture likely represents a physiologic "pop-off" valve that opens when pyelocalyceal pressures reach very high levels. With ureteral obstruction, pyelocalyceal pressures can rise from near 0 to more than 70 mm Hg in a short time. This rise leads to hydroureteronephrosis and severe renal colic. When a fornix ruptures, the pressure reduces rapidly and there is a sudden relief of symptoms, which clinically may mimic the symptoms of stone passage. Forniceal rupture is of no clinical significance as long as the high-grade obstruction does not persist for a prolonged period. Urinoma formation after spontaneous forniceal rupture caused by ureteral obstruction is uncommon. Interestingly, it is quite common to see gallbladder opacification caused by vicarious contrast material excretion hours or days after perirenal extravasation of contrast material. This finding also is of no clinical significance.

Notes

CASE 42

CT of Ovarian Dermoid Cyst

1. Dermoid cyst (mature cystic teratoma).

2. Epithelial (serous, mucinous, and endometrioid), germ cell (dermoid, dysgerminoma, endodermal sinus tumor, and choriocarcinoma), sex-cord stroma (fibroma-thecoma, granulosa cell, and Sertoli-Leydig cell tumors), and metastatic cancer.

3. There may be a greater risk of developing a germ cell malignancy in women with bilateral dermoid cysts.

4. Although malignant transformation is rare, most patients undergo surgical removal because of an increased risk of complications, including torsion and possibly rupture.

Reference

Anteby EY, Ron M, Revel A, Shimonovitz S, Ariel I, Hurwitz A: Germ cell tumors of the ovary arising after dermoid cyst resection: long-term follow up study, *Obstet Gynecol* 83(4): 605-608, 1994.

Cross-Reference

Genitourinary Radiology: THE REQUISITES, pp 278-280.

Comment

Cystic teratomas account for about 10% to 15% of all ovarian neoplasms. These tumors are composed of well-differentiated tissues from ectodermal, mesodermal, and endodermal lineage. Dermoid cysts are overwhelmingly composed of ectodermal tissues, such as hair, teeth, and sebaceous glands, which can produce oil or fat. They are most commonly discovered in young women during their reproductive years and represent two thirds of ovarian neoplasms in adolescent girls.

Torsion, perforation, and infection can occur, and rarely, sudden rupture may cause a chemical peritonitis. The risk of complications and malignant transformation is higher with larger tumors, particularly those more than 5 cm in diameter.

For the diagnosis of a dermoid cyst, CT and ultrasound findings are often pathognomonic. On CT, cystic teratomas are typically well defined, thin-walled cysts with fatty components and foci of calcification. Rarely these tumors have a nonspecific appearance of a debris-filled cyst containing proteinaceous material without calcification. On ultrasound, dermoid cysts have a varied appearance as a result of their heterogeneous internal structure. Often they appear as cysts with a fat-fluid or fat-debris level and have a highly echogenic focus that is thought to represent a mixture of matted hair and sebum. Echogenic, shadowing areas of calcification also can be identified in this benign tumor.

Notes

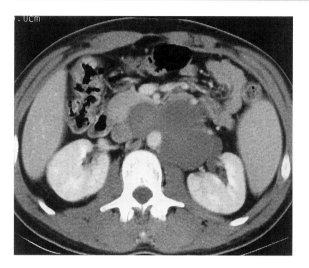 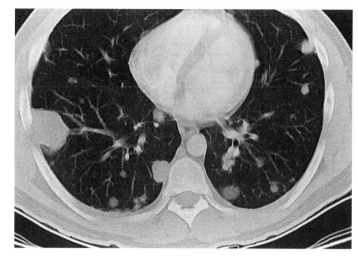

1. What is the most common route through which testicular carcinoma is spread?

2. Where is the "sentinel" node for a primary malignancy of the left testicle? Where is it for a malignancy of the right testicle?

3. What are the staging implications of testicular cancer that invades the epididymis or the scrotal wall?

4. Which testicular cancers are associated with elevated alpha-fetoprotein (AFP) levels? Which are associated with elevated human chorionic gonadotropin (hCG) levels?

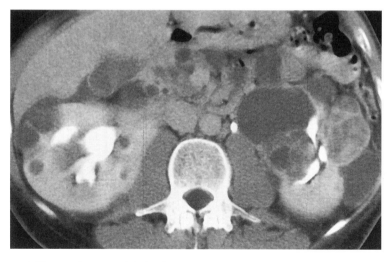 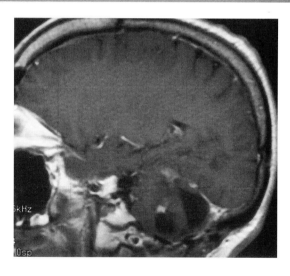

1. What is the most likely diagnosis?

2. What conditions are associated with the development of renal cysts and solid renal masses?

3. What type of central nervous system lesion is present in this case?

4. Are pancreatic cysts more commonly seen with autosomal dominant polycystic kidney disease or von Hippel-Lindau disease?

Staging of Testicular Cancer

1. Via the lymphatics to the retroperitoneal nodes first, and then hematogenously to the lungs, liver, bone, and brain.

2. Left: Renal perihilar, just inferior to the renal vein. Right: Paracaval, inferior to the right renal artery.

3. Change in the lymph nodal drainage pattern.

4. AFP: Yolk sac carcinoma, embryonal cell carcinoma, and mixed tumors (teratocarcinoma). hCG: pure seminoma, embryonal cell carcinoma, and choriocarcinoma.

Reference

Sheinfeld J: Nonseminomatous germ cell tumors of the testis: current concepts and controversies, *Urology* 44:2-10, 1994.

Cross-Reference

Genitourinary Radiology: THE REQUISITES, pp 316, 317.

Comment

The staging of germ cell testicular neoplasms is based on the tendency for these tumors to spread to the retroperitoneal nodes first, and then the mediastinal nodes and lung parenchyma. Later, hematogenous spread to the lungs, liver, bones, and brain may occur. In addition to serum assays of AFP, hCG, and lactate dehydrogenase, staging usually includes chest radiography; CT of the chest, abdomen, and pelvis; and a radionuclide bone scan. Stage I tumors have not spread from the testis, and Stage II tumors are confined to the abdominal cavity. Stage II nonseminomatous germ cell tumors have been classified into IIa (nodes less than 2 cm in diameter), IIb (nodes 2 to 5 cm in diameter), and IIc (nodes more than 5 cm in diameter). The paracaval, interaortocaval, and right common iliac node groups are considered the primary sites of spread (sentinel node groups) for right-sided tumors. For left-sided testicular tumors, interaortocaval, left paraaortic, and left common iliac nodes are sentinel nodes. Local spread of the testicular neoplasm to the epididymis may result in metastatic external iliac lymphadenopathy, and spread to the scrotal wall may result in inguinal node involvement. Stage III testicular tumor has spread to supradiaphragmatic nodal sites, viscera (lung or liver), brain, or bone.

It is important to distinguish between the seminomatous and nonseminomatous germ cell tumors (i.e., embryonal cell carcinoma, teratoma, yolk sac tumor, and choriocarcinoma) because seminomas are some of the most radiosensitive tumors, and treatment of the nonseminomatous germ cell tumors is centered on cisplatin-based combination chemotherapy. Serum markers are important for the management of testicular cancers after radical orchiectomy. AFP is produced by endodermal sinus cells of the yolk sac and has a half-life of 5 days; if the marker remains elevated 2 to 3 weeks after removal of the testis, most likely there is metastatic disease. hCG is a glycoprotein secreted by placental cells and has a half-life of 30 hours.

Notes

von Hippel-Lindau Disease

1. von Hippel-Lindau disease.

2. von Hippel-Lindau disease, tuberous sclerosis, and long-term dialysis.

3. Cerebellar hemangioblastoma.

4. von Hippel-Lindau disease.

Reference

Choyke PL, Filling-Katz MR, Shawker TH, et al: von Hippel-Lindau disease: radiologic screening for visceral manifestations, *Radiology* 174:805-810, 1990.

Cross-Reference

Genitourinary Radiology: THE REQUISITES, pp 109, 110.

Comment

von Hippel-Lindau disease is a genetic disorder inherited with an autosomal dominant pattern. The common manifestations include retinal angiomas, central nervous system hemangioblastomas, and abdominal abnormalities. Renal cysts are seen in up to 90% of patients with von Hippel-Lindau disease. Renal cell carcinomas develop in approximately 40% of these patients and in the majority of patients are multiple and bilateral. In this case there are two solid, enhancing masses that represent renal cell carcinomas in the left kidney. Even the simple-appearing cysts in the kidneys of these patients are often dysplastic and may develop into neoplasms. The second most common intraabdominal organ involved in these patients is the pancreas, which often contains multiple cysts or cystic neoplasms. This finding helps to distinguish the abdominal pattern of this disease from autosomal dominant polycystic kidney disease, which is not associated with an increased risk of renal cell carcinoma and rarely involves the pancreas. The most common cause of death in patients with von Hippel-Lindau disease relates to spread of the renal cell carcinomas.

Notes

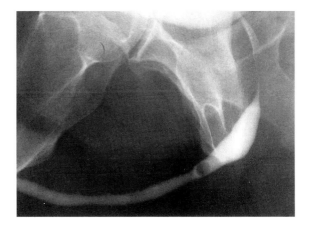
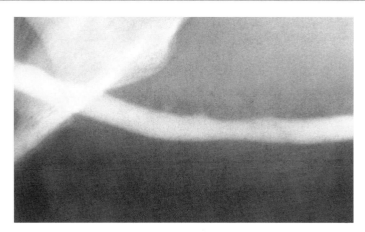

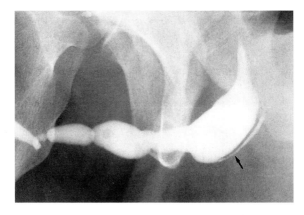

1. On the top two images, what causes the slightly irregular contour along the dorsal aspect of the anterior male urethra?

2. On the bottom image, to what structure does the arrow point?

3. Where is the gland for the structure marked by the arrow located?

4. True or False: The structure indicated by the arrow can be opacified normally on a voiding cystourethrogram or retrograde urethrogram.

Glands and Ducts of the Anterior Male Urethra

1. Contrast fills the glands of Littre.

2. Cowper's duct.

3. It is embedded in the striated urethral sphincter.

4. True.

Reference

Yaffe D, Zissin R: Cowper's glands duct: radiographic findings, *Urol Radiol* 13:123-125, 1991.

Cross-Reference

Genitourinary Radiology: THE REQUISITES, p 244.

Comment

The mucosa of the penile urethra shows many recesses, which continue into deeper-branching tubular mucous glands *(glandulae urethrales urethrae masculinae)* that are particularly numerous on the dorsal aspect. These small mucous glands were named by the French surgeon Alexis Littre (1658 to 1890) and bear his name. Although Littre's glands may sometimes opacify normally, they are more often demonstrated when the glands become inflamed and narrowed in the setting of acute or chronic urethritis (littritis).

The *glandula bulbourethralis* bear the name of the English surgeon, William Cowper (1666 to 1709). Cowper's glands are each about 1 cm in diameter (but like everything else, atrophy with age), are embedded in the substance of the sphincter of the urethra, and are located just posterolateral to the membranous part of the urethra. The excretory duct of each gland (Cowper's duct) is almost 3 cm in length and passes obliquely forward to open on the floor of the bulbar urethra. The third figure of this case shows opacification of Cowper's duct resulting from serial urethral strictures. Opacification of a minimally dilated duct on a retrograde or voiding urethrogram is of no clinical significance, but occasionally ductal stenosis may result in dilation of the more proximal duct or Cowper's gland (imperforate syringocele or retention cyst).

Notes

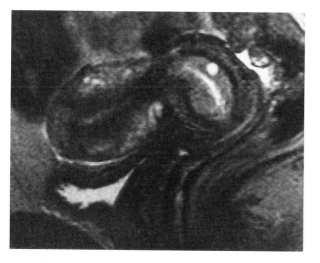 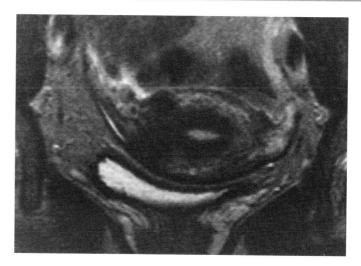

1. What is the uterine junctional zone?
2. What is the normal thickness of the junctional zone?
3. If this patient had dysfunctional uterine bleeding, would endometrial ablation be curative?
4. True or False: The ectopic endometrium in adenomyosis bleeds cyclically.

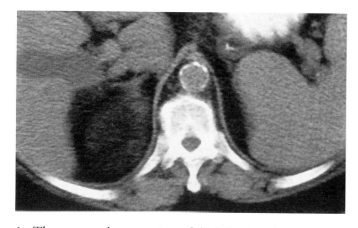 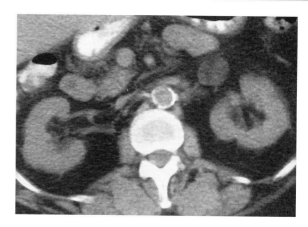

1. The measured attenuation of the left adrenal mass was −82 HU. What is the most likely diagnosis?
2. Is this lesion ever associated with hormone production?
3. What management is recommended?
4. What are the essential features of this lesion on biopsy?

CASE 46

Adenomyosis

1. The inner third of the myometrium; it is the part of the myometrium that is hypointense on a T2W image of the uterus.

2. 2 to 8 mm.

3. It may not be successful in cases of deep adenomyosis.

4. False.

Reference

Reinhold C, McCarthy S, Bret P, et al: Diffuse adenomyosis: comparison of endovaginal US and MR imaging with histopathologic correlation, *Radiology* 199:151-158, 1996.

Cross-Reference

Genitourinary Radiology: THE REQUISITES, pp 260, 261.

Comment

Adenomyosis is defined as the presence of ectopic endometrial glands and stroma within the myometrium. Islands of ectopic endometrium can be found in the inner myometrium within several millimeters of the basalis layer of the endometrium. In patients with this more superficial form of adenomyosis, endometrial ablation may be an effective treatment for menorrhagia. However, in deep adenomyosis, ectopic endometrium extends beyond the inner myometrium and is more often associated with uterine enlargement and symptoms of dysmenorrhea or dysfunctional uterine bleeding. For patients with deep adenomyosis, endometrial ablation or resection may not effectively treat symptoms, and hysterectomy may be necessary.

The diagnosis of adenomyosis on MRI relies on the demonstration of 2- to 7-mm cystic spaces (endometrial glands, endometrial cysts, or hemorrhagic foci), an abnormally thick junctional zone (endometrial stroma), or both in the uterine myometrium. Islands of ectopic endometrium or small endometrial cysts appear as multiple small, hyperintense foci in hypertrophied myometrium on T2W images. These microcystic areas enhance and in some cases are hyperintense on precontrast T1W images because of hemorrhage.

The appearance of ectopic endometrial stroma is indistinguishable from that of junctional zone tissue because both are composed of densely packed smooth muscle. Compared with the outer myometrium, the junctional zone (inner myometrium) has more compact smooth muscle, less extracellular matrix, and lower water content. Focal thickening of the junctional zone (≥12 mm), as seen in this case, or a focal spiculated mass contiguous with the endometrium is more specific than diffuse junctional zone thickening for the diagnosis of deep adenomyosis.

Notes

CASE 47

Imaging Characteristics of Myelolipoma

1. Bilateral adrenal myelolipomas.

2. Rarely. There are case reports of myelolipoma associated with Cushing's syndrome.

3. Follow up with imaging; perform surgery only if the patient is symptomatic.

4. Both mature fat and myeloid (hematopoietic) tissue.

Reference

Musante F, Derchi LE, Zappasodi F, et al: Myelolipoma of the adrenal gland: sonographic and CT features, *Am J Roentgenol* 151:961-964, 1988.

Cross-Reference

Genitourinary Radiology: THE REQUISITES, pp 360, 361.

Comment

First described in 1905 by Gierke, myelolipoma of the adrenal gland is a rare, hormonally inactive, and benign neoplasm composed of mature adipose and hematopoietic tissue. This tumor usually is discovered as an incidental mass on intravenous urography, sonography, or CT, but myelolipoma has been associated with back or flank pain and can be complicated by hemorrhage.

These tumors are well circumscribed and have various amounts of soft tissue, fat, and small calcifications. The cornerstone of the imaging diagnosis is the presence of mature fat tissue in the adrenal myelolipoma. At presentation, these masses can measure between 2 and 20 cm in diameter. Ultrasound demonstrates large areas of increased echogenicity corresponding to foci of mature adipose tissue, and on CT, areas of fat typically have measured attenuation values ranging from -30 to -115 HU. By comparison, the measured attenuation of adrenal adenoma is between -10 and $+18$ HU. False positive misdiagnosis can occur when there is partial volume averaging of normal periadrenal fat. False negative misdiagnosis may occur if contrast medium is infused; the soft tissue component may enhance and can obscure the detection of small foci of fat in the tumor. In addition, necrosis or hemorrhage may dominate the appearance if these rare complications occur.

Focal areas of mature fat can be identified in an exophytic renal angiomyolipoma, chronic adrenal hemorrhage, adrenocortical carcinoma, and retroperitoneal liposarcoma; there has even been a case report of metastatic adenocarcinoma enveloping periadrenal fat that mimicked a myelolipoma. If the diagnosis is equivocal, percutaneous needle biopsy may be used, but it is critical to identify mature hematopoietic tissue in the specimen.

Notes

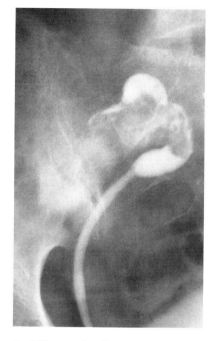

1. What is the diagnosis in this case?
2. How should the ureteral dilation in the ureter below the filling defect be described?
3. What causes this ureteral dilation?
4. Which subtype of tumor is this?

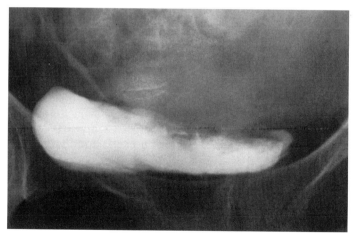 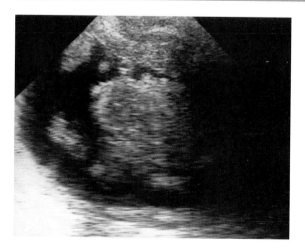

1. This patient has gross hematuria. Is it a clot or a tumor?
2. Within the bladder, what is the most common location of bladder carcinomas?
3. What is an important prognostic factor for bladder carcinoma?
4. What are the treatment options for patients with bladder carcinoma?

Transitional Cell Carcinoma with the "Goblet" Sign

1. Transitional cell carcinoma.

2. The "goblet" sign.

3. Long-standing, slowly growing polypoid mass in the ureter is repeatedly pushed into the ureter just caudal to it by peristalsis.

4. Papillary transitional cell carcinoma.

Reference

Bergman H, Friedenberg RM, Sayegh V: New roentgenologic signs of carcinoma of the ureter, *Am J Roentgenol* 86:707-717, 1961.

Cross-Reference

Genitourinary Radiology: THE REQUISITES, pp 172, 173.

Comment

Transitional cell carcinomas (TCCs) grow in either a papillary or nonpapillary form. The papillary variety tends to grow into a polypoid mass that protrudes into the lumen of the urinary tract. When this occurs in the ureter, a "goblet" sign may ensue. The term *goblet sign* describes ureteral dilation below a radiolucent filling defect. The meniscus of contrast material in the upper extent of the dilated segment outlines the inferior side of the mass and is analogous to fluid in the goblet. This sign is significant because it is nearly pathognomonic for the diagnosis of TCC. Its presence excludes nonneoplastic filling defects, such as stones, blood, or infectious debris, and indicates a long-standing, slowly growing polypoid mass, almost always a TCC. Nonneoplastic filling defects do not lead to dilation inferior to the obstruction.

A related sign is known as *Bergman's coiled catheter sign.* This sign was described by a urologist who noted that passage of a ureteral catheter in a retrograde direction sometimes led to coiling of the catheter within a dilated segment of ureter below an obstructing tumor. Neither of these signs occurs in association with nonpapillary TCC, which accounts for approximately one third of all TCCs.

Notes

Bladder Carcinoma on Urography and Ultrasound

1. Tumor.

2. Posterolateral wall near the trigone.

3. Depth of bladder wall invasion.

4. Cystoscopic fulguration, cystectomy, and chemotherapy.

Reference

Cheng D, Tempany CM: MR imaging of the prostate and bladder, *Semin Ultrasound CT MR* 19(1):67-89, 1998.

Cross-Reference

Genitourinary Radiology: THE REQUISITES, pp 197-204, 219-226.

Comment

The filling defect demonstrated on the urogram shown here is typical for a carcinoma. Of bladder neoplasms, 95% are carcinomas, and of bladder carcinomas, 90% are transitional cell carcinomas. Risk factors are industrial carcinogen exposure, smoking, and analgesic abuse. Squamous cell carcinomas account for 5% of malignant neoplasms and are seen with increased frequency in patients with vesical schistosomiasis. (Half of all bladder malignancies in patients with schistosomiasis are squamous cell carcinomas.) Squamous cell carcinoma is also commonly found in the patient with a neurogenic bladder or a chronic indwelling Foley catheter and in the patient who has had multiple episodes of cystitis. Adenocarcinomas represent 2% of bladder carcinomas, are more frequently seen in urachal remnants, and usually affect patients with the rare condition of bladder exstrophy.

Depth of bladder wall invasion continues to be one of the most important prognostic factors. Five-year survival rates for patients with tumors invading the deep muscularis of the bladder are 10% to 20%, compared with 30% to 80% for those with tumors located superficially in the bladder musculature. Superficial tumors (T_1) are usually resected transurethrally, but the recurrence rate is high (50% to 90% within 2 years). Patients with deeper invasion of the bladder musculature (T_2 or T_3) are treated by cystectomy. Patients with metastatic disease (T_4) are treated with chemotherapy, radiation therapy, or palliative cystectomy depending on the clinical circumstance.

Notes

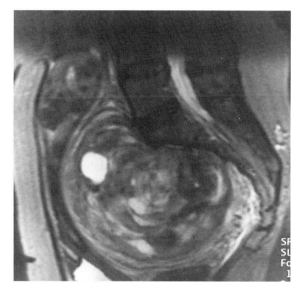 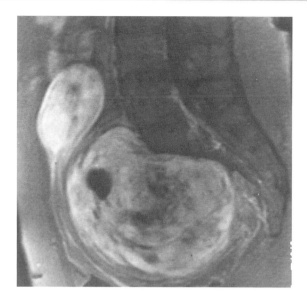

1. Where is the uterus, and is it normal?
2. True or False: Patients with this type of lesion have an increased risk of developing endometrial cancer.
3. What are some of signs or symptoms for which treatment of this lesion is indicated?
4. Name at least three different treatments for this lesion.

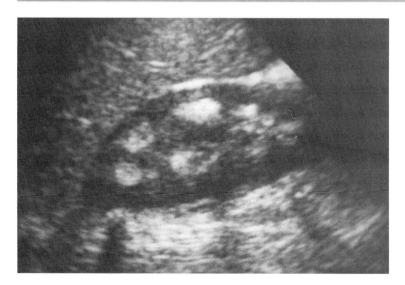

1. What are the most common causes for this finding? If the other kidney is normal, what is the most likely diagnosis?
2. What is the most common complication associated with this condition?
3. True or False: In patients with this condition, renal function is usually impaired.
4. How is this condition treated?

Degeneration of a Leiomyoma

1. The uterus, which contains multiple intramural myomas, is ventrally and superiorly displaced by a large degenerating leiomyoma.

2. True.

3. Abnormal uterine bleeding resulting in anemia, severe pelvic pain or dysmenorrhea, symptoms related to compression of the ureter or bladder, rapid increase in tumor size, and growth of the lesion after menopause.

4. Hormonal therapy, uterine artery embolization, myomectomy, myolysis, cryoablation, and hysterectomy.

Reference

Worthington-Kirsch RL, Popky GL, Hutchins FL Jr: Uterine arterial embolization for the management of leiomyomas: quality of life assessment and clinical response, *Radiology* 208:625-629, 1998.

Cross-Reference

Genitourinary Radiology: THE REQUISITES, pp 269-273.

Comment

Uterine leiomyomas are benign, estrogen-dependent tumors. As a result, they rarely develop before menarche and rarely grow after menopause. Leiomyomas may increase in size during pregnancy and when contraceptives containing high doses of estrogen are used. These tumors also occur with increased frequency in association with anovulatory states, endometrial hyperplasia, and granulosa-theca tumors of the ovary.

Uterine myomas are the most frequent cause of long-term abnormal uterine bleeding. Fibroids also can cause significant symptoms because of their bulk, which was the case in this patient with a degenerating subserosal fibroid.

Transcatheter embolization of the uterine arteries with polyvinyl alcohol particles (with or without Gianturco coils) is a viable alternative to surgical treatment of these tumors. The uterine arteries are usually enlarged and tortuous because of the hypervascular leiomyoma, and these characteristics facilitate catheterization. Embolization results in a 50% mean reduction in the size of the tumor, complete cessation or marked improvement in abnormal bleeding in 90% of patients, and reduction or relief of bulk symptoms in 90% of patients. The advantages of embolization are that uterine function (normal menses and fertility) is preserved and vaginal, laparoscopic, or abdominal surgery is averted. Postprocedural pain is a complication that can usually be controlled with nonsteroidal antiinflammatory medications, but postembolization syndrome (diffuse abdominal pain, mild fever, and leukocytosis) rarely may occur.

Notes

Medullary Nephrocalcinosis

1. Hyperparathyroidism, distal renal tubular acidosis, and medullary sponge kidney. Medullary sponge kidney is the most likely diagnosis if the other kidney is normal.

2. Urolithiasis.

3. False. However, renal insufficiency may be seen in patients with severe, long-standing hypercalcemia and renal tubular acidosis.

4. Treatment is directed to the underlying cause of the nephrocalcinosis.

Reference

Shultz PK, Strife JL, Strife CF, McDaniel JD: Hyperechoic renal medullary pyramids in infants and children, *Radiology* 181(1):163-167, 1991.

Cross-Reference

Genitourinary Radiology: THE REQUISITES, pp 69-72, 143-147.

Comment

Medullary nephrocalcinosis is calcification in the tubules of the medullary pyramids and accounts for 95% of all cases of nephrocalcinosis. It is typically bilateral and symmetric because it is often the result of a metabolic disorder, although it may be unilateral or segmental in cases of medullary sponge kidney. On ultrasound the pyramids are echogenic, and there may or may not be shadowing, depending on the size of the calcifications.

The most common causes of medullary nephrocalcinosis are hyperparathyroidism, benign tubular ectasia (medullary sponge kidney), and distal renal tubular acidosis (RTA). Other etiologies include the various other causes of hypercalcemia and hypercalciuria (e.g., sarcoidosis, milk alkali syndrome, and hypervitaminosis D), papillary necrosis, use of certain medications (e.g., furosemide and amphotericin), and diseases that cause hyperoxaluria or hyperuricosuria. Unlike cortical nephrocalcinosis, medullary nephrocalcinosis is potentially reversible. Urolithiasis is the most common complication. Progressive renal insufficiency may be found in some cases of severe, long-standing hypercalcemia or RTA.

Medullary sponge kidney is common (signs were found on 0.5% of intravenous urograms in one study), and in some cases there is an autosomal dominant inheritance pattern. It is believed to result from idiopathic dilation of the collecting ducts in the inner medulla and papillae. Bilateral renal involvement is seen in 70% of cases, but not all papillae are equally affected. Patients usually present between their twenties and forties with kidney stones, kidney infection, recurrent hematuria, or some combination of these problems.

Notes

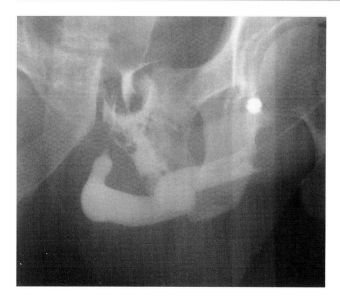

1. Name the two parts of the posterior male urethra.

2. The membranous urethra is contained within what critical anatomic structure?

3. What is the most common mechanism of traumatic injury to the posterior male urethra?

4. True or False: The posterior urethral injury demonstrated on this urethrogram is the most common type encountered after traumatic injury.

Blunt Traumatic Injury of the Posterior Urethra

1. Membranous and prostatic urethra.

2. Urogenital diaphragm.

3. Blunt traumatic injury resulting in pelvic fracture, especially those involving the anterior arch.

4. False.

References

Goldman SM, Sandler CM, Corriere JN Jr, McGuire EJ: Blunt urethral trauma: a unified, anatomical mechanical classification, *J Urol* 157:85-89, 1997.

Cross-Reference

Genitourinary Radiology: THE REQUISITES, pp 237-239.

Comment

Traumatic urethral injury (TUI) has been classified in a number of ways. Before 1977 (and even in some current urologic textbooks), TUI was divided into anterior and posterior urethral injuries. Posterior urethral tears are virtually always secondary to pelvic fractures and most often occur after motor vehicle accidents. Blunt injury of the anterior male urethra usually involves the bulbous urethra and often results from a straddle-type injury; the pelvis usually is not fractured.

In 1977 Colapinto and McCallum presented a classification system that divided urethral injuries into three types based on severity and location. In type I injuries the urethra is elongated but intact. The membranous urethra is ruptured above the urogenital diaphragm in type II injuries, and more extensive urethral injuries involving both the membranous and bulbar urethrae are classified as type III.

The most recent classification is presented in the second referenced article. Goldman and colleagues divide TUI into five types. Types I, II, and III are the same as in the Colapinto and McCallum classification. Type IV injuries involve the bladder neck and extend into the prostatomembranous urethra, and type IVA injuries involve the bladder base but spare the urethra. Type IVA was added to the classification system because on urethrography extravasated contrast material may pool in the periurethral space in type IVA injuries, thereby mimicking type IV tears. Partial or complete tears of the anterior urethra are designated as type V injuries.

This case shows a type II TUI, which was considered to be the "classic" traumatic posterior urethra injury. However, several studies have shown that only 15% of urethral injuries are type I or II, and the majority of urethral injuries are not isolated to the posterior urethra but extend into the adjacent bulbous urethra (type III).

Notes

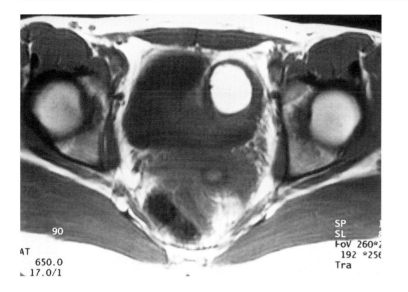

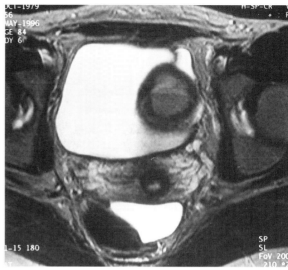

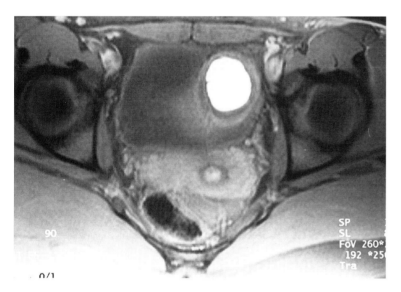

1. What is the importance of the fat-saturated T1W (upper right) image?
2. True or False: Aspiration of an endometrial cyst is contraindicated.
3. True or False: Endometrial malignancy occurs more frequently in women with endometriosis.
4. True or False: Increase in the size of an endometrioma during pregnancy indicates malignant transformation.

Endometrioma on MRI

1. It confirms that the cause of the T1-hyperintense signal is hemorrhage (or viscous proteinaceous fluid) rather than lipid.

2. False.

3. True.

4. False.

References

Togashi K, Nishimura K, Kimura I, et al: Endometrial cysts: diagnosis with MR imaging, *Radiology* 180:73-78, 1991.

Troiano RN, Taylor KJW: Sonographically guided therapeutic aspiration of benign-appearing ovarian cysts and endometriomas, *Am J Roentgenol* 171:1601-1605, 1998.

Cross-Reference

Genitourinary Radiology: THE REQUISITES, pp 258-261.

Comment

This case illustrates the classic features of an endometrial cyst (endometrioma or chocolate cyst) on MRI. On T1W images, endometrial cysts have hyperintense signal (equal to or greater than that of fat) that does not suppress with frequency-selective fat saturation or on chemical shift MRI. On T2W images, endometrial cysts are hypointense ("shaded"). With shading, the cyst can have variable hypointense signal on T2W images (i.e., they are predominantly hyperintense, with foci of lower signal intensity, or are uniformly hypointense). Shading may be related to the high iron content of endometrial cysts, which can be 10 to 20 times the concentration of whole blood. In addition, multiplicity is also common with endometriomas because cyclic perforation of endometrial cysts may generate daughter or contiguous cysts. The appearance of an endometrioma should be contrasted with that of a hemorrhagic functional cyst, which usually has higher signal intensity on T2W images because of a lower protein and iron content compared with an endometrioma.

Although malignant transformation of endometriosis has been documented, the incidence is extremely low (0.3% to 0.8%); clear cell carcinoma, endometrioid carcinoma, and mixed müllerian carcinosarcoma have been reported. Growth during pregnancy has been attributed to decidualization of ectopic endometrial tissue caused by progesterone. On color-flow Doppler ultrasound, both decidualized ectopic endometrial tissue and neoplastic endometrial tissue may appear as nodular or papillary mural excrescences with demonstrable vascularity.

A high recurrence rate has discouraged therapeutic aspiration of endometrial cysts. However, a few reports have suggested that therapeutic aspiration of an endometrioma leads to immediate symptom relief and, when combined with hormonal suppression therapy (gonadotropin-releasing hormone antagonist or noncyclic oral contraceptives), may be an effective long-term treatment.

Notes

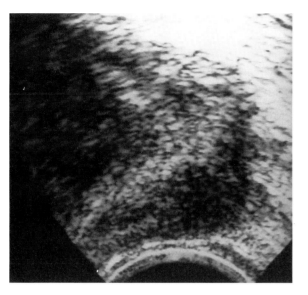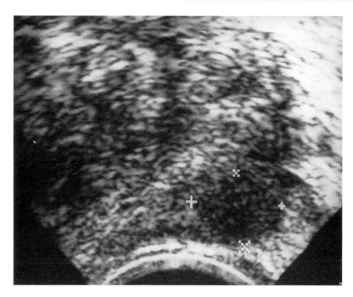

1. What is the differential diagnosis for this abnormality?
2. On transrectal prostate sonography, what percentage of hypoechoic peripheral zone lesions are malignant?
3. Where do carcinomas arise in the prostate gland?
4. In which zone does benign prostatic hypertrophy occur?

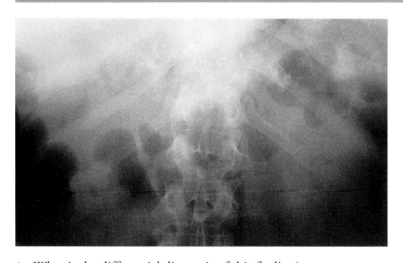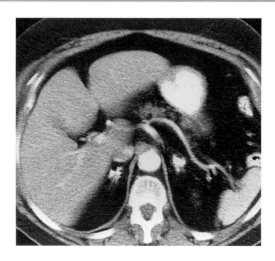

1. What is the differential diagnosis of this finding?
2. What is the expected biochemical abnormality?
3. What is the treatment for this disease?
4. Which U.S. president had this disease?

Hypoechoic Lesion on Prostate Ultrasound

1. Differential diagnosis for a hypoechoic nodule in the prostatic peripheral zone includes prostate carcinoma, atypical hyperplasia, focal prostatitis, nodule of benign prostatic hyperplasia, and prostatic cyst.

2. About 40%.

3. Of prostate carcinomas, 85% are located in the peripheral zone, 10% in the transitional zone (usually found in the chips of tissue after transurethral resection of the prostate [TURP]), and 5% in the central zone surrounding the ejaculatory ducts.

4. Transitional zone.

References

Clements R: The changing role of transrectal ultrasound in the diagnosis of prostate cancer, *Clin Radiol* 51:671-676, 1996.

Rifkin MD, Dahnert W, Kurtz AB: Endorectal sonography of the prostate gland, *Am J Roentgenol* 154:691-700, 1990.

Cross-Reference

Genitourinary Radiology: THE REQUISITES, pp 21, 22, 46, 321-323.

Comment

In the United States, prostate cancer is the most common malignancy in men and the second most common cause of cancer-related death after lung carcinoma. Along with the digital rectal examination (DRE) and serum prostate-specific antigen (PSA), transrectal ultrasound of the prostate plays an important role in the diagnosis of prostate carcinoma. Modern high frequency transducers have improved anatomic definition, and refinements in equipment have allowed for ultrasound-guided biopsy. Ultrasound guidance improves the yield of prostate needle biopsy over that of digital-guided procedures.

One limitation of transrectal ultrasound is the low specificity of a hypoechoic, peripheral zone lesion. Although prostatic adenocarcinoma can appear hypoechoic, there are benign causes, including atypical hyperplasia, focal prostatitis, and prostatic cyst. In addition, approximately 30% of prostate carcinomas are isoechoic to normal prostate gland on transrectal ultrasound and cannot be detected reliably unless there is distortion of the contour of the gland. Although 40% of hypoechoic lesions are malignant, the positive predictive value increases to 60% when there is a corresponding nodule on DRE. The positive predictive value increases to 70% when the DRE is abnormal and serum PSA level is elevated. The main role for prostatic ultrasound is to provide imaging guidance for prostatic biopsy when there is a palpable nodule or an elevated PSA level.

Notes

Adrenal Calcifications Caused by Addison's Disease

1. Granulomatous disease (e.g., tuberculosis or histoplasmosis), prior adrenal hemorrhage, and treated metastases.

2. Reduced serum levels of aldosterone and cortisol.

3. Oral supplements of cortisol and mineralocorticoids.

4. John F. Kennedy.

References

Ammini AC, Gupta R, et al: Computed tomography morphology of the adrenal glands of patients with Addison's disease, *Australas Radiol* 40(1):38-42, 1996.

Morgan HE, Austin JH, et al: Bilateral adrenal enlargement in Addison's disease caused by tuberculosis. Nephrotomographic demonstration, *Radiology* 115(2):357-358, 1975.

Cross-Reference

Genitourinary Radiology: THE REQUISITES, pp 367-369.

Comment

Addison's disease is the result of decreased production of steroid hormones by the adrenal cortex. It may be primary, when there is insufficient adrenal tissue to produce steroid hormones, or secondary, when there is insufficient adrenocorticotropic hormone (ACTH) produced by the pituitary to stimulate the adrenal glands. Primary Addison's disease has an autoimmune etiology in more than half of all cases. In these patients the adrenal glands are small on CT or MRI. Addison's disease also may result from destruction of the adrenal gland caused by hemorrhage or infection with tuberculosis, histoplasmosis, coccidioidomycosis, or cryptococcosis. Bilateral metastases are a very rare cause of Addison's disease. More than 90% of the adrenal gland must be destroyed for hypofunction to occur.

Typically, short-term involvement with an infectious process, such as tuberculosis, results in an enlargement of the adrenal glands, with or without calcification. Long-term involvement after treatment of the infection results in decreased gland size and dense calcification. Subacute and chronic insufficiency are caused by destruction of the gland as described earlier. Acute adrenal insufficiency is a separate disease process in which the adrenal glands, suppressed by exogenous steroids, are unable to secrete appropriate levels of steroid hormones. This process occurs in patients on exogenous steroids who have sepsis or are subjected to iatrogenic stress, such as surgery, burns, or severe traumatic injury.

The diagnosis of Addison's disease is made by ACTH stimulation testing but can be suggested if small adrenal glands or enlarged and calcified adrenal glands are demonstrated on CT.

Notes

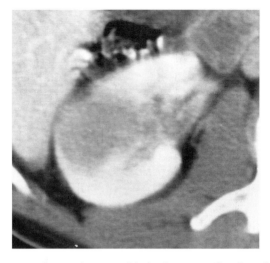 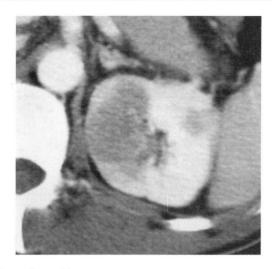

1. What is the most likely diagnosis for these bilateral renal lesions?
2. What are the common causes of solid renal masses occurring in both kidneys?
3. What neoplasms grow in the kidney in an infiltrative pattern?
4. Is the center of these lesions within the renal sinus or the renal parenchyma?

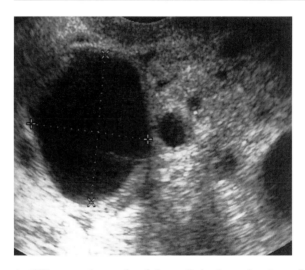 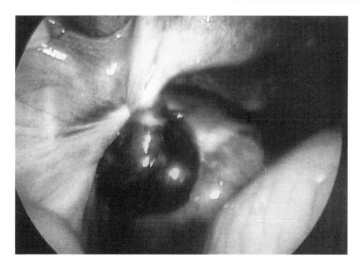

1. What are the goals of the radiologic evaluation of a suspected pelvic mass?
2. What is the most likely diagnosis in this case?
3. What are some of the risk factors for this disease?
4. What is the arterial supply to the ovaries?

Renal Lymphoma

1. Metastatic disease, including lymphoma.

2. Metastases, including lymphoma, and renal cell carcinomas.

3. Urothelial tumors; some metastases, including lymphoma; and infiltrative renal cell carcinomas.

4. Renal parenchyma.

Reference

Davidson AJ, Hartman DS, Davis CJ Jr, et al: Infiltrative renal lesions: CT-sonographic-pathologic correlation, *Am J Roentgenol* 150:1061-1064, 1988.

Cross-Reference

Genitourinary Radiology: THE REQUISITES, pp 115, 116.

Comment

This patient has bilateral solid renal lesions with a geographic, non–contour-deforming pattern. This finding indicates an infiltrative pattern. Infiltrative renal lesions fall into three main categories—inflammatory, infarction, and infiltrative neoplasm. The lesions shown are irregularly marginated, with generally rounded shapes. The center of these lesions is within the renal parenchyma, indicating that it is unlikely that they arose from the urothelium. No rim nephrogram is visible. The lesions are homogeneous.

These features suggest a diagnosis of metastatic disease. Metastases to the kidneys can lead to expansile, ball-shaped masses or infiltrative lesions. Infiltrative metastases usually result from primary squamous cell carcinomas or lymphoma. Patients usually have a known primary neoplasm, and renal metastases are typically seen late in the course of the disease. On CT, multifocal renal lymphoma cannot be distinguished from other infiltrative metastases. Sometimes the sonographic pattern is suggestive of lymphoma. Renal lymphoma is usually homogeneously low in echogenicity without significant through-transmission. The internal echogenicity of renal lymphoma may mimic that of a simple cyst, lacking only the through-transmission seen in fluid-containing masses.

Notes

Ovarian Torsion on Ultrasound and Laparoscopy

1. To determine the organ in which the mass originated; establish the size and volume of the mass; characterize the mass as a simple cyst, atypical cyst, or predominantly solid cyst; and assess for the presence of associated disease, such as ascites, adenopathy, ureteral obstruction, or liver masses.

2. Torsion of the ovary.

3. Torsion of one ovary (places the contralateral ovary at increased risk), presence of an adnexal mass, long or tortuous mesosalpinx or mesosalpingeal vessels, tubal spasm, and prior surgery.

4. Dual supply from the ovarian artery (branch of the aorta) and the adnexal branch of the uterine artery.

Reference

Lee EJ, Kwon HC, Joo HJ, Suh JH, Fleischer AC: Diagnosis of ovarian torsion with color Doppler sonography: depiction of twisted vascular pedicle, *J Ultrasound Med* 17(2):83-89, 1998.

Cross-Reference

Genitourinary Radiology: THE REQUISITES, pp 265-268, 283-287.

Comment

Ovarian torsion accounts for 3% of gynecologic emergencies and is most common during the first three decades of life. Once torsion has occurred, there is a 10% chance of contralateral torsion. The typical presentation is that of severe unilateral pelvic pain, which may have been preceded by weeks of intermittent pain. Occasionally, symptoms are nonspecific. When complete ovarian torsion is suspected, immediate surgery is necessary. Conservative laparoscopic management can be attempted if the ovary is viable, as in this case.

Not long after ovarian torsion has occurred, passive congestion occurs as a result of venous and lymphatic stasis. This congestion is soon followed by the development of venous and then arterial thrombosis and subsequent infarction. The gray scale sonographic appearance is nonspecific; the most common finding is a pelvic mass that may be cystic, complex and septated, or solid. Uniform cortical follicular enlargement (of 8 to 12 mm), which is attributed to transudation of fluid, has been reported. On color Doppler sonography, depiction of a twisted vascular pedicle is suggestive of torsion. In addition, the lack of central venous flow correlates with a nonviable, torsed ovary. However, this sign may be falsely positive because of the absence of central flow in cases of intraovarian hemorrhage and in cystic masses. False negatives can result in cases of intermittent torsion or when imaging is performed too early.

Notes

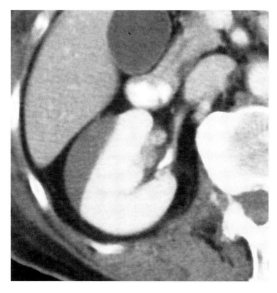

1. In what space is the low attenuation material near the right kidney?
2. How can subcapsular fluid be distinguished from perirenal, extracapsular fluid?
3. What are common causes of fluid in this location?
4. What name is given to the ischemic kidney caused by fluid in this location?

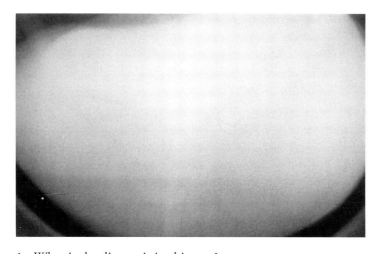 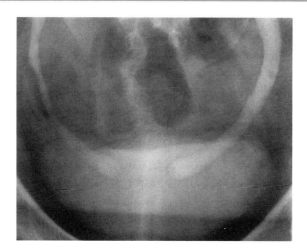

1. What is the diagnosis in this case?
2. What causes the lucent line around the bulbous segment of the ureter in the bladder?
3. What complications can be caused by the abnormality shown?
4. Failed resorption of what structure is the proposed cause of this abnormality?

Renal Subcapsular Hematoma

1. Subcapsular space.

2. Subcapsular fluid leads to deformation of the renal shape, and there is no fat plane between the kidney and the fluid.

3. Traumatic injury (including iatrogenic injury resulting from renal biopsy or percutaneous nephrostomy), vasculitis, and rupture of a vascular formation.

4. Page kidney.

Reference

Pollack HM, Wein AJ: Imaging of renal trauma, *Radiology* 172: 297-308, 1989.

Cross-Reference

Genitourinary Radiology: THE REQUISITES, p 127.

Comment

In this case there is a lens-shaped fluid collection compressing the right side of the right kidney. This patient was involved in a motor vehicle accident, and this slightly high attenuation fluid was diagnosed as a subcapsular hematoma. Blunt trauma is the most common cause of subcapsular hematoma. This finding usually indicates injury to a peripheral renal artery branch, with arterial hemorrhage into the subcapsular space. Because the capsule is a rigid fibrous layer of tissue, the enlarging hematoma compresses and deforms the renal parenchyma. Venous bleeding is not usually of sufficient pressure to cause significant subcapsular hematomas.

This entity has clinical significance because there is compression of the renal parenchyma. This compression leads to ischemia of the kidney, which may cause increased excretion of renin and the development of hypertension. When this chain of events occurs, usually within 6 months of the development of the subcapsular hematoma, the resulting kidney is described as a *Page kidney.* Compression of the renal parenchyma leading to increased renin secretion is one model of renal vascular hypertension. In the other model, called the *Goldblatt kidney,* increased renin secretion caused by underperfusion is seen in patients with renal artery stenosis.

Notes

Orthotopic Ureterocele

1. Bilateral orthotopic ureteroceles.

2. Bladder mucosa and ureteral wall herniating into the bladder.

3. Ureteral obstruction, urolithiasis, and urinary tract infection.

4. Chwalla's membrane.

Reference

Davidson AJ, Hartman DS, editors: In *Radiology of the kidney and urinary tract,* ed 2, Philadelphia, 1994, Saunders, pp 521-528.

Cross-Reference

Genitourinary Radiology: THE REQUISITES, pp 158, 159.

Comment

This case demonstrates bilateral orthotopic ureteroceles, also known as *adult-type ureteroceles.* These ureteroceles are rarely seen in children; they usually do not cause symptoms and are an incidental finding. As shown in this case, bilateral orthotopic ureteroceles are easier to see when the bladder is only partially filled and may be difficult to see when the bladder is completely filled with opacified urine. Orthotopic ureteroceles, unlike ectopic ureteroceles, are not associated with other urinary tract anomalies. Specifically they are not related to ectopic ureters. The proposed mechanism for development of orthotopic ureteroceles is incomplete resorption of Chwalla's membrane during recanalization of the fetal ureter. This incomplete resorption causes minimal stenosis of the ureteral orifice and eventual prolapse of the bulbous ureterovesical junction into the bladder. Orthotopic ureteroceles can become quite large, and the larger ones are more likely to be associated with complications. When ureteroceles are more than 2 cm in diameter, the risk of significant urinary tract stasis, with obstruction, stone formation, or infection, is increased. In addition, the appearance of a simple ureterocele must be carefully evaluated. The lucent line around the bulbous segment of the ureter is characteristic. It should be regular, smooth, and no more than 1 to 2 mm in diameter. If this outline is more than 2 mm in diameter, a pseudoureterocele (caused by an underlying pathologic condition, such as a stone or tumor) should be suspected.

Notes

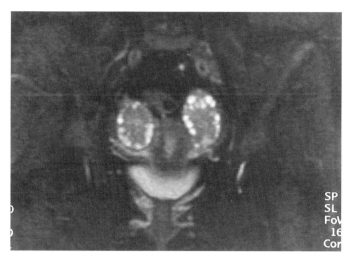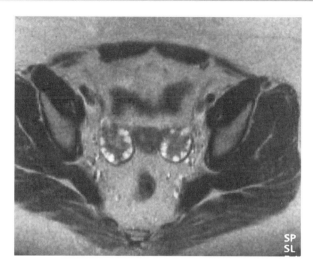

1. What are the significant findings on the T2W images in this case?
2. What is the likely clinical history in this case?
3. How is this disease diagnosed?
4. True or False: The appearance of the ovaries is pathognomonic for this disease.

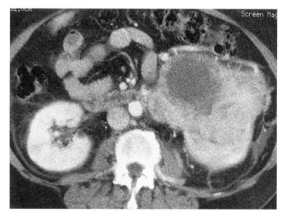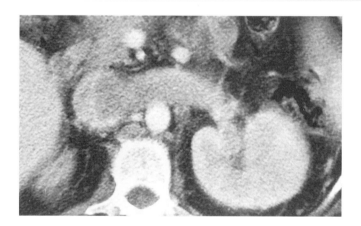

1. What is the most likely diagnosis?
2. What stage disease is shown?
3. What is the risk of a synchronous lesion in the right kidney?
4. What is the significance of the brightly enhancing tubular structures anterior to the renal mass?

Polycystic Ovary Disease

1. There are multiple small follicles along the periphery of both ovaries in this obese patient.

2. Infertility, hirsutism, obesity, and oligomenorrhea.

3. Through the combination of an appropriate clinical history and an elevated luteinizing hormone/follicle-stimulating hormone (LH:FSH) ratio. Characteristically the LH:FSH ratio is greater than 2.

4. False.

Reference

Pache T, Wladimiroff J, Hop W, et al: How to discriminate between normal and polycystic ovaries: transvaginal ultrasound study, *Radiology* 183:421-423, 1992.

Cross-Reference

Genitourinary Radiology: THE REQUISITES, pp 274, 275

Comment

Polycystic ovary disease (PCOD), or Stein-Leventhal syndrome, was originally described as an X-linked autosomal dominant disease. The fundamental pathophysiologic characteristic of this disease is chronic anovulation in the setting of acyclic estrogen production. The ovaries were originally described as being enlarged, with multiple small follicles located peripherally in the gland, but the ovary is normal in size in as many as 30% of patients. The primary abnormality in PCOD is increased production of androgens (initially from the adrenal glands and in later stages from the ovary) and its peripheral conversion to estrogen in subcutaneous fat. This conversion is facilitated in obese patients. The elevated serum estrogen level causes suppression of FSH and elevation of LH by the pituitary gland. An increased level of LH increases production of androgens by the ovarian stroma and perpetuates this cycle. The decreased level of FSH prevents ovulation and results in oligomenorrhea.

Current treatment is directed toward interrupting the cycle of excess ovarian androgen production through the use of oral contraceptives or wedge resection of the ovary. Other treatments include weight loss (to decrease the conversion of androgens to estrogens) and use of medications that promote FSH secretion (e.g., clomiphene, human menopausal gonadotropin, luteinizing hormone–releasing hormone, and purified FSH).

On ultrasound or MRI, enlarged ovaries with multiple small peripheral follicles, the so-called "string of pearls" sign, may be visible. The ovary also has been described as echogenic because of the prominent ovarian stroma. One study showed that patients with PCOD have more follicles, smaller follicles, and both larger and more echogenic ovaries.

Notes

Renal Cell Carcinoma with Extension into the Renal Vein and Inferior Vena Cava

1. Renal cell carcinoma.

2. Stage III.

3. 2%.

4. They represent collateral vessels draining or feeding the mass in the left kidney.

Reference

Zagoria RJ, Bechtold RE, Dyer RB: Staging of renal adenocarcinoma: role of various imaging procedures, *Am J Roentgenol* 164:363-370, 1995.

Cross-Reference

Genitourinary Radiology: THE REQUISITES, pp 97, 99, 100.

Comment

This patient has a large heterogeneous exophytic renal mass typical of renal cell carcinoma (RCC). RCC is hypervascular in 80% of cases. This hypervascularity often leads to enlargement of collateral arteries and veins around the kidney. RCC also has a predilection to grow contiguously into the venous system. The accurate diagnosis of venous extension of tumor is crucial for treatment planning. This diagnosis is most accurately made based on thin-section CT during bolus contrast material infusion or MRI. In this case the tumor thrombus is easily visible as a low attenuation filling defect within and enlarging the left renal vein. The tumor extends into the inferior vena cava, filling approximately one half of the vena cava lumen. This finding is diagnostic of Robson stage III disease. Tumor thrombus within the renal vein also encourages the development of venous collaterals to drain the kidney and the renal tumor. When a renal mass such as this is detected, the extent of disease must be determined, particularly with regard to regional lymph nodes, the renal vein, the inferior vena cava, and areas where metastases commonly occur (e.g., the lungs, bones, and liver). Because surgery is the conventional mode of treatment for RCC, the other kidney should be scrutinized for synchronous lesions. RCC is bilateral in approximately 1% to 2% of nonfamilial cases.

Notes

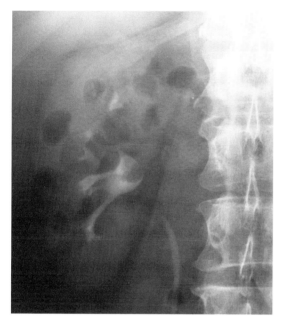 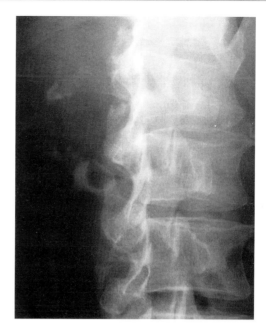

1. What is the most likely diagnosis for the filling defect shown?
2. What are the main differential diagnoses for radiolucent filling defects seen on intravenous urography?
3. What other imaging modalities could be used to better demonstrate the composition of this filling defect?
4. What chemical comprises most radiolucent urinary tract stones?

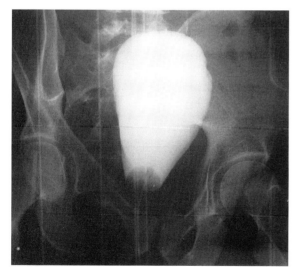 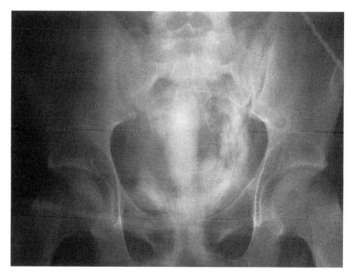

1. What is the most likely cause of the "pear-shaped" bladder in this case?
2. Name three other causes of "pear-shaped" bladder.
3. What disease causes increased pelvic radiolucency and a "pear-shaped" bladder?
4. What disease causes ureteral notching and a "pear-shaped" bladder?

Radiolucent Filling Defect

1. Radiolucent stone.

2. Radiolucent stones, transitional cell carcinoma, blood clot, infectious debris, sloughed papillae, and air bubbles.

3. Noncontrast CT or sonography.

4. Uric acid.

Reference

Fein AB, McClennan BL: Solitary filling defects of the ureter, *Semin Roentgenol* 21:201-213, 1986.

Cross-Reference

Genitourinary Radiology: THE REQUISITES, pp 184-189.

Comment

Two films from an intravenous urogram demonstrate a relatively smooth radiolucent filling defect in the right renal pelvis. On the frontal view it is difficult to determine that this defect is not an overlying gas bubble in the colon, but its position in the renal pelvis is confirmed by the left posterior oblique view of the right kidney. Radiologists should be familiar with the common causes of radiolucent filling defects seen on intravenous urography. The most common cause is a radiolucent stone. This cause is followed closely by urothelial tumors, the majority of which are transitional cell carcinomas. Less common causes include blood clots, infectious debris, sloughed papillae, and air bubbles. The significance of these filling defects must not be underestimated. Every radiolucent filling defect should be further evaluated. This evaluation can be as simple as monitoring the urine for stone passage or obtaining additional imaging studies (using CT, sonography, or endoscopy). In this patient, who had a history of gross hematuria, the sharply defined radiolucent filling defect in the renal pelvis has a somewhat innocuous appearance. However, this defect was found to be a transitional cell carcinoma, and the patient underwent right nephroureterectomy.

When further imaging evaluation of a radiolucent filling defect is necessary, CT and sonography may be helpful. On noncontrast CT performed several days after any contrast-infused study (including intravenous urography), all urinary tract stones are radiodense. CT is particularly useful when the filling defect is in the ureter, an area that is difficult to examine with sonography. Ultrasound demonstrates a stone as a hyperechoic focus with posterior shadowing in most cases. Nearly all radiolucent stones are composed of uric acid, with a small percentage formed from xanthine or nonmineralized matrix.

Notes

Pear-Shaped Bladder

1. Pelvic hematoma.

2. Lipomatosis, inferior vena cava obstruction, lymphadenopathy, and lymphocysts.

3. Pelvic lipomatosis.

4. Venous collaterals that form after inferior vena cava obstruction.

Reference

Ambos MA, Bosniak MA, Lefleur RS, Madayag MA: The pear-shaped bladder, *Radiology* 122:85-88, 1977.

Cross-Reference

Genitourinary Radiology: THE REQUISITES, pp 223, 224.

Comment

In 1950 Prather and Kaiser used the term *teardrop* to describe the bladder deformity observed after pelvic fracture and hematoma formation. Nearly 50 years later, pelvic hematoma is still the most common cause of the "pear-shaped," "gourd-like," or "inverted tear-shaped" bladder. Pelvic hematoma (resulting from fractures, traumatized muscles, or torn branches of hypogastric arteries or pelvic veins), extraperitoneal urinoma, or both may cause the symmetric bladder compression and elevation that typifies this abnormal shape of the urinary bladder.

Of course, there is a differential diagnosis. Pelvic lipomatosis is caused by the deposition of large amounts of benign adipose and fibrous tissue in the perivesical and perirectal space. Symmetric compression and elevation by excessive pelvic fat cause the bladder to become "gourd shaped"; the rectum and lower ureters also have a characteristic compressive deformity. Lipomatosis is really the only disease that compresses the bladder bilaterally and causes increased radiolucency in the pelvis. Obstruction of the inferior vena cava may also cause a pear-shaped bladder. This diagnosis should be suspected when there is bilateral peripheral edema or venous collateral vessels visible on the lower abdominal wall. Bladder distortion is the result of compression by pelvic venous collateral vessels and edema. On urography, the ureters may be notched and displaced anteriorly and medially. Rarely, massive bilateral pelvic lymphadenopathy (caused by lymphoma or leukemia) or extensive lymphocyst formation (after extensive pelvic nodal dissections) may cause the bladder to assume a pear shape.

Notes

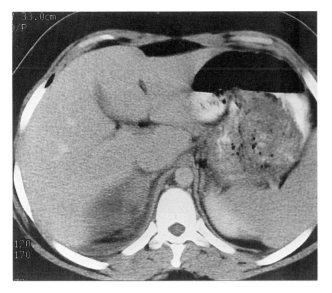
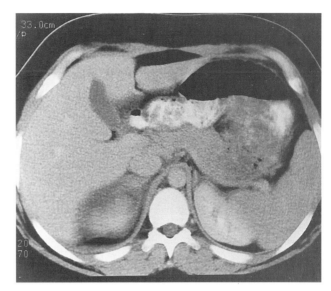

1. What is the most likely explanation for the appearance of the adrenal gland given a history of blunt trauma?
2. Which adrenal gland has a predilection for injury after blunt trauma?
3. The hemorrhage originates in what part of the adrenal gland?
4. What is the natural history of this lesion?

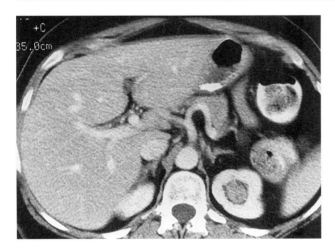
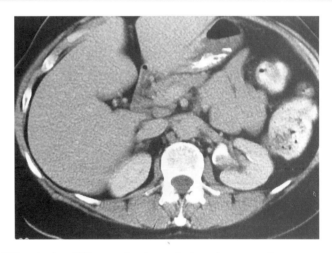

1. Two images from a CT scan of the abdomen are shown. What is the difference in the technique between these two images?
2. What is the diagnostic usefulness of the image on the right?
3. In adults, what are the three most common primary malignant neoplasms of the kidney?
4. What is the recommended treatment for this patient?

Traumatic Hematoma of the Right Adrenal Gland

1. Acute adrenal hemorrhage.

2. Right adrenal gland (see Comment for reasons).

3. Medulla.

4. Most resolve completely; in rare cases the adrenal gland may calcify or a pseudocyst may form.

Reference

Burks DW, Mirvis SE, Shanmuganathan K: Acute adrenal injury after blunt abdominal trauma: CT findings, *Am J Roentgenol* 158:503-507, 1992.

Cross-Reference

Genitourinary Radiology: THE REQUISITES, pp 357, 358.

Comment

Adrenal hemorrhage after blunt trauma usually occurs with severe multiorgan trauma and overwhelmingly involves the right adrenal gland (ratio of 8 or 9:1). The following explanations have been offered for the observed right adrenal predilection: (1) direct compression of the gland between the liver and the spine, (2) transient elevation of adrenal venous pressure caused by caval compression, and (3) shear injury of small capsular veins.

After blunt trauma, the adrenal hematoma usually presents as an ovoid mass and has measured attenuation values between 50 and 90 HU. Less often the entire gland may be enlarged, or a large suprarenal hematoma may obliterate the gland. In addition to the abnormal adrenal gland, strands of soft tissue density in the periadrenal fat and thickening of the ipsilateral diaphragmatic crus are commonly identified. Periadrenal stranding also has been reported in adrenal hemorrhage secondary to lung metastasis. Coincident injury to the liver, kidney, or both organs frequently accompanies adrenal hemorrhage after blunt abdominal trauma.

Rarely a chronic adrenal hematoma may appear as a large, heterogeneous mass and might be difficult to distinguish from an adrenocortical carcinoma on CT or MRI. Subacute adrenal hemorrhage may have a specific appearance on MRI. Focal areas of high signal or a concentric hyperintense ring may be seen on T1W images; on T2W images these same areas are hypointense.

Notes

Transitional Cell Carcinoma of the Renal Pelvis

1. The image on the left was obtained in the portal venous phase of contrast enhancement, approximately 70 to 90 seconds after the start of intravenous contrast administration. The image on the right was obtained in the pyelographic phase of enhancement, 120 to 180 seconds after the start of contrast injection.

2. Allows evaluation of the contrast-opacified renal collecting system.

3. Adenocarcinoma, transitional cell carcinoma, and squamous cell carcinoma.

4. Nephroureterectomy.

Reference

Leder RA, Dunnick NR: Transitional cell carcinoma of the pelvicalices and ureter, *Am J Roentgenol* 255:713, 1990.

Cross-Reference

Genitourinary Radiology: THE REQUISITES, pp 113-116, 135, 136.

Comment

This is a classic case of transitional cell carcinoma (TCC) of the left renal collecting system. More than 90% of urothelial neoplasms are TCCs; the remaining 10% are squamous cell carcinomas. TCC occurs in the urothelial tissue in proportion to the surface area, so the most common location is the urinary bladder, followed by the renal pelvis, and finally the ureters. In the kidney a TCC presents as a unilateral soft tissue mass in the renal sinus, as in this case. If the infiltrating mass involves the renal parenchyma, it causes obliteration of the renal sinus fat and results in the so-called "faceless kidney," a presentation of more advanced disease.

With the advent of helical CT, rapid imaging through the upper abdomen has become possible, and lesions in the kidneys can be overlooked because of the lack of sufficient renal and ureteral enhancement. For this reason, when a renal mass is suspected, delayed imaging through the kidneys during the pyelographic phase is recommended. CT performed 2 to 3 minutes after the commencement of contrast material injection increases the image contrast between a soft tissue mass and the renal cortex and collecting system. As the figure on the right shows, the soft tissue mass is outlined by radiodense contrast in the left collecting system.

TCCs frequently present with hematuria (80%). Of patients with TCC in the renal pelvis, 30% have multicentric disease. The treatment of choice for TCC is nephroureterectomy, as opposed to simple nephrectomy for renal cell carcinoma.

Notes

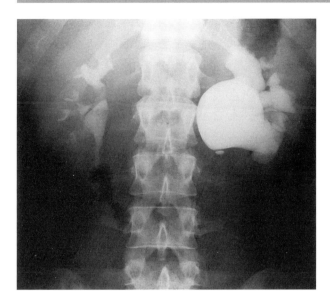

1. This condition is one of the most common causes of abdominal masses in neonates. What is the diagnosis?
2. How often are both kidneys involved?
3. What congenital urinary tract anomalies are associated with this condition?
4. How is this condition treated?

Ureteropelvic Junction Obstruction

1. Congenital ureteropelvic junction obstruction.

2. In 20% of cases.

3. Horseshoe kidney, contralateral multicystic dysplastic kidney, contralateral renal agenesis, ureteral duplication, and vesicoureteral reflux.

4. Balloon dilation, cystoscopic or antegrade endopyelotomy, or open pyeloplasty.

Reference

Park JM, Bloom DA: The pathophysiology of UPJ obstruction: current concepts, *Urol Clin North Am* 25(2):161-169, 1998.

Cross-Reference

Genitourinary Radiology: THE REQUISITES, pp 74, 75, 372-374.

Comment

Ureteropelvic junction (UPJ) obstruction can be defined as a functional or anatomic obstruction that impedes the flow of urine from the renal pelvis to the proximal ureter. This condition usually is caused by a deficiency and derangement of ureteral smooth muscle that results in a failure of normal peristalsis in the affected segment. UPJ obstruction is the most common genitourinary anomaly detected by antenatal ultrasound and is the most common cause of urinary tract obstruction in childhood.

Urography, sonography, CT, and MRI can be used to evaluate UPJ obstruction. When UPJ obstruction is equivocal or when there is a discrepancy between the symptoms and the radiologic findings, a ureteral perfusion test (urodynamic antegrade pyelography or pressure-flow study of Whitaker) or diuretic renography can be performed to assess the functional significance of the obstruction. The ureteral perfusion test is used to measure the pressure differential between the renal pelvis and the bladder. For this test, a 21-gauge needle is placed into the intrarenal collecting system and a Foley catheter is placed into the bladder. Both catheters are attached to manometers, and contrast is infused into the renal collecting system at rates of 10 ml/minute and 15 ml/minute. At a perfusion rate of 10 ml/minute, the normal differential pressure is less than 13 cm water. Mild, moderate, and severe obstruction are suggested by differential pressures of 14 to 20 cm water, 21 to 34 cm water, and more than 34 cm water, respectively.

Open pyeloplasty has been the standard treatment for obstruction in the past. However, advances in percutaneous and endourologic techniques have resulted in less invasive treatments, such as balloon pyeloplasty or endoscopic pyelotomy. The most significant risk factor for endourologic procedures is the presence of crossing vessels at the UPJ, for which preoperative imaging with CT-angiography, MR-angiography, or endoluminal sonography can be performed.

Notes

Fair Game Cases

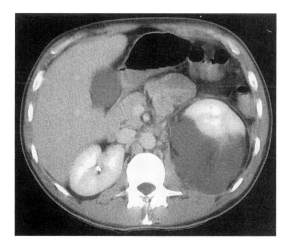

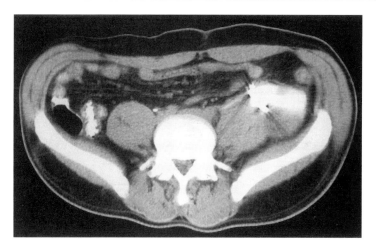

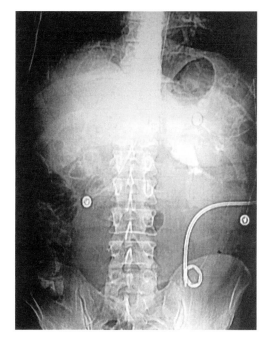

1. This patient was involved in a serious motor vehicle accident and had a partial ureteropelvic junction tear but refused treatment. At the time of this scan the patient complained of severe left flank pain and was hypertensive. What is the left perirenal mass?

2. Is this mass located in the perirenal or the posterior pararenal space?

3. What is causing hypertension in this patient?

4. Is percutaneous drainage of this mass adequate treatment?

Perinephric Urinoma

1. Urinoma.

2. Urine is contained in the perinephric space, which is surrounded by Gerota's fascia. Some of this urine is in a subcapsular location, causing deformation of the normal renal shape.

3. Hypoperfusion of the left kidney caused by the subcapsular urinoma (Page kidney).

4. No. Percutaneous drainage may result in temporary resolution of the urinoma, but ureteral stenting or percutaneous nephrostomy drainage is required to allow the ureteral laceration to heal.

Reference

McCune TR, Stone WJ, Breyer JA: Page kidney: case report and review of the literature, *Am J Kidney Dis* 18(5):593-599, 1991.

Cross-Reference

Genitourinary Radiology: THE REQUISITES, pp 189-190.

Comment

This patient developed a urinoma as a result of a ureteral laceration at the ureteropelvic junction. This segment of ureter is most commonly damaged in serious deceleration injuries that lead to complete or partial avulsion of the ureter from the renal pelvis. Urinoma development is a possible consequence of this injury. When fluid, either urine or blood, collects in a subcapsular location, it can compress the renal parenchyma. This compression leads to relative underperfusion and ischemia of the involved renal parenchyma. The kidney responds by oversecreting renin, leading to renovascular hypertension. This condition has been called the *Page kidney* and is one of two models of renovascular hypertension. The other, called the *Goldblatt kidney,* is renovascular hypertension caused by renal artery stenosis or occlusion.

Although urinomas can be easily evacuated with a percutaneously placed drain, as shown in the second and third figures in this case, other treatments may be necessary. In this case the ureteropelvic junction laceration required ureteral stenting. In addition, the formation of a urinoma greatly increases the patient's risk of developing a stricture of the damaged segment of ureter. Therefore prompt evacuation of the urinoma and stenting are recommended for proper treatment of ureteral injuries resulting in urinomas.

Notes

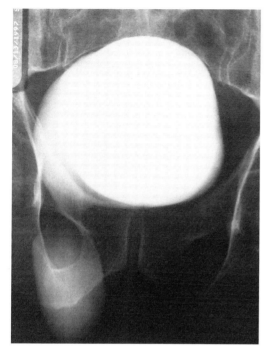 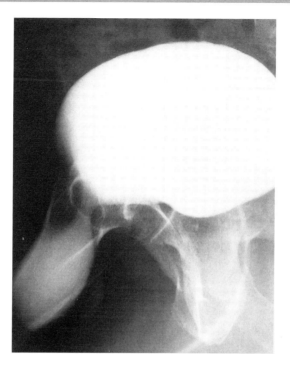

1. Through which canal is the bladder herniating?
2. What is the classic clinical voiding pattern associated with bladder hernia?
3. An indirect inguinal hernia lies lateral to which artery?
4. Name three complications of bladder hernia.

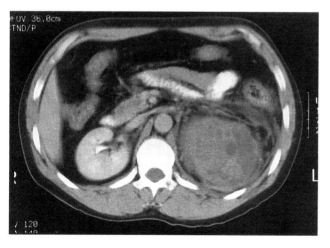 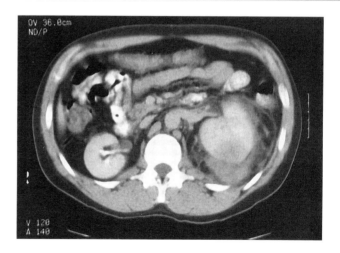

1. In what organ does this lesion originate?
2. What is the differential diagnosis?
3. What roles do other imaging modalities play with regard to this entity?
4. Does imaging-guided biopsy play a role in this patient's treatment?

Inguinal Herniation of the Bladder

1. Inguinal canal.

2. Two-stage voiding.

3. Deep inferior epigastric artery.

4. Hydronephrosis, strangulation, stone formation, vesicoureteral reflux, tumor, and inadvertent perforation during surgery.

Reference

Leibeskind AL, Elkin M, Goldman SM: Herniation of the bladder, *Radiology* 106:257-260, 1973.

Cross-Reference

Genitourinary Radiology: THE REQUISITES, p 212.

Comment

Herniations of the bladder are usually found at herniorrhaphy and are rarely discovered clinically. Large herniations may present with two-stage voiding; the patient empties the normotopic bladder initially but voids again after manually decompressing the hernia. Almost three fourths of all hernias occur through the inguinal canal and predominantly affect men. Femoral hernias are more common in women. With respect to the relationship of the hernia to the peritoneal space, the paraperitoneal hernia is most common; part of the parietal peritoneum herniates lateral to the bladder hernia, which remains extraperitoneal. Rarely the bladder can herniate into the obturator canal, ventral abdominal wall, or other abdominopelvic openings. Conditions that predispose individuals to bladder herniation include structural defects in the abdominal wall, atrophy of inguinal supportive tissues, and bladder outlet obstruction.

Unless the radiograph is centered low enough, bladder herniations are often overlooked on excretory urography. The radiologist should suspect herniation of the bladder when there is lateral displacement of the pelvic ureter or hydronephrosis (caused by traction on the trigone), an asymmetric and small bladder, and when the bladder base is not completely visible or is drawn to one side. Supine and prone radiographs are successful in demonstrating only 30% and 50% of bladder hernias, respectively. Only the erect view is uniformly successful in showing the abnormality. The herniated bladder is clearly demonstrated on cystography, whereas the hernial opening may be overlooked on cystoscopy.

Inguinal or scrotal ultrasound or CT may show the bladder herniation, although the differential diagnosis for a scrotal fluid collection includes hydrocele, varicocele, spermatocele, epididymal cyst, intestinal hernia, and ectopic ureterocele.

Notes

Adrenocortical Carcinoma

1. Left adrenal gland or possibly the upper pole of the left kidney.

2. Primary differential diagnosis is an adrenal carcinoma and an exophytic renal cell carcinoma; less likely possibilities include adrenal metastasis and hemorrhage (given the lesion's large size and low density and the lack of other lesions).

3. Ultrasound or MRI would be useful to confirm the adrenal origin of the lesion and separate it from the kidney.

4. Only if the patient has a known primary neoplasm or other site of disease. If there is only one lesion and the patient has no known primary neoplasm, biopsy probably is unnecessary and the treatment of choice would be surgical resection.

Reference

Wooten MD, King DK: Adrenal cortical carcinoma: epidemiology and treatment with mitotane and a review of the literature, *Cancer* 72(11):3145-3155, 1993.

Cross-Reference

Genitourinary Radiology: THE REQUISITES, pp 355-356.

Comment

Adrenocortical carcinoma is a relatively rare primary adrenal neoplasm; only about 2000 cases have been reported in the English medical literature. The disease has a bimodal age distribution, with peak occurrence in the first and fifth decades. There is a slight female predominance (59%), and 68% of patients have advanced nonresectable disease. Hyperfunctioning tumors are more common in children; 85% of adrenocortical carcinomas in children and 15% in adults are hyperfunctioning. Hyperfunctioning tumors present at an earlier stage than their nonfunctional counterparts, and the most sensitive biochemical assay for hormonal hyperfunction is measurement of urinary 17-ketosteroid levels. For functioning tumors the most common clinical presentation is Cushing's syndrome, whereas for nonfunctioning adrenal carcinomas it is pain resulting from local invasion and mass effect.

Adrenocortical carcinomas do not have specific imaging characteristics, although most nonhyperfunctional tumors tend to exceed 6 cm in diameter. Calcification, hemorrhage, necrosis, and heterogeneous enhancement are visible on enhanced CT. The MRI characteristics overlap with those of metastases and chronic adrenal hemorrhage. There is a limited role for percutaneous biopsy because the pathologic diagnosis can be difficult to make and the treatment for nonmetastatic disease is surgical resection.

Notes

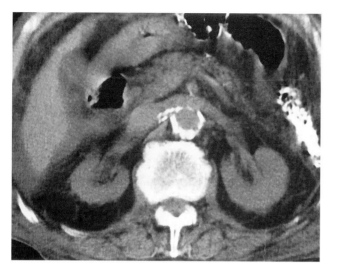 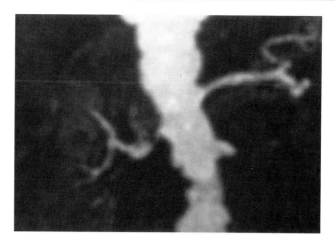

1. Given the images presented, what is the most likely cause of the small right kidney, and how does this lesion cause hypertension?

2. Describe the second image and its findings.

3. Name three imaging tests that can be used to screen for renovascular hypertension.

4. Given systemic hypertension, what is the success rate of angioplasty without stenting for ostial versus mid–renal artery stenosis?

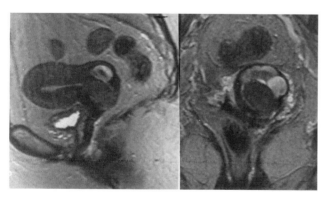 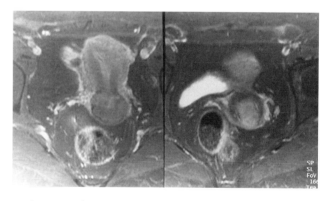

1. True or False: This case demonstrates a mass in the uterine endocervix that is completely confined to the cervix.

2. True or False: The majority of women with cervical cancer present with tumor that has already spread beyond the cervix.

3. Why is the detection of parametrial spread of cervical carcinoma important?

4. True or False: On MRI, cervical stromal tissue does not enhance.

Renal Artery Stenosis

1. Ostial renal artery stenosis (RAS), which causes glomerular hypoperfusion and primary hyperreninemic hypertension.

2. Projection image from a three-dimensional, breath-hold, contrast-enhanced MR angiogram shows a high grade stenosis of the proximal right renal artery.

3. Captopril renal scan, MR angiography, and digital subtraction angiography.

4. For ostial stenosis, angioplasty success rate is 30%; this rate is higher when intravascular stents are used. The angioplasty success rate is greater than 80% for stenoses in the mid–renal artery.

References

Mitty HA, Shapiro RS, et al: Renovascular hypertension, *Radiol Clin North Am* 34(5):1017-1036, 1996.

von Knorring J, Edgren J, et al: Long-term results of percutaneous transluminal angioplasty in renovascular hypertension, *Acta Radiologica* 37(1):36-40, 1996.

Cross-Reference

Genitourinary Radiology: THE REQUISITES, pp 124-125, 149, 395.

Comment

Arteriosclerosis is the most common cause of RAS. The site of arterial narrowing is at the ostium or proximal 2 cm of the renal artery. RAS tends to occur in patients older than 50 years of age. Fibromuscular dysplasia accounts for up to 30% of renovascular hypertension cases, tends to occur in women between ages 20 and 50, and occurs in the middle to distal renal artery.

Screening for renovascular hypertension should be performed in a select group of patients because it accounts for only 1% to 5% of cases of systemic hypertension. Renal scintigraphy with an angiotensin-converting enzyme inhibitor (ACEI) has a reported sensitivity of 90% and specificity of greater than 95%. The ACEI blocks the production of angiotensin 2 and thus unmasks the compensating mechanism of the ischemic kidney. This effect results in a significant decrease in perfusion of the kidney with RAS. Thus there is delayed function and tracer accumulation in the kidney with RAS. Catheter angiography is the gold standard for the evaluation of RAS, but it is invasive and costly and requires the use of iodinated contrast material. More recently, MR angiography has proved useful as a screening test. The most effective technique is bolus-chase, breath-hold, three-dimensional MR angiography after administration of intravenous gadolinium chelate contrast agents. This technique offers excellent spatial resolution for detecting RAS and can be used to assess the symmetry of renal perfusion and contrast excretion. Gadolinium contrast agents are not nephrotoxic and can be used safely in patients with compromised renal function.

Notes

Stage IIb Cervical Carcinoma

1. False.

2. False (in large part because of the success of Papanicolaou test screening).

3. It has implications for local staging and treatment.

4. False.

Reference

Seki H, Azumi R, Kimura M, Sakai K: Stromal invasion by carcinoma of the cervix: assessment with dynamic MR imaging, *Am J Roentgenol* 168:1579-1585, 1997.

Cross-Reference

Genitourinary Radiology: THE REQUISITES, pp 295-300.

Comment

The majority of patients with cervical cancer have stage Ib or IIa disease (tumor confined to the cervix or upper vagina), and in these patients, surgery and radiotherapy produce equivalent results. Tumors that extend beyond the cervix into the parametrium—stage IIb or higher—are primarily treated with radiation. Radiotherapy also is preferable when the growth pattern of the tumor is primarily endophytic into the cervical canal; these "barrel-shaped" tumors are particularly difficult to resect with tumor-free margins.

This case illustrates the usefulness of MRI for the staging of squamous cell carcinoma of the cervix. The uterine cervix consists of an outer stromal layer of fibrous, muscular, and elastic tissue and an inner core of columnar, squamous, or squamocolumnar epithelium. On T2W MRI, stroma appears as a hypointense rim surrounding a central core of relatively hyperintense epithelium. Parametrial extension of cervical carcinoma is suggested when, as shown in this case, the hyperintense tumor mass focally disrupts the hypointense stromal ring on a T2W MR image. Obversely, invasion of paracervical tissue can be excluded with high specificity if the low signal rim of cervical stroma completely surrounds the tumor. Dynamic, enhanced MRI also may help with the detection of invasive cervical cancer because carcinoma usually enhances earlier than or simultaneously with cervical epithelium but before cervical stroma. In this case focal tumor disruption of the cervical stroma is confirmed on enhanced T1W images.

Notes

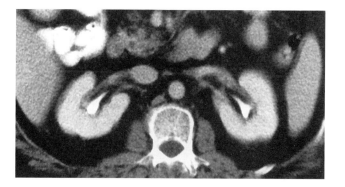
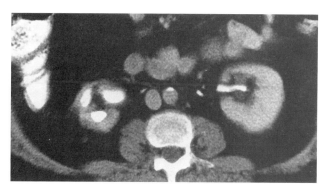
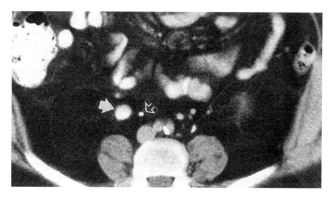

1. Three consecutive images from an abdominal CT examination are shown. In the third image, what structures are indicated by the solid and open arrows?

2. What is the significance of the size discrepancy indicated by the arrows?

3. How can the appearance of the right kidney be explained?

4. What other imaging study could be performed to confirm the diagnosis?

Reflux Nephropathy in a Duplicated Collecting System

1. Duplicated right ureters.

2. One ureter is dilated as a result of ureterovesical reflux or obstruction.

3. Reflux nephropathy in the lower pole.

4. Voiding cystourethrogram.

Reference

Cronan JJ, Amis ES Jr, Zeman RK, et al: Obstruction of the upper pole moiety in renal duplication in adults: CT evaluation, *Radiology* 161:17, 1986.

Cross-Reference

Genitourinary Radiology: THE REQUISITES, pp 157-160.

Comment

Ureteral duplications are common congenital anomalies, occurring in 1% to 10% of the population, and affect women twice as frequently as men. Duplications are described as "partial" when the two ureters join along their course and are described as "complete" when there is separate entry of each ureter into the bladder. Ureteral duplications are associated with other genitourinary tract anomalies in 30% of cases. These anomalies include ureteropelvic junction obstruction, ureterocele, hydronephrosis, and ureterovesical reflux. Atrophy of the lower pole moiety can simulate a solid renal mass; thus to avoid this diagnostic error, recognition of ureteral duplication is important.

The Weigert-Meyer rule states that the upper pole ureter inserts inferior and medial to the lower pole ureter. The upper pole ureter is subject to obstruction and at urography may result in the "drooping lily sign" (i.e., inferior displacement of the lower pole collecting system by a nonopacified upper moiety). Ectopic insertion of the upper pole ureter below the external sphincter may manifest as urinary incontinence, and insertion in the vagina can result in persistent drainage and recurrent infection. Insertion of the upper pole ureter below the external sphincter is extremely rare in men, but ectopic insertion can occur in the vas deferens or seminal vesicles. There is an increased incidence of ureteroceles at the insertion of the upper pole ectopic ureter.

Vesicoureteral reflux may occur in the lower pole moiety and is most likely the result of an aberrant insertion of the ureter into the bladder. Reflux may result in dilation of the lower pole ureter and atrophy of the lower pole cortex. If the ureteral duplication is partial, the "yo-yo" phenomenon, in which urine produced in the upper pole refluxes into the lower pole ureter and causes reflux nephropathy in the lower pole moiety, can occur.

Notes

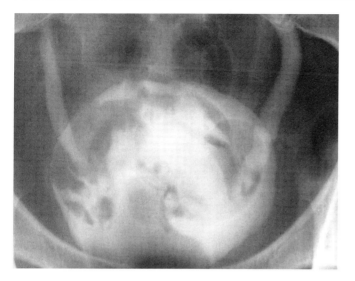 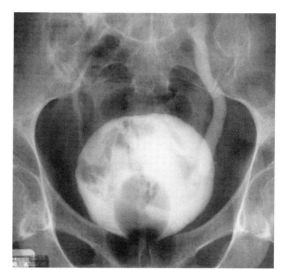

1. This patient has atraumatic, fulminant, gross hematuria. What is the most likely cause of the large filling defects in the bladder?

2. Name three causes of this disease.

3. True or False: The association of penicillin use with hemorrhagic cystitis has been linked to a urotoxic metabolite.

4. Diffuse vesical bleeding may be the initial sign of what disease? (HINT: This disease may occur in patients with long-standing rheumatoid arthritis.)

Hemorrhagic Cystitis

1. Blood clots.

2. Consumption of urotoxins, radiation therapy, and viral infection.

3. False.

4. Amyloidosis.

Reference

deVries CR, Freiha FS: Hemorrhagic cystitis: a review, *J Urol* 143:1-9, 1990.

Cross-Reference

Genitourinary Radiology: THE REQUISITES, pp 206-208.

Comment

Hemorrhagic cystitis (HC) is defined as diffuse vesical bleeding and can be either acute or insidious. The major causes of HC are (1) chemical toxins, (2) radiation therapy, (3) immune-mediated injury, and (4) idiopathic disease. Most cases of severe vesical hemorrhage are caused by radiotherapy or chemotherapeutic agents. Of the latter, oxazaphosphorine alkylating agents (e.g., cyclophosphamide and ifosfamide) are most commonly linked to HC, but busulfan and thiotepa also have been implicated. Cyclophosphamide cystitis is discussed more completely in Case 96, but an important point is that its urotoxic effects are mediated by acrolein, the aldehyde by-product of cyclophosphamide metabolism. In contrast, other drugs may cause HC through an immune-mediated mechanism that is the proposed etiology of bladder mucosal injury associated with the use of penicillin and danazol.

Radiation cystitis most commonly presents after treatment for prostate or cervical cancer and less commonly after treatment for rectal or bladder cancers. Approximately 20% of patients treated with pelvic radiation have symptoms referable to the bladder, and in one study, 9% of patients treated with full-dose radiation therapy developed HC. Hematuria may occur months to years after treatment and begins with mucosal edema, telangiectasia, and submucosal hemorrhage. Over the long term an obliterative endarteritis of the detrusor may manifest as a shrunken, fibrotic bladder.

In the middle of the 1970s, irritative voiding symptoms and gross hematuria were reported in children during several out breaks of adenovirus type 11. Subsequently, HC has been observed in bone marrow transplant recipients, presumably as a result of reactivation of a latent form of this virus. Other viruses implicated in HC include adenovirus type 21, polyoma, and influenza A.

Notes

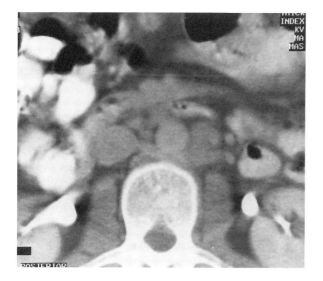
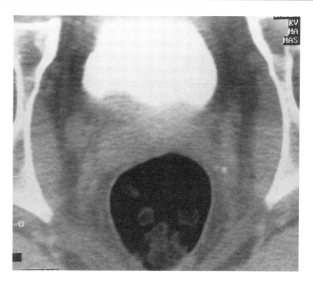
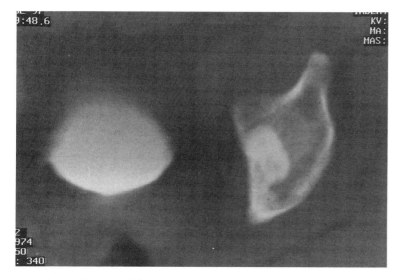

1. What is the most likely diagnosis?
2. What is the size threshold for enlarged lymph nodes in the pelvis?
3. What neoplasms are associated with osteoblastic bone metastases?
4. Would it be surprising if this patient had a PSA level of 10 ng/ml?

Staging of Prostate Cancer

1. Prostate cancer metastatic to lymph nodes and to bone.

2. Minimal axial diameter of 10 mm.

3. Prostate and breast, as well as bladder, lymphoma, lung, carcinoid, and medulloblastoma.

4. Yes, the likelihood of bone metastases with a PSA level of 10 ng/ml or less is less than 2%.

Reference

Epstein JI, Carmichael, MJ, Pizov G, et al: Influence of capsular penetration on progression following radical prostatectomy, *J Urol* 150:135-143, 1993.

Cross-Reference

Genitourinary Radiology: THE REQUISITES, pp 329-333.

Comment

The staging of prostate cancer has important implications for treatment. Microscopic and nonpalpable tumors (T_1 and A on the TNM and Jewett-Whitmore staging systems, respectively) are usually found in transurethral prostatectomy specimens or by needle biopsy as a result of elevated serum prostate-specific antigen (PSA) levels. Tumors that are confined to the gland (stage T_2 or B) may be either palpable or identified by imaging. Tumors that have already penetrated the prostatic capsule (stage T_{3a} or C1) and invaded surrounding tissues (stage T_{3b} or C2) have high rates of recurrence and morbidity. For this reason an important staging threshold for treatment is between stages T_2 (tumor confined to the prostate gland) and T_{3b} (gross or bilateral extracapsular tumor). Patients with stage T_2 or B disease are offered curative radical prostatectomy; there is some research suggesting that patients with microscopic extracapsular tumor (T_{3a}) also should be candidates for this surgery. Patients with stage T_{3b} cancer or more advanced disease are treated with external beam radiation, hormonal ablation, or both, with a palliative intent.

Patients undergo staging after the diagnosis of prostate cancer has been made, often after ultrasound-guided prostate biopsy. The serum PSA level and histologic grade (Gleason score) of the tumor may be helpful in predicting the likelihood of extraprostatic spread. For example, 75% of patients with serum PSA levels less than 4 ng/ml have prostate-confined cancer, whereas this value falls to 50% for those with PSA levels between 4 and 10 ng/ml and is only 2% when the patient's PSA level exceeds 30 ng/ml. The likelihood of lymph node metastases in prostate cancer also is correlated with the clinical T stage. For example, the chance that a patient with a poorly differentiated stage T_3 tumor has lymph node metastases is 68% to 93% but is 0% in the patient with a stage T_{1a} tumor.

Notes

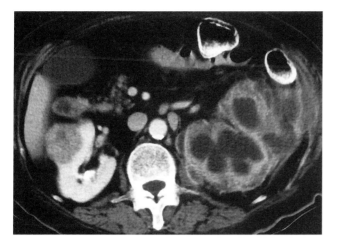 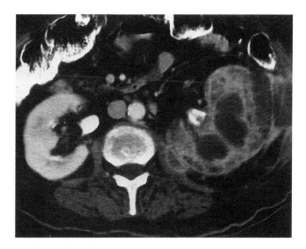

1. What is the diagnosis? What is the presumed pathophysiology of the disease involving the left kidney?

2. What organisms are most commonly involved?

3. What is the treatment for this disease process?

4. What are the findings on the image of the right kidney? Is there an association between these two entities? How should this patient be treated?

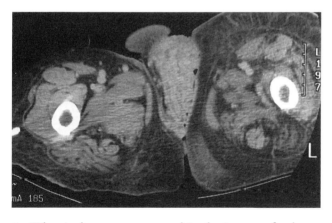 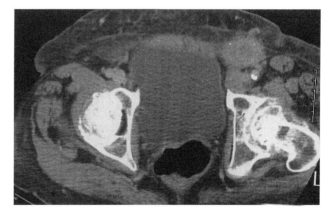

1. What is the most common histologic type of vulvar cancer?

2. What is the eponym for the paraurethral glands? What is the eponym for the major glands of the vulvar vestibule?

3. What aberrant hormonal activity has been associated with vulvar tumors?

4. Which virus causes genital warts? (BONUS QUESTION: What disease affects children whose mothers have a history of this genital problem?)

CASE 75

Xanthogranulomatous Pyelonephritis and Renal Cell Carcinoma

1. Diffuse xanthogranulomatous pyelonephritis (XGP). Recurrent upper tract infection and calculus formation cause obstruction and renal inflammation, with lipid-laden histiocytes.

2. *Escherichia coli* and *Proteus* species.

3. Nephrectomy.

4. Solid enhancing renal mass consistent with renal cell carcinoma (RCC). There is no association between RCC and XGP. The patient should be treated with right renal-sparing surgery.

Reference

Hayes WS, Hartman DS, Sesterhenn IA: Xanthogranulomatous pyelonephritis, *Radiographics* 11:485-498, 1991.

Cross-Reference

Genitourinary Radiology: THE REQUISITES, pp 103-104, 117, 132, 134-135.

Comment

Xanthogranulomatous pyelonephritis (XGP) is a rare condition that has two variant forms—diffuse and focal. XGP is believed to occur secondary to chronic urinary tract infection (most commonly with *E. coli* or *Proteus* species), which predisposes the patient to calculus formation. Of patients with XGP, 80% have a coexisting renal calculus. The presence of calculi and recurrent infections incites an inflammatory response in which lipid-laden macrophages destroy and replace normal renal parenchyma. The process causes enlargement of the kidney, and the infection can spread to the retroperitoneal fat and the psoas muscle. Typical symptoms are chronic pain, fever, and anorexia with weight loss. The disease most often afflicts middle-aged women and those with diabetes.

Focal XGP is a more localized area of inflammation and is also associated with renal calculus disease. The area of decreased enhancement indicating focal pyelonephritis may be difficult to differentiate from a solid renal mass caused by a neoplasm. There are no specific imaging findings to differentiate focal XGP from a neoplasm, and the treatment of choice is renal-sparing surgery.

This patient had diffuse XGP of the left kidney and a right RCC; however, there is no reported association between these two diseases. The treatment of choice in this case is left nephrectomy and right partial nephrectomy. A newer technique for treating RCCs is image-guided radiofrequency (RF) ablation.

Notes

CASE 76

Vulvar Carcinoma

1. Squamous cell carcinoma.

2. Skene's; Bartholin.

3. Production of a parathyroid hormone–like substance may cause hypercalcemia (in the absence of bone metastases) and has been associated with vulvar squamous cell carcinoma.

4. Human papillomavirus. (BONUS ANSWER: Laryngeal papillomatosis.)

Reference

Hacker NF, Nieberg RK, Berek JS, et al: Superficially invasive vulvar cancer with nodal metastases, *Gynecol Oncol* 15:65-72, 1983.

Cross-Reference

Genitourinary Radiology: THE REQUISITES, pp 240-241.

Comment

Squamous cell carcinoma is the most common histologic type of vulvar malignancy, but adenocarcinoma and sarcoma may occur here as well. Most tumors arise on the labia minora or majora and spread to regional lymph nodes, as in this case. The superficial inguinal nodes are the major sentinel node group, and the femoral and inguinal lymph nodes receive all of the lymphatic drainage of the vulva. Note the infiltration of dermal lymphatics in this case.

Squamous cell carcinomas, particularly the verrucous subtype, may be difficult to distinguish from condylomata acuminata. In North America the major infectious lesions of the vulva include condyloma acuminata, herpes genitalis, syphilis, and molluscum contagiosum. Condylomata acuminata are contagious, benign polyclonal neoplasms that may involve the vulva, perineal skin, urethra, vagina, and cervix. Also known as *genital warts,* this infectious tumor is caused by human papillomavirus and presents on the vulva as discrete verrucous or papillary growths.

Many adenocarcinomas of the vulva arise as primary malignant tumors of Bartholin's gland, although they can arise from sweat glands. Bartholin's glands are the major vestibular glands and are drained by a duct that exits just external to the hymenal ring on the posterolateral aspect of the vestibule. Primary adenocarcinoma of Skene's glands also has been reported. The paraurethral (Skene's) glands are distributed along the posterior and lateral aspects of the urethra, and the paired external openings of these glands are found on either side of the urethral meatus.

Notes

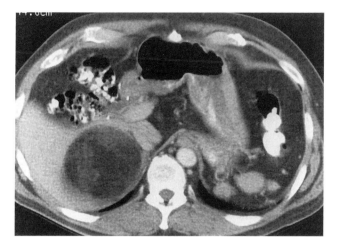 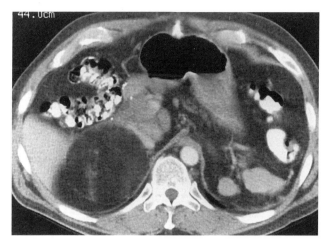

1. What suprarenal lesions may contain areas of mature adipose tissue?
2. What is the most common clinical presentation of myelolipoma?
3. Is there a correlation between tumor size and symptoms?
4. True or False: Most myelolipomas increase in size over time.

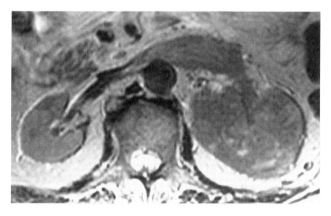 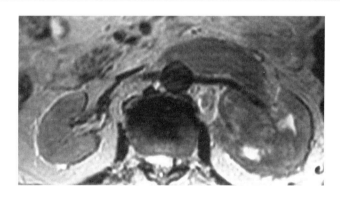

1. What is the most likely cause of this venous abnormality?
2. What are the main differential causes of renal vein thrombosis?
3. Using the Robson classification system, what stage is shown in these illustrations?
4. When there is extension into the vein, what venous landmarks are important for surgical planning?

Natural History of Myelolipoma

1. Adrenal myelolipoma, exophytic renal angiomyolipoma, retroperitoneal lipoma, retroperitoneal liposarcoma, and adrenal adenoma.

2. Incidentally discovered asymptomatic suprarenal mass.

3. No.

4. False.

Reference

Han M, Burnett AL, Fishman EK, Marshall FF: The natural history and treatment of adrenal myelolipoma, *J Urol* 157:1213-1216, 1997.

Cross-Reference

Genitourinary Radiology: THE REQUISITES, pp 360-361.

Comment

Adrenal myelolipoma is a rare benign neoplasm composed of mature adipose and hematopoietic tissues. Although there is no consensus as to the etiology of this tumor, the most widely held theory is that it is caused by adrenocortical metaplasia of reticuloendothelial cells in response to nonspecific stimuli.

Although these tumors may cause abdominal or flank pain, palpable masses, or hematuria, most adrenal myelolipomas are asymptomatic and the great majority are hormonally inactive. There have been two case reports of myelolipoma and adrenocortical adenoma in association with Cushing's syndrome. At the time of discovery, these tumors may range from several centimeters to more than 30 cm in diameter. There is no clear correlation between tumor size and symptoms relating to mechanical compression, retroperitoneal hemorrhage, or tumor necrosis. When followed over a period of up to 10 years, these tumors may increase in size, but growth is slow and is not necessarily related to the development of symptoms or hemorrhage. Growth alone therefore should not be an indication for resection.

The recommended management of adrenal myelolipoma is conservative; surgical removal is indicated only if the patient is symptomatic. Periodic imaging with CT or sonography should suffice for follow up.

Notes

Renal Cell Carcinoma with Extension into the Left Renal Vein

1. Renal cell carcinoma extension.

2. Renal cell carcinoma extension, hypercoagulable states, glomerulonephritis, and dehydration.

3. Stage III.

4. If there is extension into the inferior vena cava, it is important to determine whether it is above or below the level where the hepatic veins drain into the inferior vena cava.

Reference

Zagoria RJ, Bechtold RE, Dyer RB: Staging of renal adenocarcinoma: role of various imaging procedures, *Am J Roentgenol* 164:363-370, 1995.

Cross-Reference

Genitourinary Radiology: THE REQUISITES, pp 95, 135.

Comment

This case demonstrates a soft tissue mass in the left renal vein, with no flow in the vein. This finding indicates renal vein thrombosis. In addition, the left renal vein is markedly enlarged, suggesting that it is not just a simple blood clot but rather a neoplasm. The most common cause of renal vein thrombosis in adults is the extension of a renal cell carcinoma into the renal vein. Rarely, other renal tumors, including transitional cell carcinoma, squamous cell carcinoma, oncocytoma, and angiomyolipoma, extend into the vein. But by far the most common neoplasm to involve the renal vein is renal cell carcinoma; thus when this finding is detected, renal cell carcinoma should be the presumptive diagnosis. Extension of the tumor into the vein is important clinically. It indicates an advanced stage of the disease, at least Robson classification stage III. Interestingly, venous extension without lymph node or distant metastases is associated with a good prognosis, similar to that for stage I or II disease. A tumor thrombus usually is found within the vein lumen but does not invade the vein wall. Once tumor extension has been detected, the length of extension into the venous system should be delineated for surgical planning. It should be noted whether the tumor extends into the inferior vena cava. If it does, the radiologist should determine the cephalad extent of the tumor. When the tumor does not extend above the level of the hepatic veins, usually it can be resected with an abdominal approach. Resection of more cephalad tumors usually requires combined thoracoabdominal incisions and possibly intraoperative cardiopulmonary bypass.

Notes

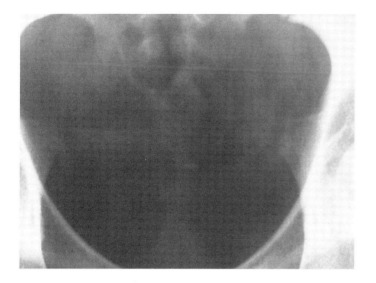
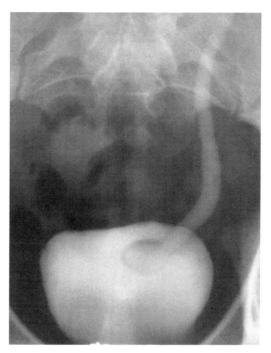

1. What name describes the bulbous portion of the lower left ureter in this case?

2. What causes this abnormality to occur?

3. What processes usually cause this abnormality?

4. To make the diagnosis of an orthotopic ureterocele, what is the maximum thickness of the radiolucent halo?

Pseudoureterocele

1. Pseudoureterocele.

2. Partial obstruction of the ureteral orifice.

3. Ureteral stone, ureteral edema from recent passage of a stone, manipulation of the ureterovesical junction, and bladder neoplasm impinging on the ureteral orifice.

4. 2 mm.

Reference

Chen MYM, Zagoria RJ, Dyer RB: Interureteric ridge edema: incidence and etiology, *Abdom Imaging* 20:368-370, 1995.

Cross-Reference

Genitourinary Radiology: THE REQUISITES, pp 158-160.

Comment

This patient has a small stone lodged in the left ureterovesical junction, causing ureteral obstruction and the appearance of a pseudoureterocele. This is described as a "pseudoureterocele" because the radiologic appearance is similar to that of an orthotopic ureterocele but the appearance is caused by an underlying pathologic condition. In this case the pathology, a stone, is visible on the scout radiograph. A pseudoureterocele is caused by partial obstruction of the ureterovesical junction with marked dilation of the lower ureteral segment and bulging of this segment into the bladder lumen. This bulging is usually accompanied by surrounding edema, which causes thickening of the "halo" of lucency around the caudal end of the ureter. As illustrated in this case, the lucent segment is considerably thickened above the pseudoureterocele. In a simple or orthotopic ureterocele the lucent line is uniform and 2 mm or less in diameter. Irregularity or thickening of the halo suggests an underlying pathologic problem, such as a stone, edema resulting from recent stone passage or manipulation, or tumor encroachment and infiltration. When the diagnosis is not apparent with urography, it may be confirmed with endoscopy. Another important finding seen in association with a pseudoureterocele is hydronephrosis. Orthotopic ureteroceles are not often associated with any significant obstruction, and therefore hydronephrosis is absent. The combination of a ureterocele-like abnormality and obstruction suggests a pseudoureterocele and an underlying pathologic problem.

Notes

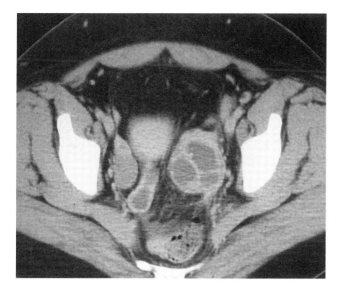
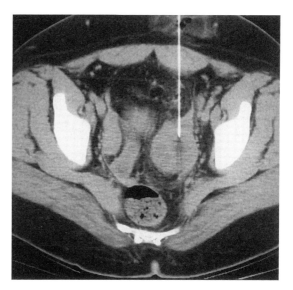
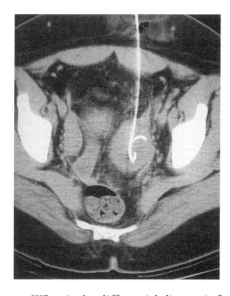

1. What is the differential diagnosis for the finding or findings in the first image?
2. True or False: The patient history and physical examination are not helpful in narrowing the differential diagnosis.
3. True or False: The treatment shown in the second and third images is the first-line treatment for this disease.
4. What alternative technique might be used to perform this procedure?

Percutaneous Drainage of a Tuboovarian Abscess

1. Tuboovarian or other pelvic abscess and ovarian neoplasm.

2. False. Patients with a tuboovarian abscess often have pain, fever, and tenderness associated with cervical motion. These symptoms are not common in patients with ovarian carcinoma.

3. False.

4. Needle aspiration using the transvaginal approach.

References

Fabiszewski NL, Sumkin JH, Johns CM: Contemporary radiologic percutaneous abscess drainage in the pelvis, *Clin Obstet Gynecol* 36:445-456, 1993.

Teisala K, Heinonen PK, Punnonen R: Transvaginal ultrasound in the diagnosis and treatment of tubo-ovarian abscess, *Br J Obstet Gynaecol* 97:178-180, 1990.

Cross-Reference

Genitourinary Radiology: THE REQUISITES, pp 264-265, 267.

Comment

A tuboovarian abscess (TOA) typically presents as a complex adnexal mass on imaging studies. Because the adnexae are well visualized and no ionizing radiation is involved, ultrasound is the initial imaging modality of choice when the diagnosis is suspected clinically. On ultrasound the radiologist typically finds a complex adnexal mass and free pelvic fluid; the specificity of the diagnosis increases if a dilated tubular structure (the distended fallopian tube) is visible within or adjacent to the mass. For the woman with nonspecific pelvic pain, tenderness, and fever, renal calculus disease and appendicitis should be considered and evaluated by ultrasound, CT, or both.

The first line of treatment for patients with a TOA is antibiotic therapy, and the majority of patients respond to this medical treatment. Percutaneous aspiration can be performed in patients who are refractory to treatment with antimicrobials. If a percutaneous procedure is performed, aspiration of the infected material is usually sufficient treatment; placement of a drainage catheter is seldom necessary. One study has shown a reduction in hospital stays and a reduction in overall cost when patients undergo percutaneous aspiration for TOA.

Although this case demonstrates CT-guided drainage, some prefer transvaginal ultrasound–guided drainage and find it technically easier and more rapid to perform. When using either technique, the clinician should perform the procedure during or after administration of intravenous antibiotics because transient bacteremia is common. Pelvic abscesses that result from perforated diverticulitis or surgery are most often drained percutaneously. Image-guided abscess drainage has a low morbidity and often results in rapid clinical improvement.

Notes

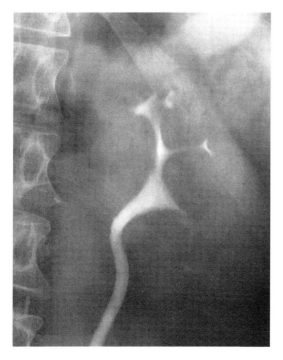

1. What abnormalities are visible on this intravenous urogram?
2. What are the main differential diagnostic considerations for this pattern of abnormality?
3. What is the best diagnostic test for confirming the diagnosis of this entity?
4. What causes the radiologic appearance of the lower pole calyx in this case?

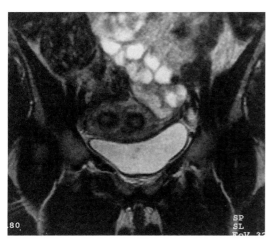 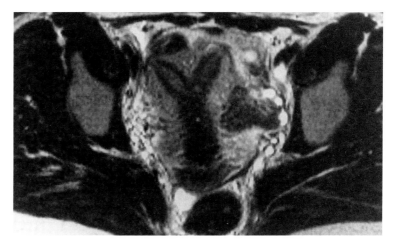

1. Based on the uterine fundal contour, what is the most likely diagnosis?
2. Based on the type of the tissue between the uterine cornua, what is the most likely diagnosis?
3. From the perspective of treatment, why is it important to identify the type of dividing tissue in patients with uterine fusion anomalies?
4. True or False: Infertility is more common in patients with septate uterus than in those with bicornuate uterus.

Calyceal Transitional Cell Carcinoma

1. Irregularity and minimal filling of lower pole calyces.

2. Transitional cell carcinoma and tuberculosis.

3. Urine cytology and bacteriology.

4. Either infiltration by tumor or inflammation of the lower pole calyx and its infundibulum.

Reference

Wong-You-Cheong JJ, Wagner BJ, Davis CJ Jr: Transitional cell carcinoma of the urinary tract: radiologic-pathologic correlation, *Radiographics* 18:123-142, 1998.

Cross-Reference

Genitourinary Radiology: THE REQUISITES, pp 113-118.

Comment

This intravenous urogram demonstrates the appearance of an "amputated" calyx. There is minimal opacification of the lower pole calyces and an apparent abrupt cutoff of the infundibulum, which should be draining these calyces. This finding almost always indicates the diagnosis of an infiltrative process involving the urothelium. The two main diagnostic considerations for this appearance are tuberculosis and transitional cell carcinoma. It is impossible radiologically to distinguish between these two entities in this type of situation. An exact diagnosis must be made after examination of renal tissue or urine. Once a diagnosis is made, cross-sectional imaging may help to better define the extent (i.e., stage) of the abnormality.

Transitional cell carcinoma can be either papillary or nonpapillary. The papillary variety tends to grow into polypoid masses and accounts for approximately two thirds of all cases of transitional cell carcinoma. The nonpapillary variety is infiltrating and leads to malignant strictures when it involves the upper tracts of the urinary system. Nonpapillary transitional cell carcinoma tends to invade through the mucosa at an earlier phase of the disease, but it is usually unifocal in the urinary tract. Papillary tumors are less invasive but more commonly multifocal.

Notes

Septate Uterus on MRI

1. Septate uterus.

2. Bicornuate uterus.

3. Septate uterus containing a fibrous septum can be treated with hysteroscopic metroplasty; bicornuate uterus is usually treated with abdominal metroplasty.

4. True.

Reference

Carrington BM, Hricak H, Nuruddin RN, et al: Müllerian duct anomalies: MR imaging evaluation, *Radiology* 176:715-720, 1990.

Cross-Reference

Genitourinary Radiology: THE REQUISITES, pp 255-257.

Comment

Both bicornuate and septate uteri represent incomplete fusion of the two müllerian ducts. When corrective surgery is contemplated, the nature of the dividing tissue is important. When a thin (typically fibrous) septum separates the endometrial cavity, excision of the hypovascular septum may be accomplished using the hysteroscope. Hysteroscopic metroplasty may be performed as an outpatient procedure. However, if unification surgery is elected to correct a uterus divided by myometrial tissue, the vascularity of that tissue necessitates metroplasty by an abdominal approach. Abdominal resection usually requires a 5- to 10-day hospital stay. Although there are diagnostic criteria for both bicornuate and septate uteri on ultrasound and hysterosalpingography, the nature of the dividing tissue is most accurately defined by MRI.

For the oral board examination it is prudent to be aware of the classic definitions of these two müllerian anomalies on MRI. However, many gynecologists believe that an accurate definition of the dividing tissue is more important than the diagnosis of bicornuate or septate uterus per se. In bicornuate uterus the fundus is typically more deeply concave, and the two horns are usually divergent. A distance of more than 4 cm separates the two horns, and the dividing tissue is isointense with outer myometrium on T2W images. However, Carrington and co-workers noted that this tissue may be hypointense at the level of the lower uterine segment in some cases. The fundal contour of the septate uterus is convex, flat, or minimally indented (less than 1 cm), and the intercornual distance is normal (2 to 4 cm). The septum has an intermediate to low signal intensity on both T1W and T2W images. More recent work has shown that some septate uteri may contain dividing tissue that is typical of outer myometrium (as in this case).

Notes

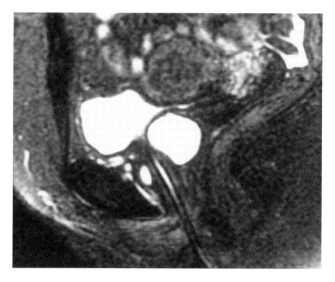 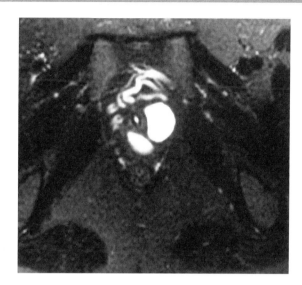

1. This patient has postvoid dribbling and dyspareunia. What is the differential diagnosis?

2. True or False: The congenital form of this lesion most often affects girls and may obstruct the urethra.

3. True or False: Urethral diverticula are much more common in African-American women.

4. True or False: Gartner's ducts are the remnants of the wolffian ducts left in the wall of the vagina, cervix, or broad ligament.

MRI of Urethral Diverticulum

1. Diverticulum of either the urethra or the bladder.

2. False. 98% occur in boys.

3. True.

4. True.

Reference

Kim B, Hricak H, Tanagho EA: Diagnosis of urethral diverticula in women: value of MR imaging, *Am J Roentgenol* 161: 809-815, 1993.

Cross-Reference

Genitourinary Radiology: THE REQUISITES, pp 244-245.

Comment

Diverticula of the urethra are uncommon but often overlooked causes of dyspareunia, postvoid dribbling, irritative voiding symptoms, and urinary tract infections in women. They are estimated to occur in 1.4% to 4.7% of women and are about 6 times more common in the African-American population. The diverticulum is believed to form after obstruction of the paraurethral glands by traumatic injury or infection. Chronic inflammation leads to a cavity that may epithelialize, producing a diverticulum.

Although they can form anywhere along the length of the female urethra, diverticula are more commonly located dorsolaterally in the middle third (in 66% of cases) and are rarely located distally (in about 10% of cases). Conventional evaluation of a suspected urethral diverticulum includes urethroscopy and contrast urethrography. For the diagnosis of female urethral diverticulum, the following studies are specific but less sensitive: urethroscopy (70% sensitivity), VCUG (65% sensitivity), and double-balloon urethrography (85% sensitivity).

Both ultrasound and MRI may be used to evaluate periurethral masses, particularly when conventional diagnostic tests are inconclusive or discrepant. Sonography can demonstrate a diverticulum that does not opacify with contrast and differentiates the diverticulum from a solid periurethral mass. Diverticula appear as septated, horseshoe-shaped, fluid-filled periurethral masses on MRI; calculi and neoplasms arising from within the diverticulum also can be demonstrated. The displaced urethra can be separated from the diverticulum, and sagittal MR images show the relationship of the mass to the vagina and bladder floor well. The size and extent of the diverticulum and the extent of periurethral inflammation can be more accurately assessed by cross-sectional imaging.

Notes

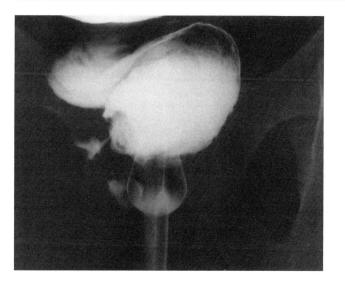

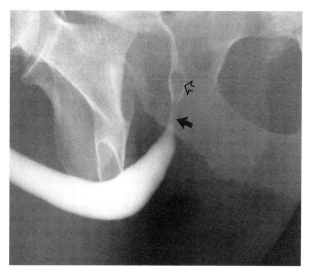

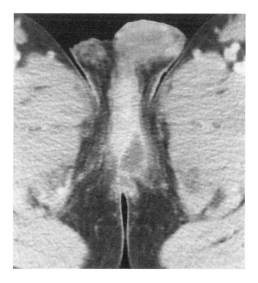

1. This patient has rectal Crohn's disease, pelvic pain, and irritative voiding symptoms. What is the diagnosis?

2. True or False: The solid arrow points to a posterior urethral stricture.

3. What is the filling defect *(open arrow)* in the posterior urethra?

4. What type of renal stones may form because of ileal Crohn's disease and fat malabsorption?

Perineal Abscess Caused by Crohn's Colitis

1. Perineal abscess.

2. False. It points to the membranous urethra.

3. Verumontanum.

4. Oxalate stones.

Reference

Shield DE, Lytton B, Weiss RM, Schiff M Jr: Urologic complications of inflammatory bowel disease, *J Urol* 115:701-706, 1976.

Cross-Reference

Genitourinary Radiology: THE REQUISITES, pp 194-195.

Comment

Shield and colleagues report urologic complications in 23% of 233 patients with Crohn's ileitis. Granulomatous enterocolitis may cause genitourinary tract disease because of the local extension of Crohn's disease, metabolic aberrations secondary to malabsorption and dehydration, or secondary local or systemic disease associated with the chronic inflammatory process (e.g., amyloidosis).

Genitourinary tract involvement by Crohn's disease is most often caused by direct extension of granulomatous enterocolitis. Regional enteritis may cause obstruction of the ureter (typically the right ureter); bladder wall lesions ("herald lesions"); or fistulas to the ureter, bladder, urethra, or vagina. Retroperitoneal fibrosis and amyloidosis caused by long-standing Crohn's disease also may have manifestations in the genitourinary tract. Of patients with Crohn's disease, 10% develop renal calculus disease. Intestinal fat, which is malabsorbed because of ileal disease, binds calcium and leads to excessive absorption of dietary oxalate. This process in turn leads to hyperoxaluria and the formation of oxalate stones. Uric acid stones may form because of dehydration and hyperuricosuria in patients with ileostomies.

This patient had rectal Crohn's disease and irritative voiding symptoms caused by a perineal abscess. Although not demonstrated in this case, fistulas to the bladder, vagina, and urethra may complicate rectal Crohn's disease. Notice the perineal gas next to the bulbous urethra on the urethrogram.

Notes

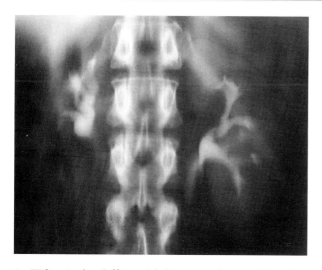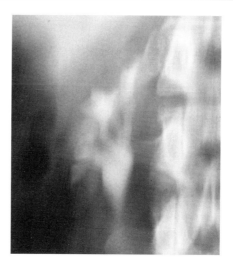

1. What is the differential diagnosis for a unilateral small, smooth kidney?
2. Which cause of a unilateral small, smooth kidney also typically causes dilated calyces?
3. What causes a unilateral small, irregular kidney?
4. What is the lower limit of normal size for either kidney?

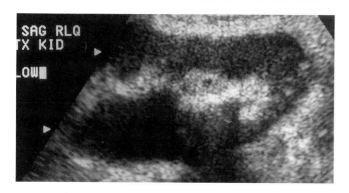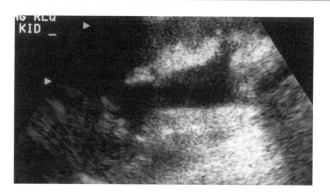

1. Sagittal sonograms of a renal transplant were performed in the perioperative period. What is the finding? What are the possible causes?
2. What normal structure can mimic the dilated collecting system, and how can the two be distinguished from one another?
3. What is the initial treatment for obstructive hydronephrosis in a recently transplanted kidney?
4. True or False: In the transplanted kidney, hydronephrosis caused by obstruction is usually painless.

CASE 85

Renal Hypoplasia

1. Chronic ischemia (e.g., caused by renal artery stenosis or chronic renal vein thrombosis), postobstructive atrophy, renal hypoplasia, chronic subcapsular hematoma, and previous radiation treatment.

2. Postobstructive atrophy.

3. Reflux nephropathy, analgesic nephropathy, or renal segmental arterial occlusions as seen in some diseases associated with preferential small vessel atherosclerosis, such as diabetes mellitus.

4. Each kidney should be no less than three lumbar vertebrae and intervening interspaces (L1-L3) in height. A height equal to four vertebral bodies and their interspaces is the upper limit of normal.

Reference

Daneman A, Alton DJ: Radiographic manifestations of renal anomalies, *Radiol Clin North Am* 29:351-363, 1991.

Cross-Reference

Genitourinary Radiology: THE REQUISITES, pp 124-128.

Comment

Unilateral renal atrophy has many causes. It is best to limit the possible diagnoses by classifying according to the pattern of atrophy. A common cause, reflux nephropathy, or chronic atrophic pyelonephritis, usually causes atrophy with marked irregularity of the cortical margin and underlying clubbed calyces. A unilateral small, smooth kidney usually is the result of renal artery stenosis, and in this case the calyces appear normal. Other findings of renal underperfusion, including delay in opacification of the kidney and calyces, also may be present in patients with renal artery stenosis. A diagnosis of renal hypoplasia should be made when there is a unilateral small, smooth kidney that excretes contrast and has normal-appearing but few calyces. When there are five or fewer calyces and all other features of a hypoplastic kidney are present, as in this case, the diagnosis should be made. The etiology of hypoplastic kidney is unknown, but it is hypothesized that in utero ischemia leads to this pathologic condition. Renal arteriography demonstrates a small but unobstructed renal artery supplying the kidney.

As illustrated in this case, compensatory hypertrophy of the contralateral kidney is a common associated finding in cases of unilateral renal atrophy. Compensatory hypertrophy can occur well into adulthood, until the sixth or seventh decade of life, and does not necessarily indicate a congenital or childhood abnormality of the other kidney.

Notes

CASE 86

Nephrolithiasis and Obstructive Hydronephrosis in a Transplanted Kidney

1. Hydronephrosis. Ureteral edema, blood clot, anastomotic stricture, or peritransplant fluid collection.

2. Enlarged, branching veins in the renal sinus can be differentiated from the collecting system on color Doppler ultrasound.

3. Percutaneous nephrostomy or placement of a nephrovesical stent.

4. True.

Reference

Reinberg Y, Bumgardner GL, Aliabadi H: Urological aspects of renal transplantation, *J Urol* 143(6):1087-1092, 1990.

Cross-Reference

Genitourinary Radiology: THE REQUISITES, pp 182-189.

Comment

The management of end-stage renal disease was changed forever with the advent of renal transplantation in the 1950s. Continuing refinements in surgical and immunosuppressive techniques over the last four decades have greatly improved long-term graft function and patient survival. Although graft rejection remains of paramount importance, transplanted kidneys are subject to many urologic complications. For the evaluation of these potential complications, ultrasound is the primary imaging modality. The complete ultrasound evaluation includes gray scale imaging and Doppler sonography. Gray scale imaging assesses parenchymal echogenicity, the size of the collecting system and its contents (e.g., calculus, clot, fungus balls), surrounding soft tissues, and fluid collections (e.g., hematoma, urinoma, lymphocele, abscess [HULA]). Color Doppler ultrasound can assess graft perfusion and vascular anatomy and permits differentiation of vascular structures from pelvocaliectasis.

Hydronephrosis is common in the postoperative period and may have many causes. Calculi are a relatively uncommon cause, accounting for less than 2% of the cases of transplant hydronephrosis. Anastomotic edema, urinomas, blood clots, lymphoceles, and ureteral sloughing are common causes of perioperative transplant hydronephrosis. Because transplanted organs are denervated, hydronephrosis is usually painless and worsening graft function is the presenting sign. Of the 18% of transplanted kidneys that have a dilated collecting system, only 9% are truly obstructed. If ultrasound findings of dilation are confined to the renal pelvis, the likelihood of obstruction is low. If dilation involves the calyces, the chance of obstruction is as high as 67%. In most cases the exact level of obstruction cannot be identified on ultrasound, and antegrade pyelography or Whitaker testing may be used for confirmation.

Notes

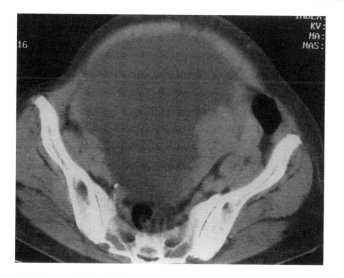 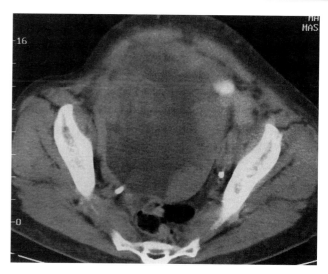

1. True or False: The majority of pelvic masses that are surgically removed because they are "suspicious" are malignant.

2. Aside from observations about the mass itself, what other findings on CT or MRI suggest that a pelvic mass is malignant?

3. Should contrast material be used to characterize a pelvic mass on CT and MRI? Why or why not?

4. True or False: MRI is more accurate than CT for staging an ovarian malignancy.

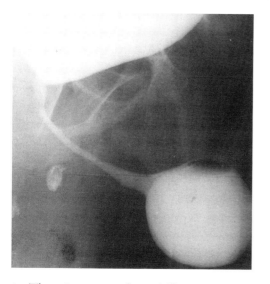 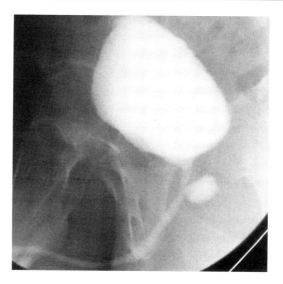

1. These images are from different patients with the same type of lesion. What is the diagnosis?

2. True or False: This lesion can be congenital or acquired.

3. Name two causes of the acquired form of this lesion.

4. Of utricular and müllerian cysts, which is usually identified in patients younger than 20 years of age?

Mucinous Ovarian Carcinoma of Low Malignant Potential

1. False.

2. Ascites; lymphadenopathy; implants on the mesentery, omentum, or peritoneum; and liver metastases.

3. Yes. Enhancement of solid tissue can help to identify solid and papillary components of a mass, delineate areas of necrosis, and identify peritoneal and omental implants.

4. True, probably. However, many gynecologic oncologists rely on surgical staging and may not perform radiologic imaging for staging.

Reference

Stevens SK, Hricak H, Stern JL: Ovarian lesions: detection and characterization with gadolinium-enhanced MR imaging at 1.5T, *Radiology* 181:481-488, 1991.

Cross-Reference

Genitourinary Radiology: THE REQUISITES, pp 283-289.

Comment

This mucinous carcinoma is of low malignant potential (of borderline malignancy). Mucinous ovarian tumors account for 20% of all ovarian tumors. The majority of mucinous ovarian tumors are benign; 15% are borderline (i.e., have a low malignant potential) or malignant neoplasms. Mucinous tumors are cystic and frequently multiloculated and range in size from 1 to 50 cm in diameter. Solid areas and raised papillary projections identify the lesion as an epithelial neoplasm and in general are more common in high grade malignancies. However, they can occur in benign (up to 20%) and borderline neoplasms. Also, adherent fibrinous clots or debris may mimic septal or mural excrescences on ultrasound, but unlike true papillary tissue, they do not enhance on CT or MRI. To stratify these three types of mucinous ovarian neoplasms, the pathologist relies more on cellular atypia, mitotic figures, and stromal invasion than on the gross appearance of the tumor.

Multiple studies have shown that one half to two thirds of all adnexal masses that are removed are benign. Is it possible to distinguish a benign ovarian mass from a malignant one on CT or MRI? Stevens and colleagues reported that five primary MRI criteria helped to accurately predict the benign nature of a pelvic mass 84% of the time. These criteria included size (benign lesions, less than 4 cm in diameter); simple cystic structure; wall and septal thickness (benign lesions, less than 3 mm); and the absence of vegetations, nodularity, and necrosis. Other criteria that, when present, support the diagnosis of a malignant mass include infiltration of the pelvic sidewall or pelvic organs; lymphadenopathy; ascites; or implants on the peritoneum, mesentery, or omentum.

Notes

Acquired Urethral Diverticulum

1. Urethral diverticulum in a male patient.

2. True.

3. Infection, trauma, and prolonged catheterization.

4. Utricular cysts.

Reference

Calenoff L, Foley MJ, Hendrix RW: Evaluation of the urethra in males with spinal cord injury, *Radiology* 142:71-76, 1982.

Cross-Reference

Genitourinary Radiology: THE REQUISITES, pp 244-246.

Comment

These cases are examples of acquired urethral diverticula in men. The first image shows a giant anterior urethral diverticulum that developed in an incontinent, paraplegic man as a result of long-term use of a penile clamp. The second image shows a posterior urethral diverticulum with a narrow neck and an off midline orifice. Recall that utricle and müllerian duct cysts are typically midline prostatic cysts.

Although occasionally discovered in men, acquired urethral diverticula are much more common in women. Diverticula may occur after urethral infection or trauma, as a result of prolonged use of an indwelling catheter, or after urethral surgery or use of other instrumentation. In some cases a periurethral abscess may drain into the urethra and thereby form a diverticulum; this process is the most common etiology of a posterior urethral diverticulum. Because of prolonged transurethral catheterization, paraplegics are particularly prone to developing urethritis and diverticula. Unlike congenital diverticula, acquired diverticula are not lined by epithelium. Although stones and carcinoma may form in diverticula of the female urethra, these complications are rare in men with acquired urethral diverticula.

When they occur after urethral instrumentation or catheterization, these focal dilations are located in areas of normal urethral narrowing (e.g., the membranous urethra and penoscrotal junction). A premonitory sign of a membranous urethral diverticulum on urethrography is the "spiral sign," a few rings of contrast material encircling the membranous urethra. This sign is usually the result of overdistention of the external sphincter during instrumentation.

Notes

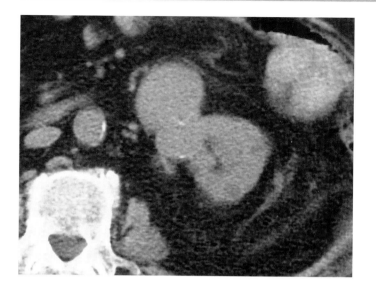
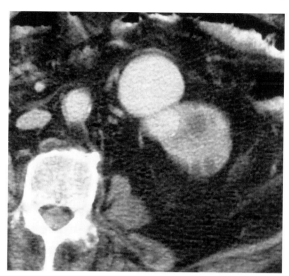

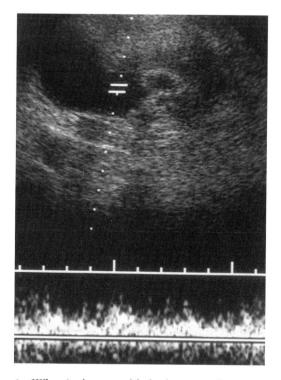

1. What is the most likely diagnosis for the mass adjacent to the lower pole of the left kidney?

2. Is this abnormality of clinical significance?

3. What CT features suggest that this is not a neoplasm?

4. How is this abnormality usually treated?

Renal Artery Aneurysm

1. Renal artery aneurysm.

2. Yes, because of the risk of rupture and renal embolization.

3. The degree of enhancement is identical to that of the aorta, and there is evidence of atherosclerotic calcification in the aorta and at the edges of the mass on the precontrast CT scan.

4. Renal artery aneurysms are usually treated surgically, although some lesions may be treated with selective endovascular obliteration.

Reference

Davidson AJ, Hartman DS, editors: *Radiology of the kidney and urinary tract,* ed 2, Philadelphia, 1994, Saunders, pp 544-557.

Cross-Reference

Genitourinary Radiology: THE REQUISITES, pp 154-155.

Comment

This patient has a 25-mm, bi-lobed mass with peripheral calcifications abutting the lower pole of the left kidney. This mass enhances to an identical degree as the aorta, and on sonography, turbulent flow is detected within the mass. These features suggest that this mass is an arterial structure. Adjacent scanning demonstrated continuity of this mass with the left renal artery. Most renal artery aneurysms are acquired and result from advanced atherosclerosis. Some develop as the result of fibromuscular disease of the renal artery, and others result from vasculitides. Even small renal artery aneurysms are significant because they may be the source of emboli to the kidney and may cause renal ischemia, oversecretion of renin, and renovascular hypertension. With increasing size, the risk of aneurysm rupture increases. When a mass in or near the kidney enhances to a degree equal to that of the arteries, an aneurysm or vascular malformation should be suspected. This diagnosis can be confirmed with conventional angiography, CT angiography, or MR angiography. Obviously, biopsy of this type of lesion should be avoided because of the risk of exsanguination. Most renal artery aneurysms are treated with renal artery bypass procedures. However, endovascular technology has been used to successfully treat some renal artery aneurysms with occlusion devices or stent–grafts.

Notes

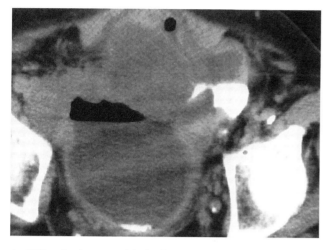 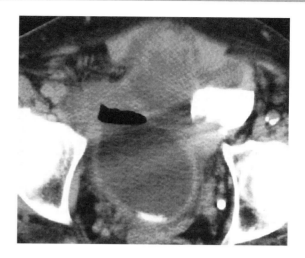

1. What is the most likely diagnosis?
2. True or False: The perivesical fat is normal.
3. Name three complications of bladder diverticula.
4. What is the most accurate cross-sectional imaging test for staging this disease?

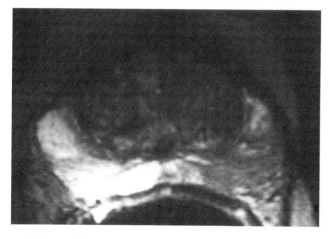 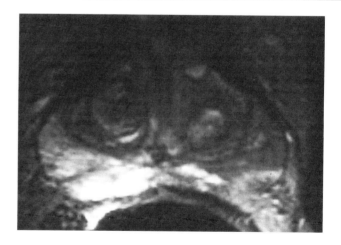

1. What is the most likely diagnosis?
2. True or False: MRI of the prostate has a role in the local staging of all patients with prostate-confined adenocarcinoma on clinical examination.
3. On endorectal coil MRI (erMRI) of the prostate, what findings correlate with poor outcome?
4. Is it important that the sign (or signs) that defines extracapsular extension is more sensitive or more specific?

CASE 90

Stage IV Bladder Carcinoma Arising from a Diverticulum

1. Locally advanced bladder carcinoma arising in a bladder diverticulum.

2. False.

3. Infection, stone formation, and neoplasm.

4. Enhanced MRI.

References

Barentsz JO, Jager GJ, van Vierzen PB, et al: Staging urinary bladder cancer after transurethral biopsy: value of fast dynamic contrast-enhanced MR imaging, *Radiology* 201:185-193, 1996.

Durfe SM, Schwartz LH, Panicek DM, Russo P: MR imaging of carcinoma within urinary bladder diverticulum, *Clin Imaging* 21:290-292, 1997.

Cross-Reference

Genitourinary Radiology: THE REQUISITES, pp 197-204, 211-212, 219-226.

Comment

This case of locally advanced transitional cell carcinoma of the bladder arose from a bladder diverticulum. The cancer has invaded the perivesical fat along the dextrolateral wall, and there is a synchronous lesion along the levolateral wall. Bladder diverticula are usually acquired secondary to bladder outlet obstruction and increased intravesical pressure. Diverticula are common, increase in incidence with age, and are associated with a higher risk (2% to 8%) of lower urinary tract infection, calculi, and neoplasm. These complications are presumably due to chronic irritation caused by urinary stasis.

The most sensitive technique for staging bladder carcinoma is enhanced MRI with dedicated surface coils. In Barentsz and co-workers' article, enhanced and T2W MRI were reported to have a staging accuracy of 84%. Notably, the accuracy of MRI in staging bladder carcinoma is highly technique-, operator-, and machine-dependent; institutions with extensive experience have reported the most accurate results. MRI is comparable to CT in detecting retroperitoneal lymphadenopathy. CT is accurate for detecting enlarged lymph nodes and direct invasion of the pelvic organs but is less accurate for predicting the depth of wall invasion because the carcinoma is isodense with the bladder wall. Ultrasound is not as sensitive as MRI or CT for detecting nodal metastases in the pelvis or retroperitoneum.

Notes

CASE 91

Extracapsular Spread of Prostatic Carcinoma: Value of Endorectal Coil MRI

1. Local spread of prostate carcinoma, arising in the left peripheral zone, beyond the capsule.

2. False.

3. Gross extracapsular extension of tumor and seminal vesicle invasion.

4. More specific.

References

D'Amico AV, Schnall M, Whittington R, et al: Endorectal coil magnetic resonance imaging identifies locally advanced prostate cancer in select patients with clinically localized disease, *J Urol* 51:449-454, 1998.

Tempany CM, Zhou X, Zerhouni EA, et al: Staging of prostate cancer: results of Radiology Diagnostic Oncology Group project comparison of three MR imaging techniques, *Radiology* 192:47-52, 1994.

Cross-Reference

Genitourinary Radiology: THE REQUISITES, pp 329-333.

Comment

Has all the initial hype and hope of the early 1990s regarding endorectal coil MRI (erMRI) been dashed by the Radiology Diagnostic Oncology Group's report of an overall 54% accuracy and a 30% variation in accuracy among radiologists, depending on their level of experience?

One of the main goals of erMRI was to assess extracapsular extension of prostate cancer. Although numerous signs had been posited, under rigorous scrutiny, few proved to be reliable signs of extracapsular extension. Length of tumor contact with the capsule, smooth capsular bulge, capsular retraction, and capsular thickening are signs that lack sensitivity and specificity. High specificity in prostate MRI is necessary to ensure that as few patients as possible are unnecessarily deprived of potentially curative radical prostatectomy because of false positive test results. On erMRI, findings of "gross extracapsular spread" of tumor (unequivocal extension into the rectoprostatic fat and neurovascular bundle) and seminal vesicle invasion are signs with sufficient specificity to warrant clinical use in the appropriate setting. D'Amico and colleagues have shown that erMRI, through the identification of extracapsular extension and seminal vesicle invasion, increases the ability to predict organ-confined prostate cancer from 65% to 82% in patients with clinically localized disease. This particular group of patients for which erMRI was most efficacious had a prostate-specific antigen level of at least 10 ng/ml (but less than 20 ng/ml), biopsy Gleason score of 7 or less, and at least 50% of the biopsies positive from a sextant sampling.

Notes

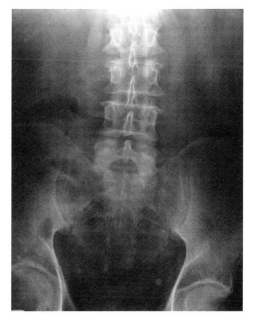 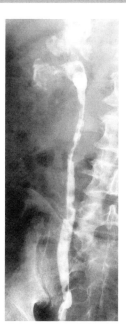

1. What are the most common causes of multiple radiolucent filling defects in the ureter?
2. Are the lesions shown more likely to be intraluminal, mucosal, or submucosal?
3. Of what substance are most radiolucent urinary tract calculi composed?
4. What is the incidence of multiple synchronous lesions in association with a papillary transitional cell carcinoma?

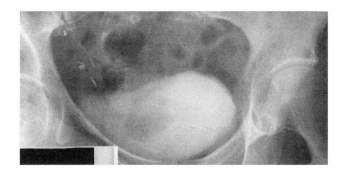 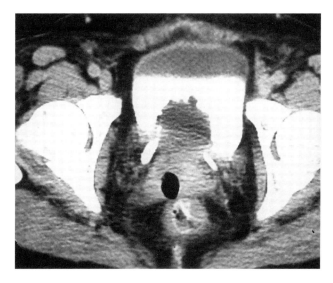

1. What is the main finding on the coned-down image of the bladder from the intravenous urogram?
2. What is the differential diagnosis for the mass?
3. What is the oval black structure in the figure on the right?
4. What stage is this tumor?

Multifocal Transitional Cell Carcinoma

1. Radiolucent stones, air bubbles, multifocal transitional cell carcinoma, blood clots, infectious debris, and sloughed papillae.

2. Mucosal.

3. Uric acid.

4. One third of patients have multifocal disease.

Reference

Williamson B Jr, Hartman GW, Hattery RR: Multiple and diffuse ureteral filling defects, *Semin Roentgenol* 21:214-223, 1986.

Cross-Reference

Genitourinary Radiology: THE REQUISITES, p 187.

Comment

The right retrograde pyelogram demonstrates multiple radiolucent filling defects in the right ureter and pyelocalyceal system. The lesions in the ureter appear to be attached to or to arise from the ureteral wall. They have acute angle margins with the ureteral wall, indicating that they are mucosal lesions rather than intraluminal or submucosal lesions. Intraluminal lesions are usually completely surrounded by contrast material, whereas submucosal lesions form obtuse angle margins with the ureteral wall. The presence of mucosal lesions strongly favors the diagnosis of transitional cell carcinoma. Other mucosal lesions include inflammatory lesions, such as forms of ureteritis, leukoplakia, and malacoplakia, and uncommon urothelial tumors, such as squamous cell carcinoma and adenocarcinoma.

Transitional cell carcinomas may grow in either a papillary or a nonpapillary form. Two thirds of transitional cell carcinomas are papillary, and one third are nonpapillary, or infiltrative. The papillary variety tends to be superficial and noninvasive but has a predilection for multifocality. One third of papillary transitional cell carcinomas, including lesions in all sites of the urinary tract, even the bladder, are multifocal. The presence of transitional cell carcinoma in the ureter increases the likelihood of synchronous or metachronous tumors to approximately 40%.

Notes

Endometrial Carcinoma Invading the Bladder

1. Irregular filling defect in the bladder.

2. Transitional cell carcinoma of the bladder, mesenchymal bladder neoplasm, cervical carcinoma, endometrial carcinoma, and metastases.

3. Vaginal tampon.

4. Stage IVb endometrial carcinoma.

Reference

Mayo-Smith WW, Lee MJ: MR imaging of the female pelvis, *Clin Radiol* 5:667-676, 1995.

Cross-Reference

Genitourinary Radiology: THE REQUISITES, pp 290-294.

Comment

An image of the bladder from the intravenous urogram demonstrates a polypoid, intravesicular filling defect originating from the right superior and lateral wall of the bladder. The most likely explanation for this mass is a transitional cell carcinoma; however, the patient initially complained only of postmenopausal bleeding. At cystoscopy an endometrial carcinoma was biopsied.

Endometrial carcinoma is the most common gynecologic malignancy, and the incidence of this tumor is increasing. Approximately 80% of the patients with this disease are postmenopausal, and the initial symptom usually is vaginal bleeding. Because of an early clinical presentation, many patients present with curable stage I disease. Therefore, even though endometrial carcinoma is more common than ovarian carcinoma, it is associated with a lower mortality rate.

A major risk factor for endometrial carcinoma is unopposed estrogen stimulation of the endometrium, which occurs in nulliparous women, obese patients, and patients treated with exogenous estrogen. The role of imaging in the work-up of the patient with suspected endometrial carcinoma is to diagnose the disease and to differentiate it from other causes of postmenopausal bleeding, such as endometrial atrophy (the most common cause of postmenopausal bleeding in patients not on hormone replacement therapy) or endometrial polyps. Ultrasound and sonohysterography are often used to evaluate patients with postmenopausal bleeding. Ultrasound differentiates atrophic endometrium (a thin endometrial stripe) from endometrial polyps, hyperplasia, and carcinoma. Biopsy is necessary to differentiate endometrial hyperplasia from carcinoma.

Notes

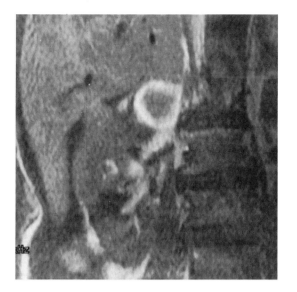
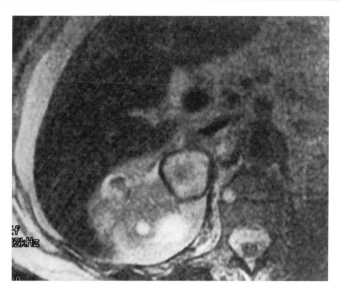

1. A coronal, T1W image and a transaxial, turbo spin-echo, T2W image of a right adrenal mass are shown. What is the most likely cause for this mass?

2. Name three iatrogenic causes for this lesion.

3. Metastasis from which primary tumor is most likely to present with this appearance?

4. What is Waterhouse-Friderichsen syndrome?

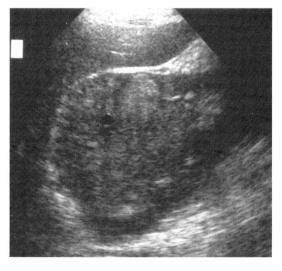
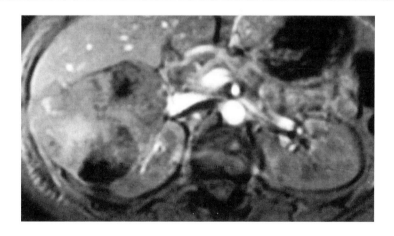

1. What is the most likely diagnosis for this renal mass?

2. Is the mass more or less echogenic than the normal kidney?

3. What are the main differential diagnostic considerations?

4. Using the Robson classification system, is this more likely a stage II or stage III tumor?

Adrenal Hemorrhage on MRI

1. Adrenal hemorrhage.

2. Adrenal biopsy, adrenal venous sampling, and orthotopic liver transplantation.

3. Bronchogenic carcinoma. There is one reported case of metastatic gastric carcinoma.

4. Hemorrhagic destruction of both adrenal glands caused by overwhelming meningococcemia that results in acute adrenocortical insufficiency.

Reference

Hoeffel C, Legmann P, Luton JP, Chapuis Y, Fayet-Boynnin P: Spontaneous unilateral adrenal hemorrhage: CT and MR imaging findings in 8 cases, *J Urol* 154:1647-1651, 1995.

Cross-Reference

Genitourinary Radiology: THE REQUISITES, pp 357-358.

Comment

There are multiple causes of adrenal hemorrhage. In neonates, hemorrhage may be the result of birth trauma, anoxia, dehydration, renal vein thrombosis, or systemic coagulopathy; the major differential diagnosis is neuroblastoma. Spontaneous adrenal hemorrhage in adults may be caused the systemic "stress" of surgery, extensive body burns, sepsis, or hypotension. Anticoagulants, disseminated intravascular coagulation, and antiphospholipid antibody syndrome may result in a bleeding diathesis that predisposes to adrenal hemorrhage. The majority of cases caused by anticoagulant administration occur within the first 3 weeks after use of the anticoagulant; patients are not necessarily overanticoagulated when bleeding complications occur.

Iatrogenic causes of adrenal hemorrhage include open and percutaneous biopsy, adrenal venous sampling, exogenous adrenocorticotropic hormone or other corticosteroid administration, and orthotopic liver transplantation. After liver transplantation, hemorrhagic infarction or hematoma of the right adrenal gland is thought to result from the ligation and division of the right adrenal vein during hepatectomy. Blunt traumatic hematoma is also more common in the right adrenal gland.

Finally, some adrenal mass lesions have been associated with "spontaneous" adrenal hemorrhage. A list of these lesions includes adenoma, metastasis, cortical adenocarcinoma, pheochromocytoma, myelolipoma, hemangioma, and adrenal cyst. A clinical point worth emphasizing is that adrenal hemorrhage can result in acute adrenal insufficiency because many cases involve both glands.

Notes

Stage II Renal Cell Carcinoma

1. Renal cell carcinoma (RCC).

2. More echogenic.

3. Oncocytoma, angiomyolipoma (without visible fat), and metastasis.

4. Stage II.

Reference

Yamashita Y, Ueno S, Makita O, et al: Hyperechoic renal tumors: anechoic rim and intratumoral cysts in US differentiation of renal cell carcinoma from angiomyolipoma, *Radiology* 188:179-182, 1993.

Cross-Reference

Genitourinary Radiology: THE REQUISITES, pp 89-100.

Comment

This sonogram demonstrates a solid, heterogeneous hyperechoic mass protruding from the middle portion of the right kidney. This finding is confirmed on the MRI scan. RCCs of the kidney generally grow by expansion, causing a ball-shaped mass that may appear hyperechogenic, isoechogenic, or hypoechogenic to normal kidney on sonography. An exophytic, solid mass arising from the kidney without visible fat is indicative of RCC in approximately 90% of cases. Other possibilities are an isolated metastasis, including lymphoma; an oncocytoma without characteristic imaging features; or an angiomyolipoma without adequate fat to be visible radiologically. In any case, unless a known primary is present elsewhere, this finding should be considered a surgical renal mass, and beyond demonstrating extent of the tumor, further imaging is unlikely to lead to additional information.

Once the mass is detected sonographically, cross-sectional imaging is of crucial importance to exclude the presence of intratumoral fat, which would indicate a benign angiomyolipoma. In addition, staging of the tumor is best accomplished with CT or MRI, both of which are essentially equivalent for this purpose. The Robson classification is a simple staging system for RCC. Radiologically, stage I and stage II tumors are difficult to distinguish from one another, but this determination is of little or no clinical significance. Stage III indicates tumor spread to regional lymph nodes or venous extension. The gradient echo image shown demonstrates a widely patent right renal vein entering the inferior vena cava. No visible lymphadenopathy is present. These findings indicate a stage I or II RCC. Stage IV indicates direct invasion of adjacent organs other than the adrenal gland, or distant metastases.

Notes

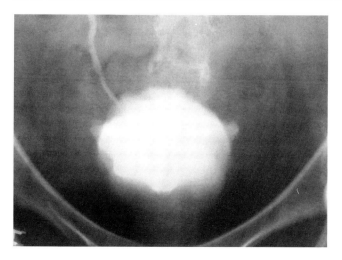 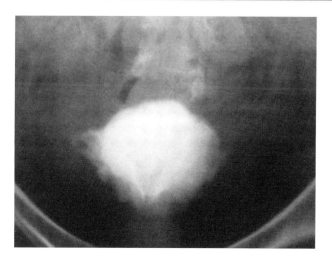

1. This patient was treated with multiple, high doses of cyclophosphamide. True or False: Cystitis secondary to cyclophosphamide administration usually occurs during or immediately after treatment is begun.

2. True or False: The prophylactic administration of mesna is effective in reducing bladder toxicity caused by the oxazaphosphorine alkylating agents (cyclophosphamide and ifosfamide) because it binds directly to the drugs.

3. What is the first-line treatment for hemorrhagic cystitis associated with cyclophosphamide toxicity?

4. True or False: The risk of invasive urothelial bladder cancer is increased in patients who have undergone prolonged cyclophosphamide treatment.

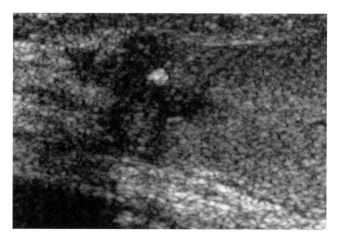 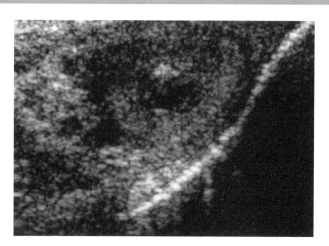

1. Two images from an ultrasound examination of the testicle are shown. What is the most likely diagnosis?

2. Name three nonmalignant causes of calcified testicular masses.

3. What is the most common extragonadal site associated with a burned-out primary testicular cancer?

4. True or False: All testicular tumors with calcification have an associated discrete mass separate from the calcification or calcifications.

Cyclophosphamide Cystitis

1. True.

2. False.

3. Forced diuresis, bladder irrigations, and mesna.

4. True.

Reference

Bramble FJ, Morley R: Drug-induced cystitis: the need for vigilance, *Br J Urol* 79:3-7, 1997.

Cross-Reference

Genitourinary Radiology: THE REQUISITES, pp 209-211.

Comment

Shortly after it was introduced for clinical use in 1958, cyclophosphamide was noted to cause frequency, urgency, dysuria, and hematuria in some patients. The reported incidence of cyclophosphamide cystitis is 2% to 4%; hemorrhagic cystitis occurs commonly and more often in patients on cyclophosphamide than in patients on other drugs that cause cystitis. Ifosfamide is a structural isomer of cyclophosphamide and has even greater urotoxicity. Symptoms usually begin during or just after treatment, and delayed hemorrhage occurs only in patients on long-term therapy. In the short term, bladder injury is manifested as mucosal erythema, inflammation, ulceration, necrosis, and oozing from small vessels. Marked bladder contraction (caused by fibrosis) and invasive bladder tumors take much longer to develop, appearing months to years after cessation of therapy. There is a 45-fold increased risk and a 5% incidence of invasive transitional cell carcinoma after prolonged cyclophosphamide use.

Urotoxicity is mediated by an aldehyde metabolite of the oxazaphosphorine alkylating agents—acrolein. Mesna (2-mercaptoethane sulfonate) was developed specifically to bind acrolein and, when prophylactically administered, can reduce the bladder toxicity but not the therapeutic effects of cyclophosphamide.

The treatment of hemorrhagic cystitis secondary to cyclophosphamide or ifosfamide begins with saline bladder irrigations, diuresis, and mesna administration. If these measures are not successful, cystoscopy and diathermy of bleeding points can be performed. Chemical cautery by intravesical administration of formalin, phenol, silver nitrate, or alum also has been advocated. If hemorrhage is life-threatening, embolization or ligation of the internal iliac arteries and even cystectomy have been performed.

Notes

Calcified Testicular Mass

1. Calcified primary testicular neoplasm, probably a non-seminomatous germ cell tumor.

2. Epidermoid cyst, resolved infection, hematoma, and infarction.

3. Most often, a regressed germ cell testicular tumor coexists with a retroperitoneal mass.

4. False.

References

Comiter CV, Renshaw AA, Benson CB, Loughlin KR: Burned-out primary testicular cancer: sonographic and pathological characteristics, *J Urol* 156:85-88, 1996.

Gierke CL, King BF, Bostwick DG, Choyke PL, Hattery RL: Large-cell calcifying Sertoli cell tumor of the testis: appearance at sonography, *Am J Roentgenol* 163:373-375, 1994.

Cross-Reference

Genitourinary Radiology: THE REQUISITES, pp 312-316.

Comment

This is a case of a teratocarcinoma of the testis containing a small focus of calcification. In contrast to seminomas, non-seminomatous germ cell tumors are more likely to be of mixed echogenicity. Teratomas and teratocarcinomas are often heterogeneous and may have well-formed multilocular cysts that contain bone, cartilage, keratin, muscle, hair, mucous glands, or neural tissue. These tumors are more common in children.

Typically a calcified testicular tumor appears as a hypoechoic mass with focal areas of shadowing hyperechogenicity. Uncommonly a focus of calcification dominates the appearance of the tumor. Two examples are burned-out primary testicular cancer and large-cell calcifying Sertoli tumors of the testis. These lesions may have greater color Doppler signal around the focus of calcification, suggesting the coexistence of a vascularized mass. Burned-out primary tumors may be associated with extragonadal germ cell tumors that typically present as ipsilateral retroperitoneal lymphadenopathy. In contrast, the majority of mediastinal and central nervous system germ cell tumors are believed to represent primary extragonadal lesions.

The differential diagnosis of calcified testicular masses includes primary malignant or benign neoplasm, either *de novo* or treated; burned-out neoplasm; testicular microlithiasis; and resolved infection, traumatic hematoma, or segmental infarction. The list of neoplasms includes teratoma and teratocarcinoma, embryonal cell carcinoma, testicular carcinoid tumor, and epidermoid cyst. Epidermoid cysts are nontender, slowly growing intratesticular cysts. A central echogenic focus represents a region of keratinization and gives the lesion its typical "target" appearance. Cyst enucleation and not orchiectomy is the treatment of choice.

Notes

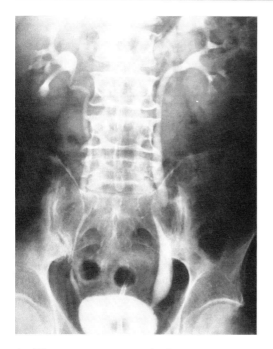 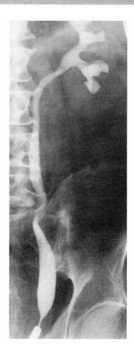

1. The pattern seen on the intravenous urogram and the retrograde pyelogram is typical of what diagnosis?

2. Is this disease usually unilateral or bilateral?

3. Is this disease more akin to Hirschsprung's disease or achalasia of the gastrointestinal tract?

4. Is there a gender predilection for this disease?

C A S E 9 8

Primary Megaureter

1. Primary megaureter.

2. Unilateral.

3. Achalasia.

4. Yes. Men are more commonly affected than are women.

Reference

Pfister RC, Papanicolaou N, Yoder IC: The dilated ureter, *Semin Roentgenol* 21:224-235, 1986.

Cross-Reference

Genitourinary Radiology: THE REQUISITES, pp 177-178.

Comment

When the ureter is dilated to more than 10 mm in diameter it is by definition a megaureter. If there is an identifiable cause for the megaureter, such as chronic ureteral obstruction, vesicoureteral reflux, diabetes insipidus, or psychogenic polydipsia, then the diagnosis is secondary megaureter. Idiopathic cases are classified as primary megaureter. Typically, primary megaureter is a unilateral process that occurs more frequently on the left and in men. Typically, primary megaureter presents with marked dilation, predominantly of the lowest one third of the ureter, as in this case. Careful evaluation of the upper tracts in this case demonstrates no evidence of increased pressure; that is, the calyces and upper ureter are not dilated. This pattern strongly suggests primary megaureter. Other causes of megaureter typically affect the entire ureter and also lead to blunting and dilation of the calyces. The intravenous urogram in this case shows completely normal, unobstructed calyceal anatomy. The etiology of primary megaureter is insufficient musculature in the segment of ureter near the ureterovesical junction and below the dilated segment. This deficiency leads to diminished peristalsis through this segment. Innervation is completely normal throughout the ureter. Therefore it is easier to understand the pathologic findings of this disease as being similar to those in patients with achalasia than those in patients with Hirschsprung's disease of the colon. The aperistaltic segment of the ureter causes delayed passage of urine and chronically increased volume just above that segment, which then results in ureteral dilation without significantly increased pressure in the ureter.

Rarely, primary megaureter can involve the entire length of the ureter and the calyces. In such cases it is difficult to distinguish this entity from ureteral obstruction.

Notes

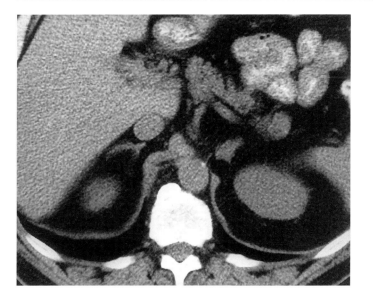
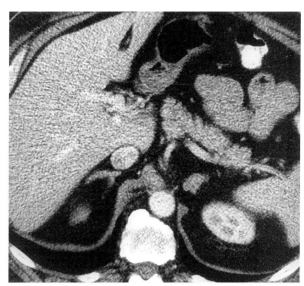
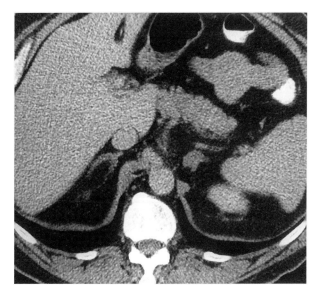

1. On a noncontrast CT of the abdomen (the first image), the left adrenal mass has an attenuation measurement of 23 Hounsfield units (HU). On noncontrast CT, what attenuation measurement HU value is used to characterize an incidental adrenal mass as an adenoma?

2. On CT performed immediately after the administration of intravenous contrast material (the second image), the measured attenuation of the left adrenal mass is 81 HU. What attenuation measurement value is used to diagnose an adrenal adenoma on early postcontrast CT?

3. The third image was performed 15 minutes after the administration of contrast medium and was used to calculate the value for the adrenal "washout" of contrast; the attenuation measurement of the left adrenal mass was 31 HU. What is the meaning of the term *adrenal washout?*

4. What percentage of adrenal washout may differentiate an adrenal adenoma from an adrenal metastasis?

Evaluation of an Adrenal Mass with Dynamic CT

1. A measurement of less than 18 HU.

2. 30 HU.

3. It refers to the relative decrease in attenuation or signal intensity in an adrenal mass on delayed imaging when compared with immediate postcontrast imaging.

4. 50%.

References

Korobkin M, Brodeur FJ, Francis IR, Quint LE, et al: CT time-attenuation washout curves of adrenal adenomas and non-adenomas, *Am J Roentgenol* 170:747-752, 1998.

Szolar DH, Kammerhuber FH: Adrenal adenomas and non-adenomas: assessment of washout at delayed contrast-enhanced CT, *Radiology* 207:369-375, 1998.

Cross-Reference

Genitourinary Radiology: THE REQUISITES, pp 346-357.

Comment

Adrenal adenomas are the most common benign tumors of the adrenal gland. They are found in up to 1.5% of autopsy cases and 1% of CT examinations. The adrenal glands also are common sites of metastases, particularly from bronchogenic carcinoma. A common clinical problem encountered by the radiologist is the evaluation of an enlarged adrenal gland on CT in a patient who has a known malignancy. Much clinical research in the past decade has been dedicated to differentiating between adrenal adenomas and adrenal metastases on CT and MRI. The histopathologic basis for differentiation is based on the relatively greater cytoplasmic lipid content of adenomas. This finding accounts for the low density of an adenoma on noncontrast CT and for signal loss on chemical shift MRI. However, most CT scans that are performed for cancer staging are completed after the administration of IV contrast. Contrast administration results in an increase in the density of the normal adrenal gland, adenoma, and metastasis. Unfortunately, there is significant overlap in the early enhancement pattern of both adenomas and metastases. Past research has focused on the measured attenuation of an adrenal mass on delayed imaging (performed 15 to 30 minutes after dynamic injection of contrast) to determine whether there is a discriminating attenuation value. The problem with this approach is that different types, concentrations, and volumes of contrast agents are used at different institutions, hence the development of the concept of adrenal washout. Adrenal adenomas enhance earlier and more intensely than do adrenal metastases. Iodinated contrast also washes out of adenomas faster than metastases. Hence the density of adenomas is lower than that of metastases on delayed enhanced CT. By comparing the density of an adrenal mass on delayed images to its density on early, enhanced images, the variation in attenuation caused by the type, concentration, and amount of contrast ad-

ministered can be minimized. Two recent studies have shown that a greater than 50% washout of contrast at 15 minutes may be more sensitive and specific for the diagnosis of adrenal adenoma than attenuation measurements on noncontrast CT. Washout or percentage loss of enhancement is calculated as follows:

$$\left[\frac{D_{early} - D_{delayed}}{D_{early}} \right] \times 100\%$$

where D_{early} is the attenuation measurement on early enhanced images (measured immediately after contrast administration) and D_{delay} is the measured density of the adrenal mass on delayed enhanced images.

Notes

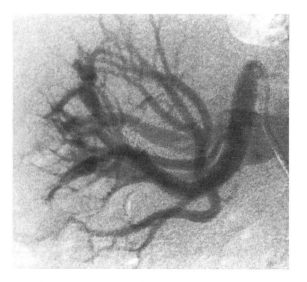 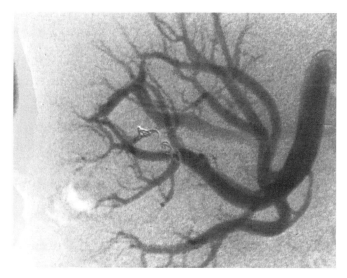

1. The image on the left is an arteriogram of a transplanted kidney after biopsy. What are the most common complications of renal biopsy?

2. What are the incidence and natural history of the lesion shown in the image on the left?

3. What are the Doppler sonographic characteristics of this lesion?

4. How is this lesion treated? (HINT: Refer to the image on the right.)

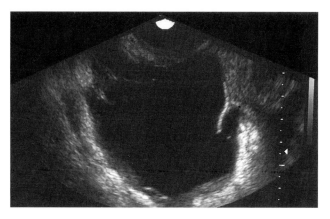 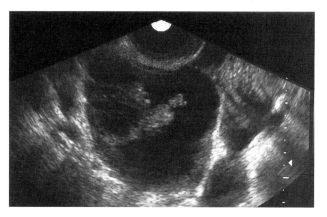

1. True or False: With respect to gray scale sonography, the presence and echogenicity of any solid element are the most important features for distinguishing between a benign and malignant ovarian mass.

2. True or False: With respect to the wall of an ovarian mass, a thickness of less than 3 mm is more typical of a benign mass.

3. True or False: With respect to Doppler sonography, the identification of flow within the wall of an ovarian mass suggests that it is malignant.

4. With respect to Doppler arterial flow patterns in an ovarian mass, define the pulsatility index (PI) and resistive index (RI).

Arteriovenous Fistula After Biopsy in a Renal Transplant

1. Hematoma at the biopsy site, hematuria, perirenal hematoma, pseudoaneurysm, and arteriovenous (AV) fistula.

2. Incidence of AV fistula is approximately 9%; 70% to 95% spontaneously thrombose.

3. High velocity and low impedance arterial flow; pulsatile, high velocity flow through the draining vein.

4. Distal, superselective embolization is necessary to minimize the loss of renal parenchyma. Steel or platinum coils are suggested to avoid the risk of systemic embolization associated with use of Gelfoam.

Reference

Shlansky-Goldberg RD: Renal transplantation. In Baum S, editor: *Abrams' angiography,* ed 4, Boston, 1997, Little, Brown and Company.

Cross-Reference

Genitourinary Radiology: THE REQUISITES, p 147.

Comment

Although many sonographic parameters have been suggested to differentiate acute tubular necrosis from cyclosporine toxicity, none are specific, and biopsy often is required. Ultrasound is the imaging study of choice for guiding renal transplant biopsy. To avoid hilar vessels, biopsy should be performed in the renal poles. AV fistulas occur in approximately 9% of patients undergoing biopsy. In this case the transplant biopsy was performed in the middle of the kidney, which may account for the formation of the fistula.

Renal transplant angiography is reserved for the investigation of either vascular complications of biopsy or hypertension resulting from suspected renal artery stenosis. The image on the left demonstrates a catheter in the transplant renal artery and early opacification of the renal vein. These findings are diagnostic of an AV fistula. Although most AV fistulas close spontaneously, there is the risk that thrombus may form. In a transplant kidney, thrombus may result in ischemia, acute tubular necrosis, or both, and early intervention is indicated. It is important for the radiologist to determine the type of vascular anastomosis before performing angiography. If an end-to-end anastomosis has been performed, arterial access should be attempted from the contralateral femoral artery. If an end-to-side anastomosis was performed, either an ipsilateral or a contralateral femoral approach is appropriate.

Notes

Ultrasound Evaluation of the Ovarian Mass

1. True.

2. True.

3. False.

4. $PI = \dfrac{\text{peak systolic velocity} - \text{end-diastolic velocity}}{\text{mean velocity}}$

   $RI = \dfrac{\text{peak systolic velocity} - \text{end-diastolic velocity}}{\text{peak systolic velocity}}$

Reference

Brown DL, Doubilet PM, Miller FH, et al: Benign and malignant ovarian masses: selection of the most discriminating gray-scale and Doppler sonographic features, *Radiology* 208:103-110, 1998.

Cross-Reference

Genitourinary Radiology: THE REQUISITES, p 284.

Comment

What sonographic features suggest that an ovarian mass is malignant? One of the better studies that attempts to answer this question is referenced above. Brown and co-workers used stepwise logistic regression to select gray scale and Doppler sonographic features that best discriminated between 28 malignant and 183 benign masses. Among several features, four were found most discriminant. By a factor of 10, the "presence and nature of a solid component" were most important. Masses without a solid component or with a markedly hyperechoic solid component (consistent with a teratoma) were benign. For masses with a nonhyperechoic solid component, the presence and location of flow were the next most valuable features. Sixty percent of malignant masses had flow in a septation or solid component, and only 9% had no flow or flow within the wall alone. Any free intraperitoneal fluid was considered abnormal in postmenopausal women, but in premenopausal women, free fluid was considered abnormal only when it filled the cul-de-sac or extended around the ovaries, above the uterus, into the paracolic gutters, or into the upper abdomen. Finally, the presence and thickness of any septation were considered important. The absence of any septation had a stronger association with malignancy than did the presence of a thin septation (3 mm in diameter); a thick septation had intermediate value.

In this retrospective study, other features, such as wall thickness, fluid echogenicity, and both average and lowest resistive and pulsatility indexes, were significantly associated with histopathologic findings but did not add to the discriminant value of the four aforementioned features. Also, this study excluded women beyond the tenth day of the menstrual cycle to avoid low resistance flow associated with the corpus luteum. By the way, the mass shown in this case was a chronic hematoma.

Notes

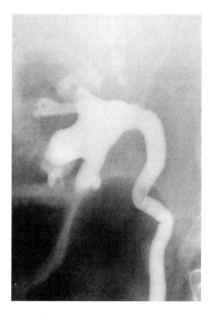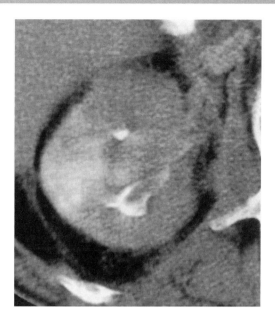

1. What is the most likely diagnosis?
2. What is the likely cause of the filling defect seen in the posterior calyx?
3. What name is used to describe the appearance of solid soft tissue replacing the normal renal sinus fat?
4. Which neoplasms involve the kidney with an infiltrative pattern, as illustrated in this case?

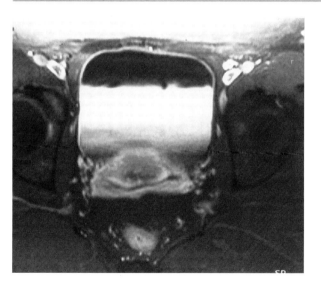

1. True or False: Gadolinium-diethylene triamine pentaacetic acid (Gd-DTPA) is eliminated exclusively in the urine.
2. True or False: After the intravenous administration of Gd-DTPA, the trilaminar appearance of urine in the bladder is visible on T1W images but not on T2W images.
3. At 1.5 T, what is the ratio of T1:T2 relaxation times for most tissues?
4. What is the ratio of T1:T2 when very high concentrations of Gd-DTPA are found in the urinary bladder?

Transitional Cell Carcinoma of the Kidney: the Faceless Kidney

1. Transitional cell carcinoma.

2. Blood clot.

3. "Faceless" kidney.

4. Urothelial tumors (transitional and squamous cell carcinomas); some metastases, including lymphoma; and the uncommon infiltrative renal cell carcinoma.

Reference

Gash JR, Zagoria RJ, Dyer RB: Imaging features of infiltrating renal lesions, *Crit Rev Diagn Imaging* 33:293-310, 1992.

Cross-Reference

Genitourinary Radiology: THE REQUISITES, pp 113-116, 135-136.

Comment

This case demonstrates a typical appearance of transitional cell carcinoma of the pyelocalyceal system called the *"faceless" kidney.* This term describes a solid mass proliferating in the renal sinus and obliterating the normal renal sinus fat. In this case the mass has infiltrated the renal parenchyma, causing decreased contrast enhancement. The area of marked enhancement represents unaffected normal renal parenchyma. The appearance of a faceless kidney strongly suggests the diagnosis of transitional cell carcinoma. However, squamous cell carcinoma, which is much less common, can have an identical appearance. Approximately one fourth of transitional cell carcinomas arising in the renal pelvis or calyx invade the renal parenchyma. When invasion of the renal parenchyma occurs, it has an infiltrative pattern radiologically, meaning there is maintenance of the normal shape of the kidney (without formation of a ball-shaped mass) and an ill-defined interface between the normal kidney and the lesion. This pattern, in combination with extensive soft tissue in the renal sinus, strongly suggests transitional cell carcinoma. Renal tuberculosis, which is a much less common diagnosis in North America, can have an identical appearance. Definitive diagnosis requires histologic or bacteriologic studies.

The intraluminal filling defect in the posterior calyx has an appearance typical of a blood clot or infectious debris. It has conformed to the shape of the calyx, suggesting soft, pliable material. This blood clot is most likely secondary to the primary transitional cell carcinoma in this patient.

Notes

The Parfait Sign: MRI of the Bladder after Intravenous Gadopentetate Administration

1. True.

2. False.

3. Ranges from 5 to 10.

4. Approximately 1.3.

Reference

Elster AD, Sobol WT, Hinson WH: Pseudolayering of Gd-DTPA in the urinary bladder, *Radiology* 174:379-381, 1990.

Cross-Reference

Genitourinary Radiology: THE REQUISITES, pp 30-32.

Comment

All radiologists have noticed the trilaminar appearance of urine in the bladder on MRI after gadopentetate administration. Why is there no gradual change in signal intensity similar to the density change shown on enhanced CT? The T1 and T2 relaxation times of urine are approximately 7 seconds and 900 ms, respectively. With increasing concentrations of gadopentetate, the T1 and T2 relaxation times of urine–gadopentetate mixtures decrease from 500 and 300 ms, respectively, at a gadopentetate concentration of 0.5 mmol/L to 27 and 21 ms, respectively, at a concentration of 10 mmol/L.

From top to bottom in the urinary bladder lumen there is a gradual increase in the concentration of gadopentetate in the supine patient, but three distinct "pseudolayers" are visible. The top layer represents pure urine with long T1 and T2 values relative to the repetition and echo times used in T1W and T2W spin-echo pulse sequences. The bottom layer of fluid represents urine with concentrations of Gd-DTPA in excess of 5 mmol/L. The T2 value of the gadopentetate–urine mixture is very short, which accounts for the dark signal of the mixture on T2W images. On T1W images the lowest layer is intermediate in signal intensity because of the opposing effects of a short T1 (increased signal intensity) and a short T2 value.

The relatively hyperintense middle layer is present when the concentration of Gd-DTPA in the mixture is between 0.5 and 5 mmol/L. On T1W spin-echo images the T1 value of the mixture is still relatively short and the T2 values are very long compared with the echo time. Thus on T1W images the middle layer appears hyperintense.

Notes

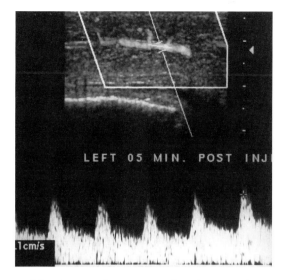 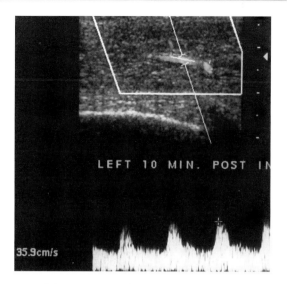

1. Two images from a Doppler ultrasound examination of the penis are shown. Spectral analysis reveals a peak systolic velocity of 36 cm/second and an end-diastolic velocity of 16 cm/second. What vessel is being investigated?

2. Is there an abnormal finding? What is it?

3. Name four causes of erectile dysfunction.

4. What are the two main causes of vasculogenic erectile dysfunction?

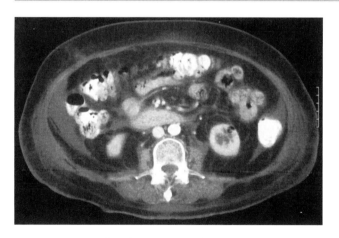 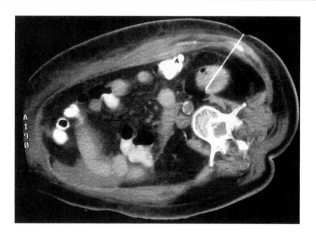

1. A contrast-infused CT in an elderly patient with urosepsis is shown. What is the most likely diagnosis?

2. Is involvement of the left kidney localized or diffuse?

3. What systemic disease usually predisposes patients to this type of urinary tract infection?

4. What type of bacteria usually cause this disease?

CASE 104

Vasculogenic Erectile Dysfunction

1. One of the two cavernosal arteries.

2. Yes. Abnormally high diastolic flow.

3. Erectile dysfunction can be endocrinologic, neurogenic, pharmacologic, psychogenic, or vasculogenic in nature or can occur after surgery.

4. Arterial inflow disease and venous incompetence.

Reference

Rosen M, Schwartz A, Levine F, et al: Radiologic assessment of impotence: angiography, sonography, cavernosography and scintigraphy, *Am J Roentgenol* 157:923-931, 1991.

Cross-Reference

Genitourinary Radiology: THE REQUISITES, pp 336-341.

Comment

Erection of the penis occurs when smooth muscle of the cavernosal arteries and sinusoids relaxes, causing distention of both corpora cavernosa. This distention leads to compression of the draining emissary veins, which limits venous outflow. The combination of increased arterial inflow and limited venous outflow results in penile erection.

Vasculogenic causes have been estimated to account for up to 37% of cases of erectile dysfunction. For the Doppler ultrasound examination of the penis, the diameter and velocities of flow in both cavernosal arteries are measured. Then 30 mg of papaverine is injected into one of the corpus cavernosa with a 27-gauge needle. Papaverine is a smooth muscle relaxant that causes dilation of the cavernosal arteries and sinusoids of the corpus cavernosa. Injection of this medication usually results in an erection. The diameter of the cavernosal arteries and the arterial and venous velocities are measured every 5 minutes for up to 20 minutes after the injection of papaverine. A normal response is an increase in the diameter of the cavernosal artery by more than 75% compared with the baseline size and a peak systolic velocity of 35 to 60 cm/second. A peak systolic velocity of less than 25 cm/second indicates arterial inflow disease. The peak diastolic velocity should be less than 3 cm/second. As illustrated in this case, diastolic velocity exceeding 3 cm/second in the presence of adequate arterial inflow reflects malfunction of the venous occlusive mechanism. Patients with arterial inflow disease may undergo selective angiography of the pudendal artery to determine whether atherosclerotic disease or a focal (often posttraumatic) stenosis can be treated with angioplasty or vascular surgery.

Notes

CASE 105

Localized Emphysematous Pyelonephritis

1. Emphysematous pyelonephritis.

2. Localized.

3. Diabetes mellitus.

4. A strain of *Escherichia coli.*

Reference

Rodriguez-de-Velasquez A, Yoder IC, Velasquez PA, Papanicolaou N: Imaging the effects of diabetes on the genitourinary system, *Radiographics* Sept 15(5):1051-1068, 1995.

Cross-Reference

Genitourinary Radiology: THE REQUISITES, p 399.

Comment

This elderly patient with diabetes mellitus had septicemia and evidence of a urinary tract infection. The contrast-infused CT scan demonstrates ascites resulting from chronic congestive heart failure. More importantly there is an inhomogeneous appearance of the lower pole of the left kidney. Centrally there is a small fluid collection with a locule of air clearly visible within the renal parenchyma. In a patient with urinary tract infection, gas within the renal parenchyma is diagnostic of emphysematous pyelonephritis. This infection is an aggressive variant of acute pyelonephritis and is seen almost exclusively in patients with diabetes mellitus. It is most commonly caused by an unusual strain of *E. coli.* However, strains of *Proteus* and *Klebsiella* species and some fungi can also lead to gas production within the renal parenchyma. Until recently, conventional treatment for emphysematous pyelonephritis in the United States consisted of radical nephrectomy. Radical nephrectomy was performed to remove the source of infection and because the kidney was often irreversibly damaged by the aggressive infectious process. Since the widespread application of cross-sectional imaging techniques, some refinements in diagnosis and treatment of this disease have occurred. When this infectious process involves only one area within the kidney, it can be classified as localized emphysematous pyelonephritis. On numerous occasions this condition has been treated successfully with a combination of percutaneous drainage and systemic antibiotic therapy. When applying percutaneous treatment for renal infections, the clinician must ensure that ureteral obstruction, if co-existing, is resolved to facilitate antibiotic treatment combined with infection drainage.

Untreated localized emphysematous pyelonephritis can progress very rapidly to a diffuse renal infection. Cases of diffuse emphysematous pyelonephritis almost always require radical nephrectomy, and this procedure carries a significant associated risk of morbidity in these severely ill patients.

Notes

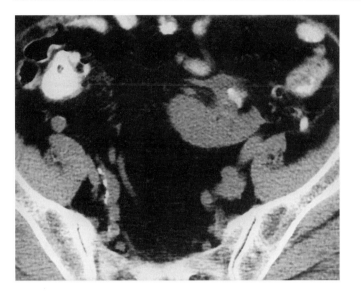 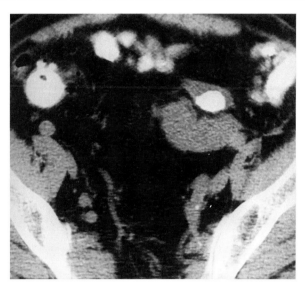

1. What findings are evident on these images?
2. What is the normal path of renal migration during development?
3. What complications are associated with this condition?
4. Which radiologic examination may be helpful before surgery is performed on patients with this condition?

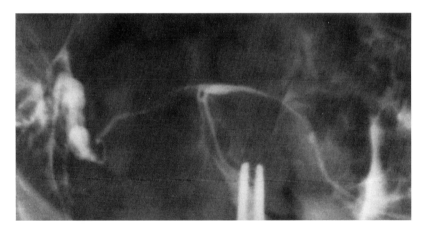

1. For what malignancy are patients with this abnormality at risk?
2. Is this abnormality associated with complications during pregnancy? If so, what complications?
3. What is the single best method of diagnosis in patients at risk for this abnormality?
4. Is this abnormality associated with abnormalities of the urinary tract?

Nephrolith in a Pelvic Kidney

1. Left pelvic kidney with a renal pelvis calculus.

2. Ureteral bud develops at the S1 level and migrates cranially to the L2 level.

3. Obstruction, vesicoureteral reflux, and stone formation.

4. Angiography, because the vascular supply to a pelvic kidney may be quite variable.

Reference

Daneman A, Alton DJ: Radiographic manifestation of renal anomalies, *Radiol Clin North Am* 29:351, 1991.

Cross-Reference

Genitourinary Radiology: THE REQUISITES, p 56.

Comment

Both the ureteral bud and the metanephric blastema are necessary for the normal development of a kidney. The kidneys develop from the ureteral bud and metanephric blastema between the fourth and eighth weeks of gestation. The kidney starts developing at approximately the S1 vertebral level and migrates cranially to the L2 level. Any arrest in this cranial migration results in renal ectopia. Pelvic kidney, as illustrated in this case, has an incidence of approximately 1 per 1000 live births. Most patients with a pelvic kidney have no symptoms. However, some may have symptoms resulting from vesicoureteral reflux or obstruction; ureteropelvic junction obstruction is particularly common. In this case there is a renal pelvis stone, presumably caused by urinary stasis. Pelvic kidneys are usually maloriented and are often smaller than their normal counterparts. Renal function also may be decreased.

It is important to confirm that a pelvic "mass" is a pelvic kidney to avoid unnecessary surgery. Imaging of the upper abdomen at the time a reniform pelvic mass is discovered confirms the diagnosis of ectopic kidney if the ipsilateral renal fossa is empty. If surgery is planned, conventional catheter angiography (or more recently CT- or MR-angiography) may be helpful because the blood supply to ectopic kidneys is variable. The arterial supply to the embryonic kidney starts with the iliac vessels, then involves the distal aorta, and finally arises from the middle aorta at the L1-2 level. As new vessels develop, the caudal vessels usually regress. However, a duplicated arterial supply is common.

Notes

Uterine Hypoplasia Secondary to Diethylstilbestrol Exposure

1. Clear cell adenocarcinoma of the vagina.

2. Yes. Premature delivery, ectopic pregnancy, and cervical incompetence.

3. Hysterosalpingography. MRI can identify uterine constrictions in 60% of patients and T-shaped uterus in 25% of diethylstilbestrol (DES)-exposed patients who have confirmed abnormalities on a hysterosalpingogram. Transvaginal ultrasound has no role in identifying uterine constrictions or T-shaped uterus in DES-exposed patients.

4. No.

References

Hatch EE, Palmer JR, Titus-Ernstoff L, et al: Cancer risk in women exposed to diethylstilbestrol in utero, *JAMA* 280: 630-634, 1998.

Kipersztok S, Javitt M, Hill MC, Stillman RJ: Comparison of magnetic resonance imaging and transvaginal ultrasonography with hysterosalpingography in the evaluation of women exposed to diethylstilbestrol, *J Reprod Med* 41(5):347-351, 1996.

Cross-Reference

Genitourinary Radiology: THE REQUISITES, pp 254, 257-258.

Comment

Between 1945 and 1971 in the United States, as many as 3 million pregnant women with threatened abortion were prescribed DES, a synthetic estrogen, to prevent miscarriage. Multiple abnormalities of the female genital tract have been linked to in utero DES exposure since an association with clear cell adenocarcinoma of the vagina was reported in 1971. The most common abnormalities demonstrated on hysterosalpingography after in utero (particularly first trimester) DES exposure are (1) a T-shaped uterine cavity, with marked narrowing of the lower uterine segment; (2) annular constrictions of the uterine horns or body; (3) an irregular shaggy outline of the entire uterine cavity; (4) a widened, boxlike lower uterine cavity often accompanied by flaring triangular uterine horns; and (5) decreased size of the uterine cavity.

In addition to uterine anomalies, in utero DES exposure is associated with vaginal and cervical adenosis (glandular epithelial metaplasia, which usually disappears over time without treatment), dysmorphic fallopian tubes, and clear cell adenocarcinoma of the vagina. There is no known association with müllerian duplication anomalies or urinary tract abnormalities. The effect of in utero DES exposure on male offspring is still unknown.

Notes

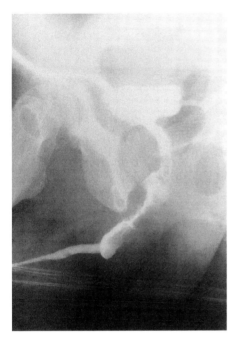 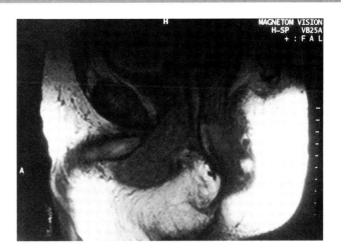

1. What is the differential diagnosis for this urethral lesion?
2. Name three benign urethral lesions that can mimic a urethral neoplasm.
3. What is the most commonly cited risk factor for squamous cell carcinoma of the urethra?
4. What findings should alert the clinician to the presence of urethral carcinoma after urethroplasty?

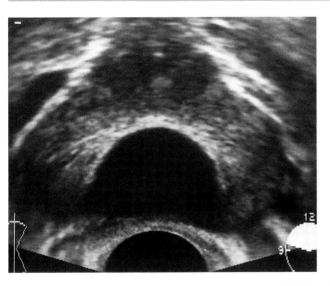 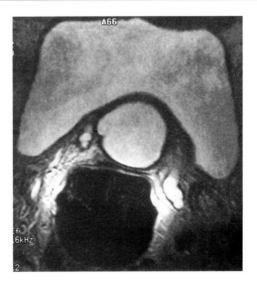

1. An axial transrectal prostatic ultrasound and a T2W MR image from two patients with the same diagnosis are shown. What are the causes for a midline prostatic cyst?
2. What is the most common cause of a prostatic cyst?
3. Which type of prostatic cyst is associated with hypospadias and undescended testis?
4. True or False: Cysts derived from müllerian duct remnants may contain sperm.

Squamous Cell Carcinoma of the Male Urethra

1. Tumor and tumorlike conditions of the urethra. Malignant tumor is most likely.

2. Papillary urethritis, nephrogenic adenoma, and inflammatory polyp can mimic a benign urethral tumor. Condylomata acuminata, amyloidosis, sarcoidosis, and balanitis xerotica obliterans can mimic a more aggressive malignant tumor.

3. Chronic urethral stricture of any cause.

4. Recurrence of stricture or urethral obstruction, fistula or abscess formation, and induration or ulceration.

References

Hricak H, Marotti M, Gilbert TJ, et al: Normal penile anatomy and abnormal penile conditions: evaluation with MR imaging, *Radiology* 169:683-687, 1998.

Cross-Reference

Genitourinary Radiology: THE REQUISITES, p 243.

Comment

Carcinoma of the urethra is at least twice as common in women as in men. These uncommon tumors are discovered in men older than 50 years of age. Common clinical presentations include a palpable mass or induration in the perineum or urethra, obstructive voiding symptoms, a urethral fistula, and a periurethral abscess.

The major histologic types of urethral malignancy include squamous cell carcinoma (80%), transitional cell carcinoma (15%), adenocarcinoma (4%), and undifferentiated tumor (1%). The major risk factor for squamous cell carcinoma is chronic urethral irritation secondary to urethral stricture, and it has been suggested that urethroplasty reduces the risk of carcinoma associated with urethral stricture. Approximately 60% of urethral squamous cell carcinomas occur in the bulbomembranous urethra, and 34% arise in the distal bulbar or penile urethra. The prognosis for anterior urethral carcinoma is much better than that of the posterior urethra (5-year survival rate of 43% versus 14%, respectively).

Carcinoma should be suspected when a urethral stricture is associated with multiple, irregular filling defects. A stricture with ill-defined margins is suspicious. Diverticula, fistula, or perineal abscess formation may be associated. MRI may demonstrate the full extent of the stricture-associated mass, as well as local invasion of the corporal bodies or perineum and lymphatic metastases.

Notes

Midline Prostatic Cyst

1. Most commonly, utricular cyst and müllerian cyst.

2. Benign prostatic hyperplasia.

3. Utricular cyst.

4. True.

References

McDermott VG, Meakem TJ III, Stolpen AH, Schnall MD: Prostatic and periprostatic cysts: findings on MR imaging, *Am J Roentgenol* 164:123-127, 1995.

Ngheim HT, Kellman GM, Sandberg SA, Craig BM: Cystic lesions of the prostate, *Radiographics* 10:635-650, 1990.

Cross-Reference

Genitourinary Radiology: THE REQUISITES, pp 326-327.

Comment

The different causes of prostatic cysts have been classified by embryologic derivation and by location. For the imager the latter classification as midline, paramedian, and lateral prostatic cysts may be more useful. Midline cysts include utricular and müllerian cysts. Paramedian cysts include both benign prostatic hypertrophy–associated cysts and ejaculatory duct cysts. Congenital prostatic and retention cysts are usually located laterally in the prostate gland, and the seminal vesicle cyst is a lateral extraprostatic cyst. Other causes of a cystic prostate mass include pyogenic abscess, parasitic cyst, and rarely carcinoma.

The most common midline prostatic cysts, the utricular and müllerian duct cysts, are derived from remnants of the paramesonephric (müllerian) duct system. In men the only derivatives of this duct system are the müllerian tubercle, which gives rise to the prostatic utricle, and the appendix testis. In addition to embryologic development and location, other similarities between these two types of cysts include a rare association with renal agenesis and prostatic carcinoma. Notably, up to 3% of these cysts may be associated with endometrial, clear cell, or squamous cell carcinomas of prostate. There are several important differences. The utricular cyst maintains a connection with the posterior urethra and may be associated with other genital tract anomalies. The müllerian duct cyst can be large and sometimes extends cephalad to the prostate, whereas the utricular cyst is intraprostatic. Stones may be found in müllerian duct cysts but not in utricular cysts. Finally, utricular cyst fluid may contain sperm, but fluid aspirated from the müllerian duct does not.

Notes

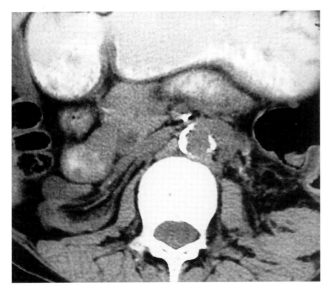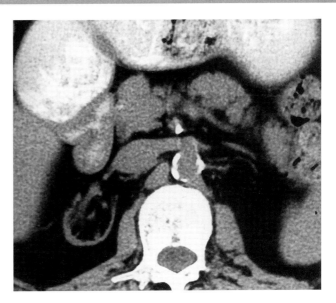

1. On the image on the left, given the appearance of the kidneys, what may have caused the right renal cyst to form?
2. What treatments may have been performed after the first and before the second CT scan?
3. True or False: Patients on hemodialysis have an increased risk of renal cell carcinoma.
4. True or False: Dialysis is a contraindication to the use of iodinated contrast media for CT.

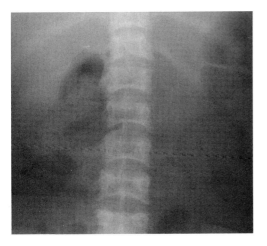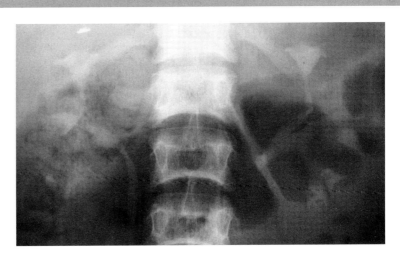

1. What is the cause of gross hematuria in this pediatric patient?
2. What underlying disease is present?
3. What are common causes of bilateral papillary necrosis?
4. What special precaution should be taken before intravenous contrast media injection in this patient?

Renal Cystic Disease Secondary to Hemodialysis

1. Cyst is either idiopathic in nature or the result of dialysis.

2. Left nephrectomy and renal transplantation.

3. True. Of patients on long-term hemodialysis, 7% develop renal cell carcinoma.

4. False.

Reference

Levine E, Slusher SL, Grantham JJ, Wetzel LH: Natural history of acquired renal cystic disease in dialysis patients: a prospective longitudinal CT study, *Am J Roentgenol* 156:501, 1991.

Cross-Reference

Genitourinary Radiology: THE REQUISITES, pp 87-89, 108-111, 142, 389.

Comment

Renal cysts are common and increase in prevalence with age. Half of all individuals older than 50 years of age have a renal cyst. The etiology of the cyst is believed to be obstruction of a renal tubule and subsequent dilation of the more proximal tubule with serous fluid. Cysts most often occur in the renal cortex and do not communicate with the collecting system. On ultrasound a cyst is anechoic and has increased through-transmission of sound posterior to the cyst. No mural or central enhancement is visible on intravenous urography or CT. Fluid in a simple renal cortical cyst is isodense with water and should measure less than 15 Hounsfield units (HU) on noncontrast CT.

This patient had end-stage renal disease secondary to diabetic nephropathy. A right renal cortical cyst developed while the patient was on hemodialysis, and this cyst resolved after renal transplantation. Multiple renal cysts are common in patients on long-term dialysis. The number of cysts increases with the duration of hemodialysis or peritoneal dialysis. After 3 years of dialysis, 10% to 20% of patients develop renal cysts. Up to 90% of patients acquire renal cysts after 5 to 10 years of dialysis. The mechanism is not known, but one theory implicates the accumulation of nephrotoxins to cyst formation. Dysplasia may develop in the epithelial wall of these cysts, and 7% of patients on long-term dialysis develop a solid renal neoplasm (i.e., adenoma, oncocytoma, or adenocarcinoma). Renal adenocarcinoma that develops in the patient on dialysis tends to be less aggressive and metastasizes less frequently than conventional renal carcinoma. The treatment is nephrectomy, unless the patient has a short life expectancy.

Iodinated contrast can be administered to patients on dialysis who produce no urine or who have been on dialysis for longer than 6 months. Nephrotoxicity is not an issue because damage to the renal parenchyma has already occurred.

Notes

Papillary Necrosis Caused by Sickle Cell Anemia

1. Papillary necrosis.

2. Sickle cell anemia.

3. Sickle cell anemia, hepatic cirrhosis or pancreatic disease, analgesic abuse, and diabetes mellitus.

4. Hydration.

Reference

Davidson AJ, Hartman DS, editors: *Radiology of the kidney and urinary tract,* ed 2, Philadelphia, 1994, WB Saunders, pp 177-189.

Cross-Reference

Genitourinary Radiology: THE REQUISITES, p 71.

Comment

The scout film and intravenous urogram on this patient demonstrate biconcave vertebral bodies, surgical clips from cholecystectomy, and bilateral renal papillary necrosis. The skeletal findings strongly suggest sickle cell anemia, and this diagnosis is supported by the secondary findings of papillary necrosis and previous cholecystectomy for gallstones. Care should be taken when administering intravenous contrast material in patients with sickle cell anemia. It is advisable to use only low osmolar contrast agents and to ensure adequate hydration before contrast media injection. Hyperosmolar agents can stimulate a sickle crisis, resulting in multifocal infarcts, which are a rare but important complication of contrast media administration. Sickle cell anemia also can cause papillary necrosis, probably as a result of occlusion of small vessels in the renal medulla caused by red cell sickling and resulting ischemia. This patient demonstrates the "lobster claw" appearance of the calyces in the middle of each kidney. Elongation of the angles of the calyces is caused by necrosis and sloughing of the margins of the renal papilla, leading to apparent elongation of the calyceal angles. Other common appearances of papillary necrosis include the "ball on tee" and "signet ring" patterns. Other causes of bilateral papillary necrosis include analgesic abuse, diabetes mellitus, and rarely hepatic cirrhosis or pancreatic disease. Phenacetin, once commonly used in the United States, is the analgesic most closely associated with papillary necrosis. It has been speculated that other agents, such as ibuprofen and acetaminophen, when used for an extended period in large doses, may also cause papillary necrosis and eventually renal failure.

Notes

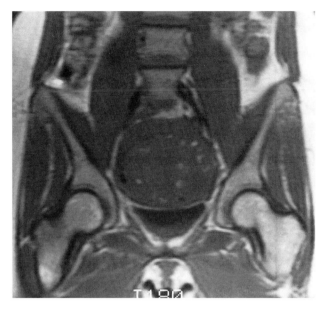 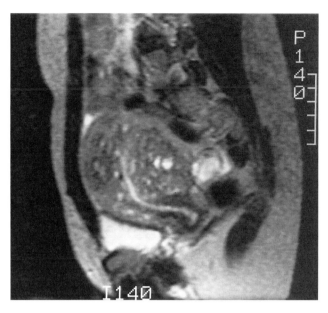

1. What is the most likely diagnosis? What findings support this diagnosis?

2. Name the two morphologic forms of this disease.

3. What is the main differential diagnosis for the focal form of this disease?

4. What does high signal intensity on T1W MR images represent?

Diffuse Adenomyosis

1. Diffuse adenomyosis. There are numerous small areas of abnormal signal (high signal intensity foci on T1W and T2W images) that are consistent with small hemorrhages in the myometrium.

2. Focal and diffuse.

3. Leiomyoma.

4. Tiny hemorrhages in ectopic endometrial tissue.

Reference

Reinhold C, McCarthy S, Bret P, et al: Diffuse adenomyosis: comparison of endovaginal US and MR imaging with histopathologic correlation, *Radiology* 199:151-158, 1996.

Cross-Reference

Genitourinary Radiology: THE REQUISITES, pp 258-261.

Comment

Adenomyosis is a benign disease in which there is ectopic endometrial tissue located within the myometrium. It can be focal or diffuse in form and has an autopsy incidence of 10% to 15%. Often presenting in 40- to 60-year-old women, the disease has nonspecific symptoms, including pelvic pain, menorrhagia, and dysmenorrhea. Adenomyosis is a challenging clinical diagnosis, and imaging can play a critical role.

On endovaginal sonography the uterine walls may appear thickened or asymmetric. The myometrium may be increased or heterogeneous in echotexture and may contain multiple tiny cysts. In less severe forms of the disease, findings may be very subtle, and the diagnosis may be overlooked unless specifically sought. Recent studies have shown that MRI is the most accurate imaging modality for establishing the diagnosis. The ectopic endometrial glands and stroma have high signal intensity on T2W images and are surrounded by hypointense tissue on both T1W and T2W images. The latter finding is presumably hyperplastic smooth muscle. In some cases hemorrhage may be present in ectopic myometrium and is manifested by small foci of increased signal on T1W MR images, as in this case. Diffuse adenomyosis lacks specific characteristics and may appear only as thickened junctional zone. A junctional zone thicker than 12 mm is considered abnormal. Uterine myoma may mimic focal adenomyosis; however, leiomyomata usually are spherical with smooth, well-defined borders and have greater mass effect on the surrounding uterine tissue.

Adenomyosis is less responsive to hormonal stimulation than is endometriosis because the endometrial rests usually are not functional. There have been reports of clinical improvement after treatment with gonadotrophin-releasing hormone and danazol (a synthetic steroid with androgenic activity). However, patients with recalcitrant symptoms usually undergo hysterectomy.

Notes

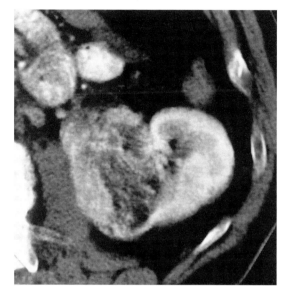 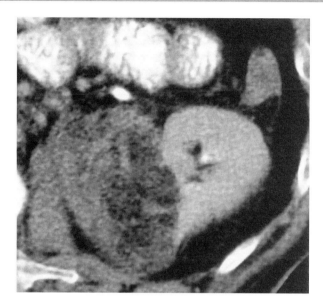

1. What is the most likely diagnosis for the renal mass shown?

2. What renal masses may present with internal renal fat?

3. What is the major complication associated with the type of mass shown?

4. What is the risk of distant metastases with the lesion shown?

Renal Angiomyolipoma

1. Angiomyolipoma.

2. Angiomyolipoma or rarely lipoma, liposarcoma, Wilms' tumor, and renal cell carcinoma.

3. Spontaneous hemorrhage.

4. None.

Reference

Bosniak MA: Angiomyolipoma (hamartoma) of the kidney: a preoperative diagnosis is possible in virtually every case, *Urologic Radiol* 3:135-142, 1981.

Cross-Reference

Genitourinary Radiology: THE REQUISITES, pp 106-108.

Comment

The patient shown has a fat-containing, heterogeneous exophytic mass extending from the left kidney. The presence of fat in a renal mass should be considered diagnostic of angiomyolipoma. Rare lesions that may contain fat include renal lipoma, liposarcoma, dedifferentiated Wilms' tumor, and renal cell carcinoma that grows to engulf renal sinus or perinephric fat. Other than angiomyolipoma, fat-containing lesions are exceedingly rare and should not be considered unless there are features suggesting an alternative diagnosis. Angiomyolipomas are benign hamartomas of the kidney comprised of vascular, smooth muscle, and fatty components. Approximately 90% of angiomyolipomas contain an adequate amount of fat to be visualized with CT. The major complication associated with angiomyolipoma is spontaneous hemorrhage. This complication is rare when lesions are smaller than 4 to 4.5 cm in diameter. Smaller asymptomatic angiomyolipomas usually are not treated and may be followed with periodic sonographic monitoring. Larger lesions may be treated with surgery or prophylactically embolized.

Of patients with angiomyolipomas, 20% suffer from tuberous sclerosis. These patients usually develop multiple angiomyolipomas and also may develop simple renal cysts. Angiomyolipomas in tuberous sclerosis patients often grow rapidly and may become large. The remaining angiomyolipomas are considered idiopathic, and they tend to grow very slowly, if at all. Rapid increase in the size of a fat-containing tumor suggests an alternative diagnosis or evidence of complication related to the angiomyolipoma and may lead to surgical resection.

Notes

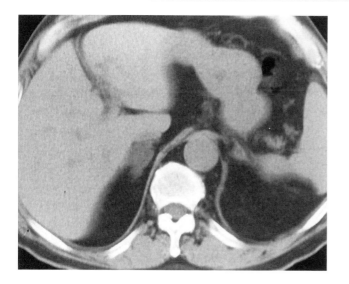
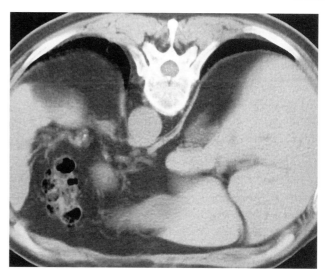
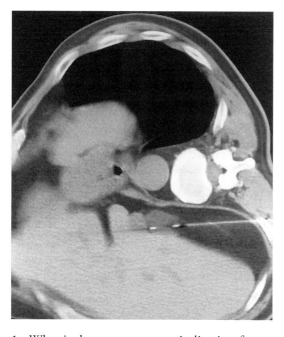

1. What is the most common indication for percutaneous adrenal biopsy (PAB)?

2. Which occurs more often, a false-positive or false-negative PAB?

3. What are some of the complications of PAB?

4. Is it more cost-effective to perform chemical shift MRI or PAB after an incidental adrenal mass is discovered on CT?

Percutaneous Adrenal Biopsy: Approach and Pitfalls

1. Presence of an adrenal mass in a patient with a history of bronchogenic carcinoma.

2. False-negative.

3. Flank pain, hematoma, and pneumothorax.

4. Chemical shift MRI.

References

Silverman SG, Mueller PR, Koenker RM, Seltzer SM: Predictive value of image-guided adrenal biopsy: analysis of results of 101 biopsies, *Radiology* 187:715-718, 1993.

Welch TJ, Sheedy PF, Stephens DH, Johnson CM, Swensen SJ: Percutaneous adrenal biopsy: review of a ten-year experience, *Radiology* 193:341-344, 1994.

Cross-Reference

Genitourinary Radiology: THE REQUISITES, pp 361-364.

Comment

The number of PABs performed has decreased in recent years in part because of the excellent performance characteristics of CT and chemical shift MRI for adrenal mass characterization. Yet PAB still has an important role (1) when a specific tissue diagnosis of metastatic disease is necessary for management decisions and (2) when there are discordant results on CT and chemical shift MRI.

There are several approaches to PAB. First, either CT or ultrasound can be used to guide the procedure. Second, fine needles (20 to 22 gauge) and 18-gauge cutting needles are used. The right adrenal mass can be biopsied from a transhepatic approach, direct posterior approach, or right side down decubitus position. Left adrenal mass biopsies can be performed with a direct posterior approach or a left side down decubitus position. In the authors' experience, CT is the imaging modality of choice. The authors use a coaxial technique to obtain a core biopsy and prefer to have the patient lie in the decubitus position with the enlarged adrenal in the dependent position. The dependent lung does not expand as much as the nondependent lung, and thus the lung rarely has to be transgressed to obtain an adequate specimen. This point is illustrated in the images accompanying this case. With the patient in the prone position, the position of the lungs is such that access to the adrenals is difficult. With the patient in the decubitus position, the dependent lung is hypoinflated, which creates a good window for a biopsy. Complications have been reported in 3% to 9% of biopsies and do not appear to be related to needle size.

Notes

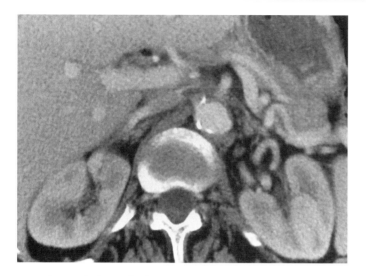
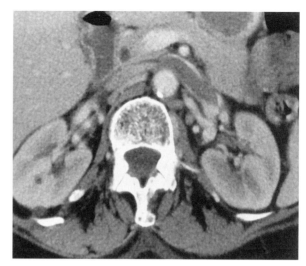

1. What radiologic findings are present?

2. How sensitive and specific is CT for detection of this abnormality?

3. What might the intravenous urogram show?

4. Name three complications of this condition.

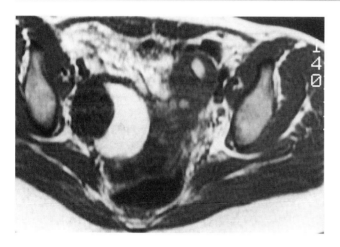
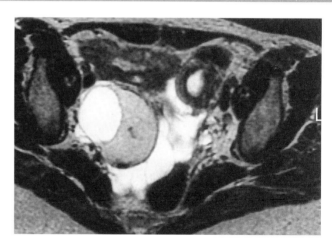

1. What is the differential diagnosis for a T1 hyperintense adnexal mass?

2. What is the Rokitansky protuberance?

3. What percentage of dermoid cysts are bilateral?

4. True or False: The most common complication of a dermoid cyst is slow leak of keratinaceous debris with a granulomatous reaction.

Renal Vein Thrombosis

1. Enhanced CT demonstrates an enlarged left renal vein that contains a filling defect. Perivenous inflammation is visible. The left kidney is swollen and poorly perfused.

2. 92% sensitive and 100% specific.

3. Enlargement of the kidney, with moderately to markedly delayed excretion.

4. About one third of patients with renal vein thrombosis (RVT) develop pulmonary embolism. Other complications include renal atrophy and papillary necrosis.

Reference

Zucchelli P: Renal vein thrombosis, *Nephrol Dial Transplant* 7(Suppl) 1:105-108, 1992.

Cross-Reference

Genitourinary Radiology: THE REQUISITES, pp 95, 126, 135, 138.

Comment

The cause of RVT is multifactorial and depends on the age of the patient and the existence of any comorbid disease. Primary RVT occurs because of a hypercoagulable state. In children, RVT is often the result of dehydration, and in adults, nephrotic syndrome is a frequent cause. Other less common causes include sickle cell disease, vasculitis, amyloidosis, and systemic lupus erythematosus. Causes of secondary RVT include renal or extrarenal tumors that either grow into or compress the renal vein, infection (e.g., acute pyelonephritis, abscess, tuberculosis, sepsis), trauma (accidental and iatrogenic), and extension of caval thrombus. RVT constitutes 5% of all renal transplant complications.

Renal vein thrombosis has variable imaging findings, depending on the age of the thrombus. In RVT of recent onset the intravenous urogram may show enlargement of the kidney with moderately to markedly delayed excretion. In long-standing RVT there is characteristic ureteral notching caused by the development of periureteral venous collaterals. Late in the course of the disease, the urogram may show a small, poorly functioning kidney. CT may demonstrate an enlarged renal vein containing a central filling defect, poor parenchymal perfusion, and delayed contrast material excretion. Similarly, MRI can directly demonstrate the thrombus. In the acute phase of the disease, ultrasound may demonstrate an enlarged kidney, absence of the venous Doppler signal, and a high-resistance arterial waveform with reversal of diastolic flow.

Notes

Mature Cystic Teratoma of the Ovary

1. Dermoid, hemorrhagic ovarian cyst, endometrioma, lipoma, or liposarcoma.

2. A solid mass that typically contains bone or teeth, hair, and solid fat and protrudes into the cavity of a dermoid cyst.

3. 8% to 15%.

4. False.

Reference

Stevens SK, Hricak H, Campos Z: Teratomas versus cystic hemorrhagic adnexal lesions: differentiation with proton-selective fat-saturation MR imaging, *Radiology* 186:481-488, 1993.

Cross-Reference

Genitourinary Radiology: THE REQUISITES, p 279.

Comment

Almost all lipid-containing masses in the adnexae are teratomas. Mature cystic teratoma (i.e., dermoid cyst, dermoid, adult cystic teratoma, and benign cystic teratoma) is the most common type of ovarian teratoma and the most common ovarian germ cell neoplasm. These common germ cell tumors are usually discovered during the child-bearing years. Parthenogenesis is the currently accepted theory of pathogenesis and holds that the dermoid cyst arises from a primordial germ cell, usually after the first meiotic division.

The appearance of dermoids on ultrasound and MRI is variable and depends on the presence of fat (in solid or liquid form), hemorrhage, dental elements, bone, and hair. Within the tumor, arising from its wall and projecting into its cavity, there is often a protuberant mass that varies in size from a small nodule to a rounded, elevated mass; this mass has been termed the *dermoid plug* or *nipple,* or *Rokitansky protuberance.*

Almost all ovarian dermoid cysts (mature cystic teratomas) contain either sebum (liquid fat) or solid adipose tissue; this characteristic allows these tumors to be differentiated from other adnexal masses. Several techniques help characterize fat-containing tissues in the pelvis. These include chemical shift misregistration, proton-selective fat saturation, short tau inversion recovery, and chemical shift imaging using gradient echo techniques. By demonstrating fat–water phase cancellation, in-phase and opposed-phase chemical shift MRI can demonstrate smaller amounts of lipid in a mass than can frequency-selective fat saturation. However, because in-phase and opposed-phase imaging does not show as much qualitative signal loss in the majority of dermoids, frequency-selective fat saturation is the preferred MRI technique.

Notes

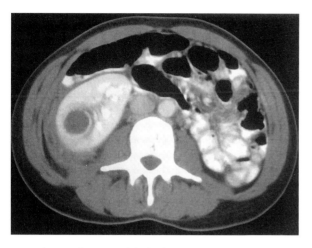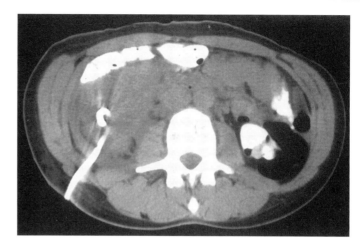

1. What is the most likely diagnosis in this patient with right flank pain and fever lasting 1 week?
2. Is this renal lesion usually symptomatic?
3. What treatment is best for patients with this disease?
4. What is the likely cause of this lesion?

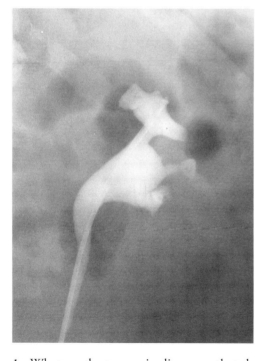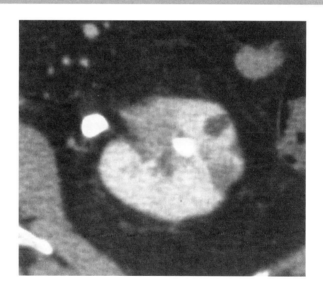

1. What are the two main diagnoses that should be considered in this patient with an abnormal left kidney?
2. What is the name of the line that connects the lateral edges of the laterally oriented calyces?
3. What causes calyceal amputation?
4. What percentage of patients with calyceal transitional cell carcinoma (TCC) develop synchronous or metachronous tumors?

Percutaneous Drainage of a Renal Abscess

1. Renal abscess.

2. Yes.

3. A combination of systemic antibiotics and percutaneous drainage.

4. Acute pyelonephritis (often if inadequately treated).

Reference

Siegel JF, Smith A, Moldwin R: Minimally invasive treatment of renal abscess, *J Urol* 155(1):52-55, 1996.

Cross-Reference

Genitourinary Radiology: THE REQUISITES, p 390.

Comment

In a patient with signs and symptoms of acute pyelonephritis and a complex fluid collection within the kidney, the diagnosis of renal abscess should be made. The patient shown has a complex, thick-walled cystic mass in the right kidney, thickening of Gerota's fascia, perinephric fluid, and stranding. Heterogeneous enhancement of the right kidney indicates associated pyelonephritis. Renal abscesses generally develop in patients who have pyelonephritis. In turn the pyelonephritis usually results from an ascending infection from the bladder. In a minority of cases renal abscesses develop as a result of hematogenous spread of infection. Renal abscesses, like abscesses elsewhere in the body, usually do not resolve with simple antibiotic management. Percutaneous drainage of renal abscesses combined with systemic antibiotics has become the standard treatment.

The second image demonstrates placement of a pigtail catheter in this renal abscess. Typically, using CT or ultrasound guidance, the radiologist places a needle percutaneously in the fluid collection. Fluid is aspirated and usually confirms the diagnosis of abscess. Then, using either the trocar or Seldinger technique, the radiologist places a drainage catheter. The abscess should be evacuated and flushed at the time of drainage. Renal abscesses usually resolve in less than 1 week after initiation of treatment with percutaneous drainage and systemic antibiotics. After resolution of symptoms and cessation of drain output, the percutaneous drain can be removed.

Notes

Calyceal Transitional Cell Carcinoma

1. TCC and tuberculosis.

2. Interpapillary line.

3. Obstruction of a major calyx, usually resulting from infiltration by tumor or from inflammation.

4. 25%.

Reference

Wong-You-Cheong JJ, Wagner BJ, Davis CJ Jr: Transitional cell carcinoma of the urinary tract: radiologic-pathologic correlation, *Radiographics* 18:123-142, 1998.

Cross-Reference

Genitourinary Radiology: THE REQUISITES, pp 113-116.

Comment

This case demonstrates calyceal amputation. Notice on the retrograde pyelogram that the calyces subtending the lower pole of the left kidney are not filling. The interpapillary line that connects the most lateral aspects of the marginal calyces should parallel the peripheral margin of the renal contour. Also, every lobe of the kidney should be drained by a calyx, with a similar distance from the marginal calyces to the edge of the kidney in all regions, which clearly is not so in this case. The CT scan demonstrates a soft tissue mass filling the renal sinus and invading the renal parenchyma. There is also a small simple cyst adjacent to this mass. These findings strongly suggest the diagnosis of either TCC or tuberculosis. Other much less common causes include squamous cell carcinoma and infiltrative renal cell carcinoma. It is unlikely that this mass represents a renal parenchymal process because it is clearly centered in the renal sinus and there is infiltration of the major calyx. Renal tuberculosis and TCC cannot be reliably distinguished from one another with imaging, and definitive diagnosis should be based on histologic or bacteriologic studies. However, radiology can be used, as in this case, to demonstrate the abnormality, suggest the correct diagnosis, and delineate the extent of the disease. Calyceal TCC accounts for approximately 9% of urinary tract TCCs, and 90% of them occur within the bladder. Presence of an upper tract TCC indicates a high risk of multifocal TCC.

Notes

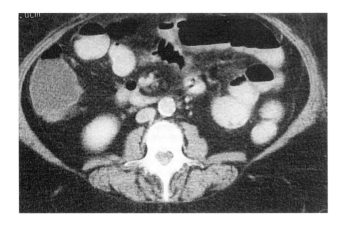 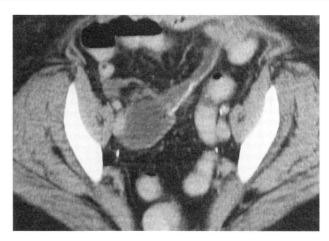

1. What procedure has been performed on this patient?
2. What are the indications for this procedure?
3. What are the advantages of this procedure over the traditional ileal loop?
4. What is an appropriate CT protocol for evaluating this type of patient?

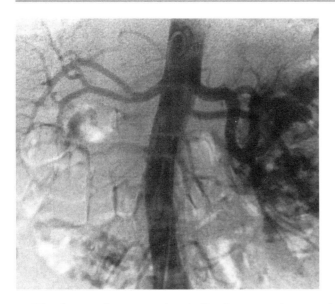 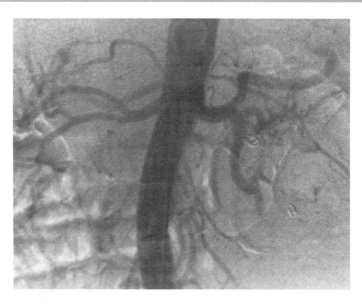

1. Two images from a renal embolization procedure are shown. In this case why was this procedure performed?
2. What is the time interval between this procedure and definitive surgery?
3. What are the other indications for this procedure?
4. What are the potential complications of this procedure?

CASE 119

Indiana Pouch

1. Urinary diversion with an Indiana pouch formed from cecum and distal terminal ileum.

2. Prior cystectomy to treat carcinoma, a neurogenic bladder, or incapacitating urinary incontinence.

3. Larger reservoir, decreased reflux, and a continent ostomy.

4. Give either oral contrast alone or intravenous contrast alone. In this way the diversion can be separated reliably from the gastrointestinal tract.

Reference

Amis ES, Newhouse JH, Olsson CA: Continent urinary diversions: review of current surgical procedures and radiologic imaging, *Radiology* 168(2):395-401, 1998.

Cross-Reference

Genitourinary Radiology: THE REQUISITES, pp 233-235.

Comment

In the past two decades, multiple new surgical procedures have been developed for the creation of continent urinary diversions. With continent diversions, the conduit is made of either small bowel alone or a combination of a terminal ileum and cecum. Egress from these loops can be to the skin through a continent ostomy or, if the sphincter and urethra are intact, to the proximal urethra. The latter procedure is called a *bladder replacement* or *orthotopic diversion.* To undergo an orthotopic diversion, patients must have unifocal bladder cancer with no involvement of the prostatic urethra. The goal of continent urinary diversions is to prevent reflux and to provide urinary continence. This technique obviates the need for an ostomy bag and provides sufficient capacity so that self-catheterization is required only every 3 to 6 hours.

The various types of continent diversions use different portions of the bowel and different types of anastomoses. For the Camey and Kock pouches, small bowel is used exclusively. Continent ostomy devices also can be created from terminal ileum and cecum (e.g., the Indiana, Mainz, Penn, and King techniques). For these procedures the cecum acts as a reservoir.

Postoperative complications of this procedure include extravasation of urine, infection, stone or fistula formation, and obstruction. Radiologic studies for the evaluation of continent urinary diversions include a loopogram to assess for leakage at the anastomosis site and an intravenous urogram to evaluate for urinary tract obstruction. CT is the study of choice to evaluate for abscess. In these patients it is usually preferable to use either oral or intravenous contrast material but not both. In this way the loop can be differentiated reliably from the bowel.

Notes

CASE 120

Embolization of a Renal Cell Carcinoma

1. To reduce blood loss during nephrectomy performed to treat renal cell carcinoma.

2. Generally, nephrectomy is performed only hours after the embolization.

3. Selective total renal ablation is indicated to reduce blood loss in patients undergoing nephrectomy.

4. Complications include renal abscess formation, transient elevation of blood pressure, temporary or irreversible renal failure, and embolization of nontarget tissues.

Reference

Bakal CW, Cynamon J, Lakritz PS, Sprayregan S: Value of preoperative renal artery embolization in reducing blood transfusion requirements during nephrectomy for renal cell carcinoma, *J Vasc Interv Radiol* 4:727-731, 1993.

Cross-Reference

Genitourinary Radiology: THE REQUISITES, pp 86, 89-99.

Comment

The intent of renal artery embolization is to reduce blood loss in patients undergoing a nephrectomy to treat large hypervascular renal cell carcinomas. The technique of renal artery embolization and the embolic material used largely depend on the indications for the procedure. In most cases ablation with absolute (98%) ethanol is performed, and the entire arterial tree is embolized. Considerable controversy has surrounded this procedure and, although many urologists have abandoned preoperative renal ablation, citing the lack of proved efficacy, others still request it. Less commonly, renal artery embolization may be performed as a palliative treatment for inoperable and symptomatic cancer, cancer in patients with high surgical risk, or cancer in the solitary kidney. (In the latter case subselective embolization of the feeding branch is performed, and the rest of the branches are preserved.)

Embolization of the renal artery also is used to treat uncontrollable hematuria after incidental or iatrogenic trauma, which may result in arterial laceration or the formation of a pseudoaneurysm, arteriovenous fistula, or arteriocaliceal fistula. In these cases Gelfoam is used and is often supplemented with use of coils in larger vessels or in fast-flowing arteriovenous fistulas. Embolization also is performed in transplanted kidneys that develop arteriovenous fistulas after percutaneous biopsy.

Notes

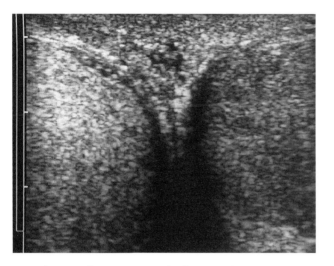
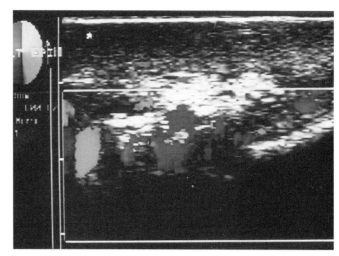

1. What are the important findings in this case? What is the most likely diagnosis?
2. What is the most common cause of this disease?
3. What age group is most commonly affected?
4. What is the differential diagnosis?

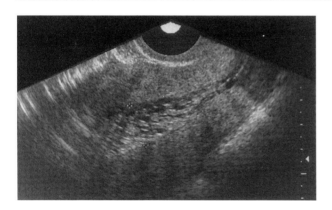
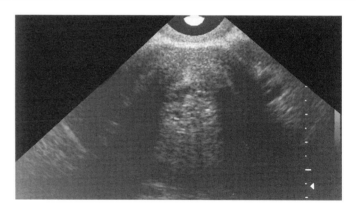

1. During which phase of the menstrual cycle is the endometrium normally thickest? What is the range of thickness (in millimeters) during this phase?
2. True or False: In women treated with tamoxifen, endometrial hyperplasia is the most common histopathologic abnormality resulting in abnormal endometrial thickening.
3. True or False: The relative risk of tamoxifen use leading to endometrial cancer is not dose dependent.
4. True or False: The prevalence of abnormal endometrial thickening depends on the duration of tamoxifen use.

Epididymoorchitis

1. Left testicle is hypoechoic with increased flow in the left epididymis. Epididymoorchitis.

2. Infection by *Escherichia coli, Staphylococcus aureus,* or *Proteus mirabilis* is most common cause.

3. Sexually active men between the ages of 20 and 30.

4. Focal orchitis may be indistinguishable from an intratesticular neoplasm.

Reference

Frush DP, et al: Diagnostic imaging of pediatric scrotal disorders *Radiographics* 18(4):969-985, 1998.

Cross-Reference

Genitourinary Radiology: THE REQUISITES, pp 309-312.

Comment

Epididymitis is the most common inflammatory process involving the scrotum in postpubertal men. The majority of cases are caused by retrograde infection, typically from the bladder or prostate. Epididymitis and epididymoorchitis rarely occur in children. The most common pathogens are *E. coli, S. aureus,* and *P. mirabilis. C. trachomatis* and *N. gonorrhoeae* should be considered in the younger age group. Unilateral orchitis is a common complication of mumps infection, occurring in 25% of cases. Rarely, epididymitis or orchitis may be caused by tuberculosis or syphilis.

Patients with epididymitis typically experience fever and increasing scrotal pain and swelling over 1 to 2 days. The scrotum may be erythematous and exquisitely tender to palpation, particularly over the epididymis. Pyuria is present in 95% of cases. Dysuria and frequency are common complaints.

Sonography demonstrates an enlarged, hypoechoic epididymis and spermatic cord, and hypervascularity is notable on color-flow Doppler imaging. Other imaging features include an ipsilateral reactive hydrocele and scrotal skin thickening. The presence of a complex extratesticular fluid collection may indicate a pyocele. When the condition is long lasting, the inflamed epididymis may be hyperechoic and may contain calcifications. An inflamed testicle may be uniformly decreased in echogenicity relative to the normal side or may be normal in appearance. Duplex sonography may demonstrate an increase in the visible number of vessels per unit area of testicle. Focal orchitis may be difficult to distinguish from a testicular neoplasm; neoplasia typically distorts the testicular contour, whereas a focal orchitis may not. When the acute inflammation resolves, the involved testicle may atrophy.

Notes

Endometrial Changes in Patients Treated with Tamoxifen

1. Secretory phase; between 8 and 12 mm.

2. False.

3. False.

4. True.

Reference

Hann LE, Giess CS, Bach AM, Tao Y, et al: Endometrial thickness in tamoxifen-treated patients: correlation with clinical and pathologic findings, *Am J Roentgenol* 168:657-661, 1997.

Cross-Reference

Genitourinary Radiology: THE REQUISITES, p 289.

Comment

Tamoxifen is a synthetic estrogen antagonist that has been used in the treatment of breast cancer. Paradoxically, tamoxifen has estrogenic effects on the endometrium. The association between tamoxifen treatment and endometrial cancer was first reported in 1985. When compared with historical controls, the relative risk ratio of endometrial cancer is 2.2 when tamoxifen is given at a dose of 20 mg/day, and the risk ratio increases to 6.4 with a dose of 40 mg/day.

In the study referenced above, Hann and her colleagues found that about half of 91 postmenopausal patients being treated with tamoxifen (20 mg/day) had an endometrial thickness of 8 mm or more on transvaginal sonography. Histologic abnormalities, including polyps (both endometrial and endocervical) and carcinoma, were found in about half of these patients; other studies have found subendometrial cysts and hyperplasia as well. Endometrial polyps were the most frequent abnormality. There was no association between abnormal endometrial thickness and postmenopausal bleeding, and more than half of the women with endometrial histologic abnormalities were asymptomatic. This finding underscores the importance of transvaginal sonography in the follow up for these patients. The authors found a correlation between duration of tamoxifen use and increased endometrial thickness; patients on tamoxifen for less than 5 years had a median endometrial thickness of 5 mm, whereas those receiving tamoxifen for 5 years or more had a median endometrial measurement of 14 mm.

Multiple studies suggest that the incidence of endometrial carcinoma is increased in patients treated with tamoxifen, but the incidence is less than 1%. It appears that the risk increases as the duration of tamoxifen use increases, particularly when use exceeds 5 years. In contrast to patients with endometrial abnormalities other than carcinoma, many women with endometrial carcinoma who are on tamoxifen have abnormal uterine bleeding.

Notes

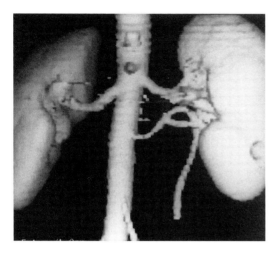 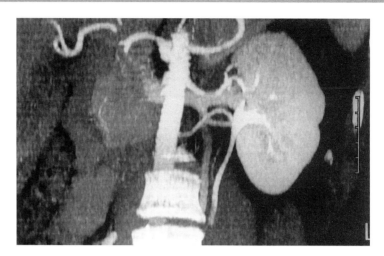

1. Identify this examination. What are the indications for this study?
2. What is the significance of the renal arterial anatomy in this renal donor?
3. What imaging parameters (collimation, pitch, and reconstruction interval) are usually chosen for this study?
4. What contrast type, concentration, and rate of injection are usually chosen for this study?

CT Angiography of Duplicated Renal Arteries

1. CT angiography. Often performed to evaluate potential renal transplantation donors; performed less frequently to diagnose renal artery stenosis.

2. Duplicated left renal artery means that the right kidney will be chosen as the donor kidney.

3. Collimation of 3 mm, pitch of 1 to 2, and reconstruction interval of 2 mm.

4. Low osmolar contrast medium at a concentration of 300 mg iodine/ml; injection rate varies from 3 to 5 ml/second.

Reference

Platt JF, Ellis JH, Korobkin M, Reige KA, et al: Potential renal donors: comparison of conventional imaging with CT, *Radiology* 198:419, 1996.

Cross-Reference

Genitourinary Radiology: THE REQUISITES, p 24.

Comment

Renal transplantation is the treatment of choice for end-stage renal disease. Donor kidneys can come from living, related donors or from unrelated cadavers. HLA matching, better immunosuppression, and improvements in transplant surgical technique have resulted in a 75% to 90% 1-year graft survival rate.

The objectives of the pretransplant evaluation of the renal donor are to determine that there are (1) two viable kidneys without intrinsic disease, (2) no vascular abnormalities (arterial or venous) that might contraindicate transplantation or leave the donor with a single compromised kidney, and (3) no ureteral abnormalities that might contraindicate surgery. Duplication of the renal arteries or renal veins is estimated to occur in up to 35% of the healthy population. Duplication of renal arteries may be a contraindication to renal transplant, depending on the size and number of duplicated vessels. In general, small hypoplastic renal arteries can be sacrificed without a significant loss of renal function. The finding of multiple renal arteries of a similar size necessitates multiple anastomoses, which lengthens the transplant surgery and increases the likelihood of postoperative complications. The same caveat applies for duplicated renal veins. In general the left kidney is preferred for transplantation because the longer renal vein facilitates vascular anastomosis.

Historically the radiologic evaluation of a potential renal transplant donor included excretory urography and catheter angiography. Helical CT angiography and MR angiography have replaced conventional angiography for the evaluation of renal transplant donors at most institutions. Helical CT provides accurate information regarding the number, location, and size of renal arteries and veins. Experienced radiologists are more than 95% accurate in identifying accessory renal arteries and veins.

Notes

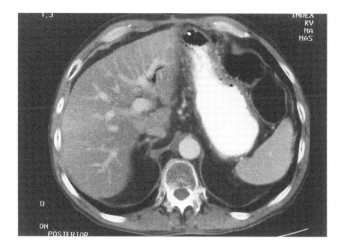

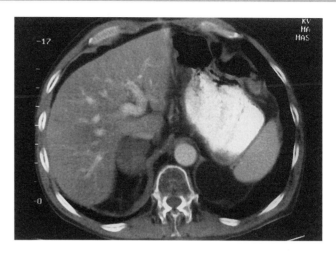

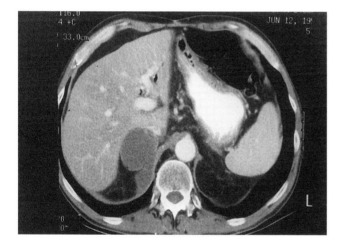

1. Three abdominal CT scans, each performed 2 months apart, are shown. What is the diagnosis? What is the cause of this abnormality?

2. Which primary adrenal tumors may present as a predominantly cystic mass?

3. What are some indications for surgical removal of an adrenal cyst?

4. How can the radiologist determine whether a large upper abdominal cyst arises from the adrenal gland?

Adrenal Pseudocyst

1. Adrenal pseudocyst; it is secondary to hemorrhage.

2. Adenoma and pheochromocytoma. There have been only six reported cases of cystic adrenal carcinoma.

3. Symptoms that can be attributed to the size of the cyst, endocrinologic hyperfunction, hemorrhage, infection, or possibility of malignancy.

4. Through analysis of cystic fluid. Adrenal cyst fluid may have a high concentration of cortisol and androgen precursors and may contain cholesterol crystals.

Reference

Gaffey MJ, Mills SE, Fechner RE, Bertholf MR, et al: Vascular adrenal cysts: clinicopathologic and immunochemical study of endothelial and hemorrhagic (pseudocyst) variants, *Am J Surg Pathol* 13:740-747, 1989.

Cross-Reference

Genitourinary Radiology: THE REQUISITES, pp 357-359.

Comment

Adrenal cysts can be divided into several pathologic subtypes—true cysts, pseudocysts, and infectious cysts. Some "true" adrenal cysts arise from endothelium; of this type, lymphangiomatous cysts are much more common than adrenal hemangiomas. Epithelial cysts are the other type of "true" adrenal cyst and are divided into retention, embryonal, and adenomatous types. Infectious cysts are the least common, and the majority of infectious adrenal cysts are echinococcal in origin.

Adrenal "pseudocysts" are so named because the wall in these types of cysts does not have a benign endothelial or epithelial lining. Instead, the pseudocyst wall has variable composition depending on its etiology; pseudocysts can be the sequela of chronic adrenal hemorrhage (as in this case), a hemorrhagic complication of benign vascular neoplasm or malformation, or cystic degeneration of a primary or metastatic tumor. Benign primary adrenal tumors that can present as pseudocysts include cystic adenomas, pheochromocytomas, adenomatoid tumors, and schwannomas. Many cysts with attenuation values in excess of 30 HU have evidence of organizing hemorrhage pathologically; intracystic proteinaceous debris or calcification also may account for an attenuation higher than that of water.

Notes

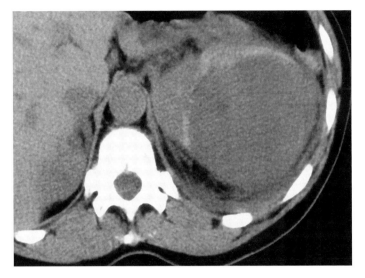 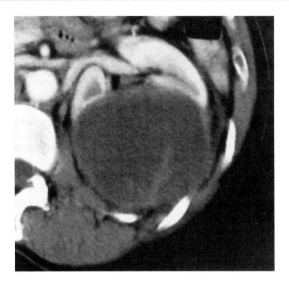

1. What is the material layering posteriorly in the left perinephric space?

2. Is spontaneous perinephric hemorrhage usually idiopathic?

3. What is the most likely diagnosis of the left renal mass?

4. What causes the internal enhancement in this mass?

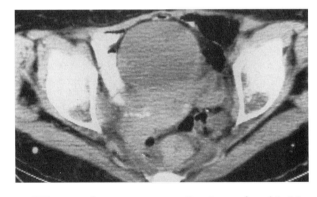 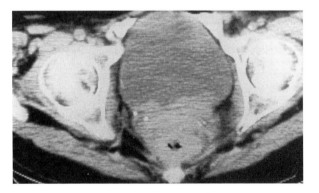

1. What are the treatment implications when bladder cancer invades through the bladder wall?

2. Which pelvic primary tumors may secondarily invade the urinary bladder?

3. What is a "herald" lesion?

4. True or False: All forms of bladder invasion by extravesical inflammation or tumor can be detected by cystoscopy.

Renal Cell Carcinoma with Spontaneous Perinephric Hemorrhage

1. Hemorrhage.

2. No. In nearly all cases there is an underlying abnormality, most commonly neoplasm.

3. Renal cell carcinoma.

4. Enhancing septa.

Reference

Zagoria RJ, Dyer RB, Wolfman NT: Radiology in the diagnosis and staging of renal cell carcinoma, *Crit Rev Diagn Imaging* 31:81-115, 1990.

Cross-Reference

Genitourinary Radiology: THE REQUISITES, pp 93-94.

Comment

Spontaneous perinephric hemorrhage indicates hemorrhage into the perirenal and pararenal spaces unrelated to trauma. Although this hemorrhage is spontaneous, it is not idiopathic. In nearly all cases an identifiable underlying cause can be found. In approximately 60% of cases the underlying cause is neoplasm. The neoplasm may be either a renal cell carcinoma or an angiomyolipoma, both of which have a predilection for bleeding. Other causes of spontaneous perinephric hemorrhage include complicated renal cysts, vasculitis, renal infarction, and renal infection. Therefore spontaneous perinephric hemorrhage alone should lead the clinician to carefully and thoroughly investigate an underlying cause. When CT scanning does not help identify a cause, angiography may be useful to detect underlying vascular lesions.

In this patient the cause of bleeding is obvious. There is a large cystic mass. It is ball shaped, without visible fat. It is not a simple cyst because there are numerous septa that enhance, and there is clearly a thick rind of tissue at the circumference of the mass. These features alone suggest a neoplasm, either renal cell carcinoma or multilocular cystic nephroma. In combination with the perirenal hemorrhage, the diagnosis of renal cell carcinoma is more likely. In either case this abnormality represents a surgical renal mass. It was resected and found to be a papillary renal cell carcinoma.

Notes

Invasion of the Urinary Bladder by Uterine Cervical Carcinoma

1. Complete resection of the tumor may not be possible; radiation therapy may be necessary.

2. Neoplasms of the uterine cervix, prostate, urethra, and rectum.

3. A bladder mucosal lesion with inflammatory features that results from extravesical tumor or inflammation.

4. False.

Reference

Kim SH, Han MC: Invasion of the urinary bladder by uterine cervical carcinoma: evaluation with MR imaging, *Am J Roentgenol* 168:393-397, 1997.

Cross-Reference

Genitourinary Radiology: THE REQUISITES, p 197.

Comment

Mucosal invasion of the urinary bladder or rectum by uterine cervical cancer is designated stage IVa disease and is treated with chemotherapy and radiation therapy. Chemotherapy that reduces a locally advanced tumor can improve the effectiveness of radiation therapy or reduce the size of a tumor sufficiently to make surgery feasible. In studies of cisplatin-based regimens administered to patients with locally advanced cervical carcinoma, response rates of 90% have been reported.

"Herald" lesions are vesical mucosal lesions caused by extravesical tumor or inflammation. On cystoscopy a sessile and shaggy mucosal lesion surrounded by telangiectasia, bullous edema, or hemorrhage may be visible. However, endoscopy may not identify all forms of bladder wall invasion by perivesical lesions; local invasion of the bladder that is confined to the serosa or muscular wall may go undetected and has treatment implications similar to mucosal disease.

Cross-sectional imaging is useful in staging locally advanced cervical carcinoma. Discrete masses protruding into the lumen of the bladder or sessile nodularity of the posterior bladder wall contiguous with a uterine cervical mass should suggest the diagnosis on CT or MRI. In addition, on MRI, abnormally high signal within the posterior bladder wall (which is normally hypointense on T2W images) and strands of abnormal soft tissue signal in the uterovesical space are other clues to stage IVa disease. However, abnormal signal or contrast enhancement of the uterovesical space may not indicate serosal invasion by tumor but a desmoplastic or inflammatory response to the cervical tumor.

Notes

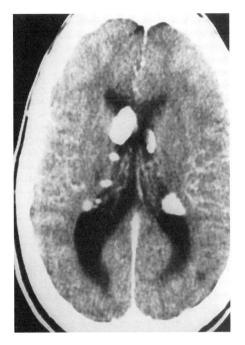
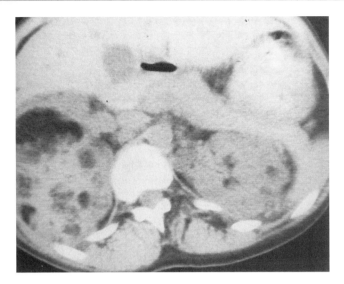

1. Of the three-tiered diagnostic criteria for this disease, there are six "primary" features. Name three of them.
2. What is the most common presenting symptom of this disease, and how does it impact the likelihood of another common feature of this disease?
3. Name two of the three skin lesions that are associated with this disease.
4. What combination of renal lesions is characteristic for this disease?

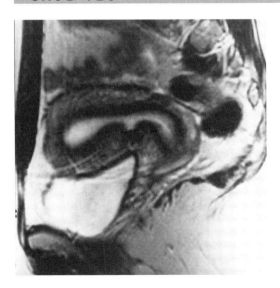
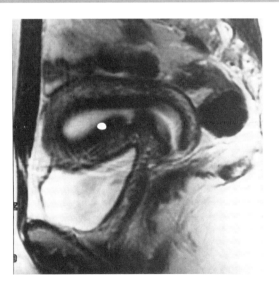

1. What pulse sequence was employed in these T2W images?
2. What is the name of the inner third of the myometrium?
3. What abnormality is present?
4. True or False: The thickness of the myometrium changes during the menstrual cycle.

Angiomyolipoma and Tuberous Sclerosis

1. Facial angiofibromas, multiple ungual fibromas, cortical tuber, subependymal nodule or giant cell astrocytoma, multiple calcified subependymal nodules protruding into the ventricle, and multiple retinal astrocytoma.

2. Myoclonic seizures that begin in infancy or early childhood. Patients who manifest seizures before the age of 5 years are more likely to have mental impairment than those who develop seizures at a later age.

3. Adenoma sebaceum (adenofibroma), nevus depigmentosus (ash leaf spots), café au lait spots.

4. Multiple angiomyolipomas together with renal cystic disease.

References

Seidenwurm DJ, Barkovich AJ: Understanding tuberous sclerosis, *Radiology* 183:23-24, 1992.

Takahashi K, Honda M, Okubo RS, et al: CT pixel mapping in the diagnosis of small angiomyolipomas of the kidneys, *J Comput Assist Tomogr* 17:98-101, 1993.

Cross-Reference

Genitourinary Radiology: THE REQUISITES, pp 111-112, 142.

Comment

Within the genitourinary system, the most common and characteristic manifestation of tuberous sclerosis is the renal angiomyolipoma. Of patients with tuberous sclerosis, 80% develop angiomyolipomas, and they are frequently multifocal lesions. Angiomyolipomas have a tendency to hemorrhage spontaneously when larger than 4 cm in diameter. Even though the finding of a discrete echogenic renal mass on ultrasound likely represents an angiomyolipoma, CT is still recommended because there have been reports of small echogenic renal cell carcinomas. Thin-section CT using 5 mm collimation through the renal mass should be performed. In equivocal cases a pixel histogram through the mass that demonstrates three contiguous pixels measuring less than –10 HU is diagnostic for fat within an angiomyolipoma. Patients with tuberous sclerosis also develop renal cysts, and the findings of renal cyst and renal angiomyolipoma strongly suggest the diagnosis of Bourneville's disease.

The presence of an angiomyolipoma alone does not imply tuberous sclerosis because 80% of these hamartomas are discovered in middle-aged adults who do not have tuberous sclerosis. In this cohort the majority of patients are women, the tumor is often asymptomatic, and the hamartoma is usually solitary. Symptoms resulting from local mass effect or hemorrhage may occur if the mass enlarges. Renal hemorrhage from an angiomyolipoma can be treated with arterial embolization.

Notes

Cesarean Section Scar

1. Fast spin-echo or turbo spin-echo.

2. Junctional zone.

3. A focal disruption in the junctional zone along the ventral uterine corpus.

4. True.

Reference

Mayo-Smith WW, Lee MJ: MR imaging of the female pelvis, *Clin Radiol* 50:667-676, 1995.

Cross-Reference

Genitourinary Radiology: THE REQUISITES, pp 28-30, 36-38, 288-301.

Comment

This is an "Aunt Minnie" case of a uterine scar resulting from a cesarean section performed several years earlier. There is focal thinning of the inner myometrium in the lower ventral uterus with an focal outpouching of the endometrial cavity, which appears hyperintense on this T2W sequence. The dark band superficial to the endometrium is called the *junctional zone* and represents the inner third of the myometrium. It is believed to be relatively hypointense because of an increased nuclear-to-cytoplasmic ratio or a relative decrease in the amount of free water. Thickening of the junctional zone has been described with both focal and diffuse adenomyosis. The junctional zone can be disrupted by invasive endometrial carcinoma, invasive cervical carcinoma, or postoperative scarring. The junctional zone also can be distorted by a uterine leiomyoma, and the direction of the distortion can act as a clue to the site of origin. Distortion of the junctional zone toward the uterine cavity implies an intramural or subserosal fibroid; distortion away from the endometrial cavity implies a submucosal fibroid.

The development of pelvic phased array coils and faster imaging techniques such as fast (turbo) spin-echo has led to increased spatial resolution when imaging the female pelvis. The HASTE (*h*alf-Fourier *s*ingle-shot *t*urbo spin-*e*cho) sequence should permit further increases in spatial resolution while providing sufficient contrast and suppressing motion artifacts because of its rapid acquisition time.

Notes

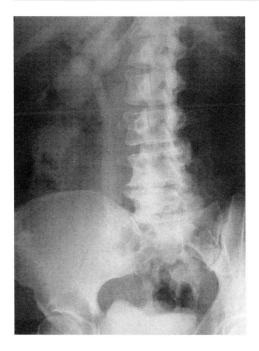
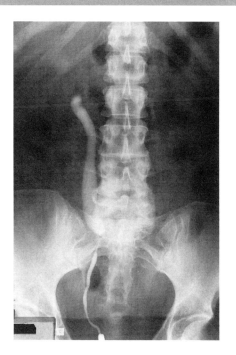

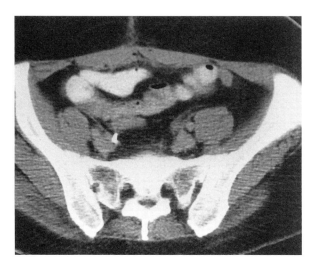

1. This patient has a history of cervical cancer treated with hysterectomy, lymph node dissection, and radiation therapy. Name the three studies that were performed.
2. What is the differential diagnosis?
3. What are the treatment options for this patient?
4. In this case, what is the indication for retrograde pyelography?

Ureteral Stricture Resulting from Retroperitoneal Surgery

1. Intravenous urogram, retrograde pyelogram, and noncontrast CT.

2. Extrinsic ureteral compression by tumor, iatrogenic stricture, ureteral infection (tuberculosis or schistosomiasis), and periureteral inflammation (endometriosis, inflammatory bowel disease, appendicitis, or diverticulitis).

3. Stent placement, balloon dilation, and surgical resection of the stricture.

4. To further evaluate the obstructed right ureter, particularly the distal ureter, which is not visible on the excretory urogram.

Reference

Winalski CS, Lipman JC, Tumeh SS: Ureteral neoplasms, *Radiographics* 10:271-283, 1990.

Cross-Reference

Genitourinary Radiology: THE REQUISITES, pp 170-182, 388-389.

Comment

This patient had a history of cervical carcinoma and had a hysterectomy with pelvic lymph node dissection and pelvic radiation 2 months before these imaging studies. She had no evidence of hydronephrosis before the surgical procedure. The intravenous urogram demonstrated right hydronephrosis and hydroureter extending down to the pelvis. The distal ureter could not be visualized on the intravenous urogram. The retrograde pyelogram demonstrated a short stricture and a normal distal ureter. The contrast-enhanced pelvic CT demonstrated enhancement of the right ureter but no adjacent soft tissue mass. The etiology of this stricture is believed to be iatrogenic (i.e., secondary to a right pelvic lymph node dissection with postoperative scarring adjacent to the ureter).

Ureteral narrowing has many different etiologies. As with most tubular structures, the causes of obstruction can be classified as intrinsic or extrinsic. Intrinsic causes of ureteral obstruction, such as a transitional cell carcinoma, tend to cause mucosal irregularity, which is not present in this case. Extrinsic causes of ureteral stricture occur from adjacent tumor (e.g., prostate cancer, cervical carcinoma, or lymphoma) or extrinsic masses (e.g., retroperitoneal fibrosis, endometriosis, inflammatory bowel disease, appendicitis). Extrinsic causes of ureteral obstruction are best demonstrated with cross-sectional imaging studies, such as CT. CT was helpful in this case because it demonstrated a normally opacified ureter but no mass adjacent to the stricture. Even though this patient received radiation therapy, a radiogenic stricture is unlikely because they typically develop 12 months or more after therapy.

Patients with strictures soon after surgery tend to respond well when treated with a balloon dilation and stent placement. These patients have a better than 50% chance of complete resolution of the stricture. Long-standing strictures or those from malignant etiologies do not respond as well and may require other therapies. The ureteral stricture in this case was successfully treated with balloon dilation and stent placement.

Notes

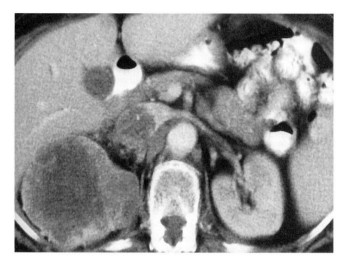 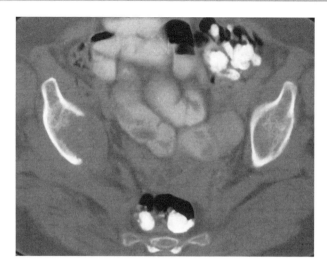

1. What is the most likely diagnosis?
2. What is the stage of this disease?
3. How does the radiologist differentiate caval invasion by tumor from inflow phenomenon?
4. How would you obtain a histologic diagnosis on this patient?

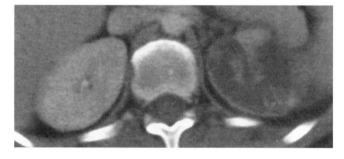 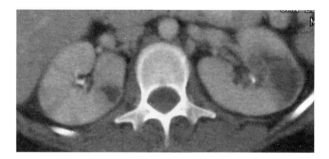

1. What term describes the nephrographic pattern shown in the area of the multiple renal abnormalities?
2. What artery is supplying the outer cortex of these kidneys?
3. What pathologic conditions should be considered when bilateral renal lesions with this shape are present?
4. What is the most likely diagnosis in this patient?

Metastatic Renal Cell Carcinoma

1. Renal cell carcinoma (RCC) associated with inferior vena cava invasion and osteolytic metastasis to the right ilium.

2. Stage IV.

3. Continuity of filling defect with ipsilateral renal vein, expansion of inferior vena cava, and persistent filling defect on delayed imaging.

4. CT-guided biopsy of iliac lesion.

Reference

Zagoria RJ, Bechtold RE, Dyer RB: Staging of renal adenocarcinoma: role of various imaging procedures, *Am J Roentgenol* 164:363-370, 1995.

Cross-Reference

Genitourinary Radiology: THE REQUISITES, pp 89-100.

Comment

Every year in the United States 20,000 new cases of renal adenocarcinoma are diagnosed. Men are afflicted twice as often as women, and the incidence peaks between the ages of 50 and 70 years. The terms *clear cell carcinoma* and *hypernephroma* were used in the past because of the similarity of the lesion's histologic characteristics to those of clear cells of the adrenal cortex and because of the original misconception that these tumors arose from the adrenal gland itself, hence the term *hypernephroma*. Renal adenocarcinoma arises from epithelial cells of the proximal tubules and often develops in the upper or lower poles of the kidney.

The appearance of RCCs on CT varies, depending on the size of the lesion and the phase of contrast enhancement. Approximately 90% are exophytic masses, and all are hypodense compared with kidney during the infusion phase of enhancement. Of RCCs, 31% display calcification on CT. The calcification is typically central, diffuse, and coarse. Although 20% of RCCs are described as cystic, the number is deceiving. The majority of cystic RCCs have peripheral nodular enhancement or thickened, calcified septa.

Helical CT enables evaluation of the liver and kidney in different stages of enhancement. With dynamic imaging performed early in the cortical phase of enhancement, subtle renal masses can be overlooked. Imaging during the nephrographic phase of enhancement (approximately 120 seconds after the injection of contrast has begun) is optimal for detecting small renal masses.

Notes

Renal Infarction

1. Rim nephrogram.

2. Renal capsular artery.

3. Renal infarctions; metastases, including lymphoma; and renal infections.

4. Bilateral renal infarctions caused by emboli or vasculitis.

Reference

Gash JR, Zagoria RJ, Dyer RB: Imaging features of infiltrating renal lesions, *Crit Rev Diagn Imaging* 33:293-310, 1992.

Cross-Reference

Genitourinary Radiology: THE REQUISITES, pp 118-119, 135.

Comment

The abnormal low attenuation lesions present in both kidneys maintain the normal shape of the kidney without significant mass effect. There is decreased perfusion to the involved areas, with a rim of normally enhancing parenchyma at the peripheral edge of the abnormal areas. This pattern is typical of renal infarction, with the cortical rim nephrogram being diagnostic of this entity. The rim nephrogram results from the occlusion of segmental renal arteries leading to renal infarction with maintenance of flow to the capsular artery, which branches proximally from the main renal artery. The renal capsular artery maintains perfusion to the outermost renal cortex in the area of infarction. Unfortunately, the rim nephrogram sign is present in only one half of renal infarctions. Abnormalities that cause infiltrative renal lesions include infiltrative neoplasms, such as transitional cell carcinoma and some metastases; renal infarctions (as shown here); and some inflammatory renal lesions, including pyelonephritis and xanthogranulomatous pyelonephritis. Of these abnormalities, only renal infarctions, bacterial pyelonephritis, and infiltrative metastases to the kidney commonly cause bilateral lesions. The presence of the rim sign is diagnostic of renal infarction.

Renal infarction may result from numerous causes of renal vascular occlusion, including embolus, dissection, thrombosis, and vasculitis. Bilateral renal infarctions suggest systemic emboli or a vasculitis. The patient shown had subacute bacterial endocarditis with multiple systemic emboli.

Notes

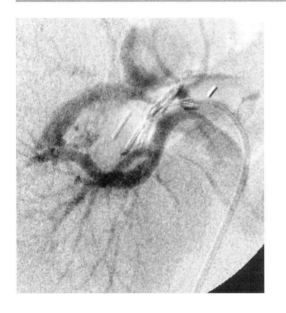
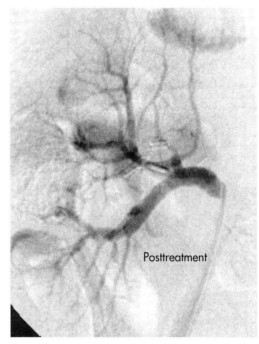

Posttreatment

1. This selective renal arteriogram of a transplanted kidney demonstrates what abnormality?
2. What is the likely cause of this abnormality in a transplanted kidney?
3. How can this abnormality be treated in the radiology department?
4. In the native kidney, what is the usual noniatrogenic cause for this type of abnormality?

Arteriovenous Fistula

1. Arteriovenous fistula.

2. Renal biopsy.

3. Superselective embolization of the fistulous connection.

4. Congenital arteriovenous malformation of the kidney.

Reference

Voegeli DR, Crummy AB, McDermott JC, et al: Percutaneous management of the urological complications of renal transplantation, *Radiographics* 6:1007-1022, 1986.

Cross-Reference

Genitourinary Radiology: THE REQUISITES, p 397.

Comment

The term *arteriovenous fistula* (AVF) describes an abnormal connection between the arterial and venous vessels. In the native kidney this abnormality usually results from congenital vascular malformations and penetrating trauma, including iatrogenic interventions. After trauma, an arterial pseudoaneurysm may develop and erode into an adjacent vein. This problem can then lead to marked arteriovenous shunting with diminished perfusion to the renal parenchyma and increased demands for cardiac outflow. Although the AVF is usually quite small, the artery and vein feeding and draining the AVF can enlarge markedly, reflecting the high flow through the AVF. Renal AVFs can be treated successfully with embolization of the fistula or of the feeding artery because the renal arteries are end arteries without significant intrarenal collateral pathways. The posttreatment angiogram in this patient demonstrates complete obliteration of the fistula, with excellent flow to the kidney.

Notes

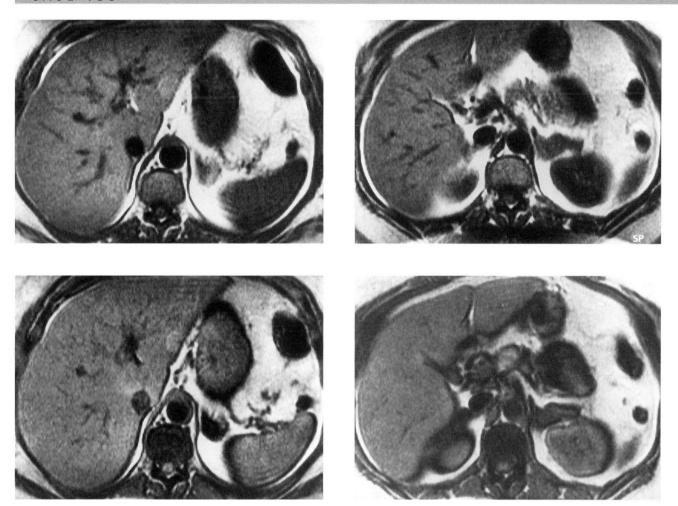

1. What two types of MR image pairs are shown?

2. What is a collision tumor?

3. What are the two most common histologic tumor types found in an adrenal collision tumor?

4. What are the implications for biopsy of an adrenal collision tumor?

Collision Tumor of the Adrenal Gland

1. In-phase and opposed-phase T1W, gradient echo images of a left adrenal mass.

2. A mass that contains two coexistent but independent neoplasms without substantial histopathologic admixture.

3. Adenoma and metastasis.

4. The component of the tumor that is more likely to be malignant should be biopsied.

Reference

Schwartz LH, Macari M, Huvos AG, Panicek DM: Collision tumors of the adrenal gland: demonstration and characterization at MR imaging, *Radiology* 201:757-760, 1996.

Cross-Reference

Genitourinary Radiology: THE REQUISITES, pp 29-30, 346-351.

Comment

Rarely, masses may consist of more than one histologic type. Three morphologic patterns of such masses—composite, combination, and collision—have been described. Composite tumors have two different cell types that are intermixed (e.g., carcinosarcoma), and in the related combination tumor a common stem cell precursor may produce these different but admixed histologic components. Collision tumors consist of two histologically different tumors that are proximate but separate. Collision tumors can occur in one organ, in adjacent organs, or as metastases from one organ to another. Some examples of collision tumors include hepatocellular carcinoma with cholangiocarcinoma, gastric adenocarcinoma with lymphoma, and squamous cell carcinoma of the esophagus with leiomyoma.

In the adrenal gland, collision tumors consisting of an adenoma and metastasis have been reported. As illustrated in this case, in- and opposed-phase T1W gradient echo pairs show a focal area of the tumor that loses signal on the opposed-phase image (suggesting a fat-containing adenoma) and another part of the tumor that does not demonstrate signal loss (and is more suspicious for metastasis). The adrenal collision tumor may be the result of two highly prevalent tumors occurring in contiguity by chance. After all, the autopsy prevalence of adrenal adenomas is 3%, and the adrenal gland is a common site for metastasis from a variety of primary tumors. As suggested by Schwartz and co-workers, collision tumors of the adrenal gland should be suspected when (1) there has been growth of a known adrenal adenoma or (2) the signal intensities of two adjacent adrenal lesions show distinctly different characteristics on MRI. In either of these cases needle biopsy of the more suspicious component of the mass (i.e., the mass that shows no signal loss on the opposed-phase, T1W gradient echo image) should be considered.

Notes

Challenge Cases

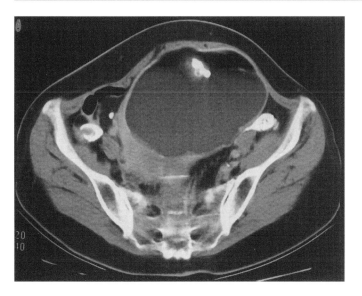 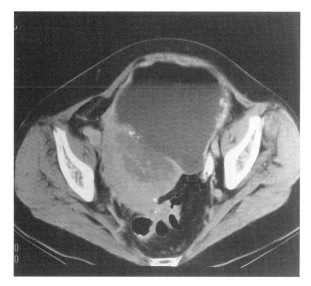

1. What is the most common complication associated with a dermoid cyst?

2. Name three other complications.

3. What is the most common malignancy associated with a dermoid cyst?

4. What findings on CT or MRI suggest malignant transformation?

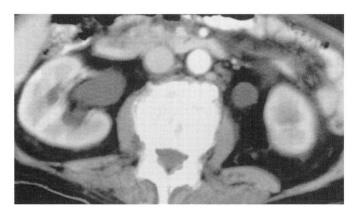 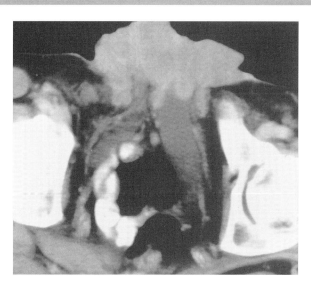

1. This patient has a congenital anomaly of the lower urinary tract. What is the fluid-filled structure entering the mass in the lower abdominal wall?

2. What abnormality of the pubic bones may accompany this congenital anomaly?

3. An unusual configuration of the distal ureters in this anomaly mimics the shape of a stick used in an Irish game. What name is given to this configuration?

4. What complication of this anomaly is illustrated by this case?

Mature Cystic Teratoma with Malignant Transformation

1. Torsion.

2. Trauma, infection, rupture or slow leak, autoimmune hemolytic anemia, perforation into a hollow viscus, and malignancy.

3. Squamous cell carcinoma.

4. Rapid growth, infiltration of adjacent tissues, extensive adhesions, and peritoneal implants.

Reference

Case records of the Massachusetts General Hospital, *N Engl J Med* 332(24):1631-1636, 1995.

Cross-Reference

Genitourinary Radiology: THE REQUISITES, p 279.

Comment

In its pure form, the dermoid cyst is always benign. However, rarely (in 2% of cases) malignant transformation occurs. This transformation occurs only in lesions larger than 5 cm in diameter. This case illustrates an ovarian squamous cell carcinoma, the most common malignancy (accounting for 80% of cases) arising from epidermal dysplasia or from squamous metaplasia of the respiratory tract epithelium in a dermoid cyst. However, any of the mature tissues in a dermoid cyst may undergo malignant transformation, which is reflected in the variety of tumors reported (i.e., adenocarcinoma of the intestinal epithelium, carcinoid tumor, thyroid carcinoma, basal cell carcinoma, malignant melanoma, leiomyosarcoma, and chondrosarcoma).

Although dermoid cysts are most often discovered in women of child-bearing age, malignant transformation usually occurs in postmenopausal women. Clinical evidence of transformation includes pain, weight loss, and rapid tumor growth. When infiltration into adjacent tissues, extensive adhesions, or peritoneal metastases are evident on imaging or at laparoscopy, malignancy should be suspected. Note the eccentric, necrotic mass along the dextrolateral wall of the cystic teratoma in this patient. Occasionally, paraaortic and pelvic lymphadenopathy are reported, but hematogenous metastasis is rare. Poor prognostic factors include ascites, rupture, and malignant invasion of the dermoid wall. Overall, the 5-year survival rate is 15% to 31%.

Notes

Bladder Exstrophy Complicated by Adenocarcinoma

1. A dilated left ureter.

2. The pubic bones are separated more than 1 cm at the symphysis. Also note the everted left pubic bone in this case.

3. Hurley stick appearance.

4. Bladder carcinoma.

Reference

Vik V, Gerharz EW, Woodhouse CRJ: Invasive carcinoma in bladder exstrophy with transitional, squamous and mucus-producing differentiation, *Br J Urol* 81:173-174, 1998.

Cross-Reference

Genitourinary Radiology: THE REQUISITES, pp 197-204.

Comment

Exstrophy of the bladder and epispadias represent the two ends of a spectrum of abdominal wall defects caused by abnormal cloacal membrane closure. Bladder exstrophy (which means "turned inside out") occurs in 1 of every 30,000 to 40,000 live births, is twice as common in men, and is 3 times more common than epispadias. In exstrophy the ventral bladder wall and the remaining bladder are everted and protrude through a defect in the lower anterior abdominal wall. A short penis, epispadias, and chordee are present. Affected girls may have vaginal stenosis or müllerian anomalies of uterovaginal fusion, but the uterus, tubes, and ovaries are usually unaffected. Characteristically the pubic bones are widely separated at the pubic symphysis, the iliac bones are rotated outward along the fulcrum of the sacroiliac joints, and each pubic bone is rotated outward at its junction with the ilium and ischium.

The mucosa of the bladder may be normal, metaplastic, or ulcerated. Squamous metaplasia may be found at the apex, or glandular metaplasia (cystitis glandularis) may occur at the bladder base. The risk of developing carcinoma is increased 200-fold. Adenocarcinoma has been found in 70 of the 82 reported cases of carcinoma complicating bladder exstrophy. The pathogenesis of this unusual type of bladder cancer may be glandular metaplasia, ectopic rectal mucosa displaced during cloacal division, or proliferation of an uncommitted epithelial stem cell.

Notes

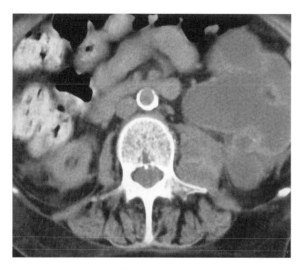 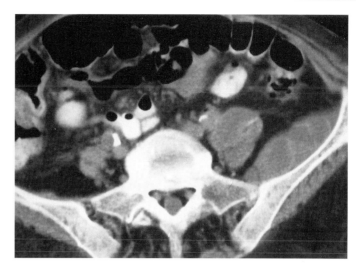

1. What abnormal findings are shown on these images?
2. What group of patients is typically afflicted by this disease?
3. What is the classic urographic triad seen in these patients?
4. What complications are associated with this disease?

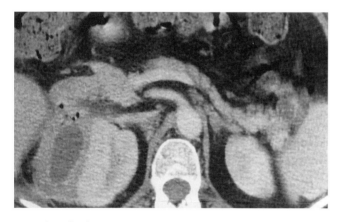 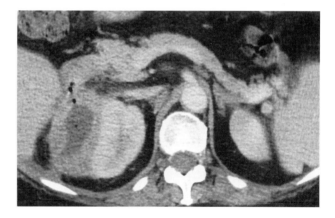

1. What finding is evident?
2. Which spaces of the retroperitoneum are involved?
3. What is the differential diagnosis?
4. What is the significance of the normal renal cortical enhancement?

CASE 136

Xanthogranulomatous Pyelonephritis Complicated by Iliopsoas Abscess

1. Marked enlargement of the left kidney, possibly resulting from chronic obstruction; left ureteral stone; and enlargement and hypodensity of left psoas and iliacus muscles.

2. Middle-aged (45-65 years) women with a history of repeated urinary tract infections.

3. Nephromegaly, markedly diminished or absent renal function, and nephrolithiasis.

4. Extrarenal extension and renal-cutaneous or renal-enteric fistula formation.

Reference

Eastham J, Ahlering T, Skinner E: Xanthogranulomatous pyelonephritis: clinical findings and surgical considerations, *Urology* 43(3):295-299, 1994.

Cross-Reference

Genitourinary Radiology: THE REQUISITES, pp 103-104, 117-118, 132, 134-135.

Comment

Xanthogranulomatous pyelonephritis (XGP) is an uncommon form of renal inflammation in which a chronically infected and obstructed kidney is infiltrated with lipid-laden macrophages. A renal calculus is present in at least 80% of patients. In addition to the urographic findings described, diffuse XGP has typical imaging features on both ultrasound and CT. Ultrasonography usually demonstrates a renal pelvic calculus, reniform enlargement of the kidney, and generalized loss of corticomedullary differentiation. On CT the kidney is enlarged; has a thin rim of enhancing parenchyma; contains multiple hypoattenuating, cystic areas (attributed to necrosis rather than to hydronephrosis); and has a central calculus. The appearance of the last two CT features listed has been likened to a bear's paw print. Another useful finding is fragmentation of the staghorn calculus, referred to as the *fractured calculus sign.* On the basis of the CT examination, correct preoperative diagnosis can be made in 87% of patients.

Extrarenal extension of XGP is common and is accurately identified on CT. Extension into the perinephric fat, Gerota's fascia, and the ipsilateral psoas muscle is common. Renal-cutaneous and renal-enteric fistulas rarely develop.

Focal or tumefactive XGP accounts for only 15% of the total number of cases. This form is difficult to differentiate from a renal tumor because the imaging findings are less specific. Findings include a hypofunctioning focal mass on intravenous urography, an echogenic mass on ultrasound, and a nonspecific solid or cystic mass (often associated with a renal calculus) on CT. Perinephric inflammation often is evident on CT. Both the focal and diffuse forms are irreversible and therefore are managed with surgery.

Notes

CASE 137

Perinephric Abscess Caused by Perforated Duodenal Ulcer

1. A perinephric fluid collection that exerts mass effect on the right kidney.

2. Anterior pararenal space and perinephric space.

3. Perinephric abscess, necrotic renal tumor, and perforated duodenal ulcer.

4. Normal cortical enhancement is unusual in pyelonephritis.

Reference

Lowe LH, Zagoria RJ, Baumgartner BR, et al: Role of imaging and intervention in complex infections of the urinary tract, *Am J Roentgenol* 163:363-367, 1994.

Cross-Reference

Genitourinary Radiology: THE REQUISITES, pp 133-135, 390.

Comment

This patient had fever, leukocytosis, and pyuria. The abdominal CT was performed to determine the source of infection. This case is an example of a perinephric abscess. The most common cause of an abscess in this area is spread from a renal infection (e.g., pyelonephritis). Pyelonephritis has typical imaging findings evident on CT, including unilateral renal enlargement, heterogeneous enhancement with wedge-shaped areas of decreased perfusion and enhancement, and perinephric inflammation. Pyelonephritis can be diffuse or focal.

Treatment of renal infections depends on the patient's clinical condition, underlying diseases, and extent of infection. Patients with pyelonephritis alone are treated with antibiotics alone. Patients with a focal perinephric collection can be treated with intravenous antibiotics and percutaneous drainage. Patients with emphysematous pyelonephritis require intravenous antibiotics and either nephrectomy or percutaneous drainage. Percutaneous drainage is preferable if the gas collection is localized. In patients treated with percutaneous drainage, the radiologist should be certain that the ipsilateral collecting system is not obstructed by a calculus or tumor. If there is ureteral obstruction, the obstructed collecting system should be drained by a ureteral stent or percutaneous nephrostomy.

The illustrated case is a perinephric abscess resulting from a perforated duodenal ulcer that extended posteriorly to the perinephric space. Clues to the correct diagnosis include the following: (1) the renal enhancement is normal, (2) there is no ureteral obstruction, (3) the fluid collection is contiguous with the decompressed duodenum, and (4) there is air between the duodenum and the perinephric collection. This patient was treated with CT-guided percutaneous abscess drainage, placement of an nasogastric tube, intravenous antibiotic therapy, and extensive antiulcer therapy.

Notes

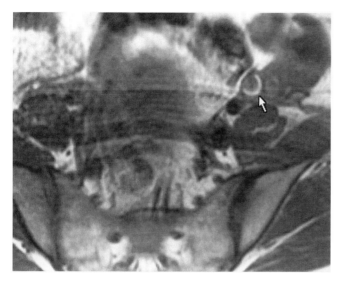 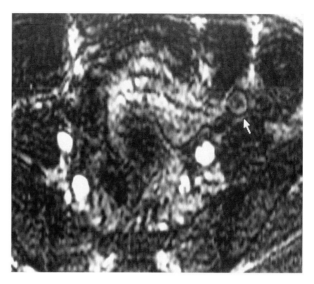

1. Name three complications of puerperal (postpartum) metritis.

2. Of ultrasound, CT, and MRI, which modalities are most sensitive for the detection of puerperal metritis complications?

3. Can enhanced MRI be safely performed in the puerperium?

4. What is the treatment for this disease?

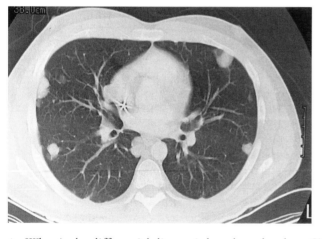 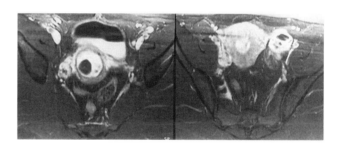

1. What is the differential diagnosis based on the chest CT?

2. What is most likely cause of the endocervical mass?

3. True or False: Endometrial carcinoma metastasis to the lungs is uncommon in the absence of metastatic lymphadenopathy.

4. True or False: After the administration of gadopentetate dimeglumine, most endometrial carcinomas enhance.

MRI of Puerperal Ovarian Thrombophlebitis

1. Septic thrombophlebitis, pelvic abscess, parametrial phlegmon, and dehiscence of the uterine incision after cesarean section.

2. Enhanced CT and MRI are equally sensitive and more sensitive than ultrasound.

3. It is safe, but some authorities caution against breast-feeding for 48 hours after the intravenous administration of gadolinium chelates.

4. Septic ovarian thrombophlebitis is treated with antibiotics; anticoagulation is controversial.

Reference

Twickler DM, Setiawan AT, Evans RS, et al: Imaging of puerperal septic thrombophlebitis: prospective comparison of MR imaging, CT, and sonography, *Am J Roentgenol* 169: 1039-1043, 1997.

Cross-Reference

Genitourinary Radiology: THE REQUISITES, pp 261-264.

Comment

Postpartum infections occur in up of 20% of high-risk cesarean deliveries, and serious complications occur in up to 10% of women with puerperal metritis. Septic thrombophlebitis usually becomes apparent in the first week after delivery. Predisposing factors for puerperal thrombosis include venous stasis after childbirth, increased circulation of clotting factors during pregnancy, and vascular damage. Thrombosis of the right ovarian vein is more common because of the long length of the vein, multiple incompetent valves, and absence of retrograde venous blood flow. If untreated, ovarian vein thrombophlebitis may extend into renal veins or the inferior vena cava and result in pulmonary embolism.

Ultrasound and CT are the mainstays of evaluation, but ultrasound is not as sensitive for the detection of thrombophlebitis as CT or MRI. Because of the difficulty in identifying ovarian veins, ultrasound detected only half of the cases of ovarian thrombophlebitis diagnosed by CT and MRI in the study referenced above. Ovarian or iliac thrombosis is diagnosed on unenhanced CT when a hyperdense or isodense thrombus is identified in the lumen of an enlarged vessel. On enhanced CT, thrombophlebitis is diagnosed when there is a hypodense filling defect within the enhancing walls of the enlarged vein. Venous tortuosity and perivascular edema are common findings.

On MRI an acute venous thrombus may appear as a hyperintense filling defect on T1W images and has moderate signal on proton-density or T2W images. On two- or three-dimensional time-of-flight MR venography, absent filling of a large and tortuous puerperal ovarian vein is a sign of thrombosis.

Notes

Benign Metastasizing Leiomyoma

1. Lung metastases, fungal disease, septic pulmonary emboli, and vasculitis.

2. Endometrial carcinoma.

3. True.

4. True.

Reference

Martin E: Leiomyomatous lung lesions: a proposed classification, *Am J Roentgenol* 141:269-272, 1983.

Cross-Reference

Genitourinary Radiology: THE REQUISITES, pp 269-273.

Comment

Martin classifies smooth muscle–containing pulmonary lesions into three general groups. The first group is primary leiomyoma of the lung, which is a benign fibroleiomyomatous hamartoma. The second group is metastatic leiomyoma that arises from extrauterine sites; growth of these tumors is not responsive to hormones, and they may represent low grade sarcomas. The third group of lesions is exemplified by this case of benign metastasizing leiomyoma (BML).

In this case the uterine mass was an endocervical leiomyoma. Women with uterine leiomyoma have a higher prevalence of endometrial carcinoma. Malignant dedifferentiation of a leiomyoma rarely occurs. An even rarer occurrence is metastasis of histologically benign myomas to pelvic lymph nodes, the abdominopelvic peritoneum, the heart, and the lungs. Approximately 50 cases of BML have been reported in the medical literature, and multiple pulmonary nodules are the most common radiologic presentation. Other reported radiologic patterns include miliary nodules and a giant cystic mass obstructing the mainstem bronchus. The pulmonary lesions of BML are fibroleiomyomatous tumors containing variable mucinous glands. The tumors lack histologic features of malignancy (i.e., nuclear atypia, mitoses, or vascular invasion), and most have both estrogen and progesterone receptors. The clinical course of the disease parallels the estrogen status of the patient. In premenopausal women the disease progression may be difficult to control, but in postmenopausal women the course tends to be more indolent.

Notes

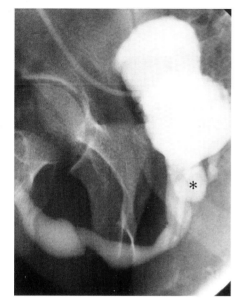
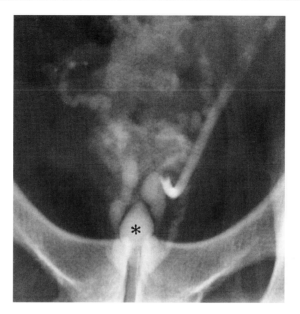

1. What is the most likely cause of the structure denoted by the asterisk in both figures?
2. Name two congenital anomalies associated with this structure.
3. What genital ducts are opacified in the image on the right?
4. What is the most likely explanation for the abnormal appearance of the anterior urethra?

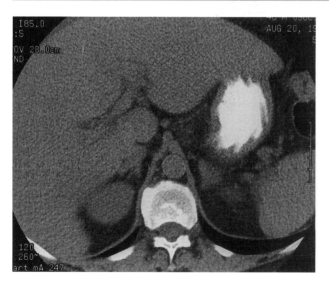
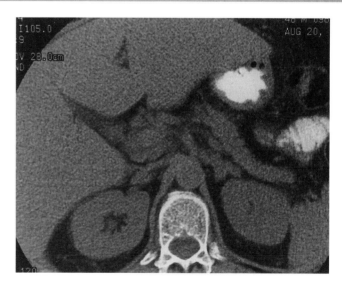

1. Given the clinical history of insulin-dependent diabetes, autoimmune thyroiditis, and Addison's disease, what is the most likely diagnosis?
2. What are some of the clinical manifestations of Addison's disease?
3. What is the differential diagnosis for adrenal enlargement and Addison's disease?
4. In idiopathic Addison's disease, what are the primary autoantigens?

Large Prostatic Utricle

1. Prostatic utricle.

2. Hypospadias, ambiguous genitalia, undescended testis, and congenital urethral polyp.

3. Deferent and ejaculatory ducts.

4. Hypospadias repair.

Reference

Ikoma F, Shima H, Yabumoto H: Classification of enlarged prostatic utricle in patients with hypospadias, *Br J Urol* 57:334-337, 1985.

Cross-Reference

Genitourinary Radiology: THE REQUISITES, pp 326, 327.

Comment

Before or after surgical correction, boys with hypospadias are not routinely evaluated radiologically. However, suspected postoperative complications, such as urethrocutaneous fistula or urethral obstruction, often are investigated with contrast urethrography. In this case the patient was evaluated because of recurrent epididymitis after hypospadias repair of the anterior urethra.

Although all males have a small prostatic utricle (utriculus masculinus), it is visible on cystourethrography only in those individuals with hypospadias, ambiguous genitalia, undescended testis, or congenital urethral polyps. Four types of congenitally large prostatic utricles are recognized and have been assigned grades 0 to III. Grades 0, I, and II utricles open in the center of the verumontanum. The grade 0 utricle does not extend above the verumontanum, the grade I utricle extends above the verumontanum but below the bladder neck, and a grade II utricle extends above the bladder neck. The Grade III congenitally large utricle arises from the bulbous urethra. In this case a grade I utricle communicates with the ejaculatory ducts, which explains the patient's recurrent epididymitis. Other complications of a prostatic utricle include stone formation and recurrent infections. Also note that the prostatic utricle has a dome-shaped fundus. A filling defect in the fundus of the diverticulum suggests vagina masculina (i.e., a cervix or uterus is attached).

In patients with hypospadias the prostatic utricle is more likely to be large, as in this case. The grade of the utricle is related to the severity of the hypospadias. For instance, patients with penile hypospadias usually have utricles of grade 0 or I, whereas those with perineal hypospadias usually have grade III prostatic utricles.

Notes

Schmidt's Syndrome

1. Polyglandular syndrome, type 2 (Schmidt's syndrome).

2. Asthenia (weakness and fatigue), arterial hypotension, abnormalities of gastrointestinal function (anorexia with weight loss, pain, nausea, vomiting, and diarrhea), and hyperpigmentation.

3. Subacute granulomatous adrenalitis, adrenal hemorrhage, metastatic disease, lymphoma, sarcoidosis, and amyloidosis.

4. Enzymes involved with steroidogenesis (17-alpha hydroxylase, 21-alpha hydroxylase, and side-chain cleavage enzymes).

References

Baker JR Jr: Autoimmune endocrine disease, *JAMA* 278(22): 1931-1937, 1997.

Vita JA, Silverberg SJ, Goland RS, Austin JHM, Knowlton AI: Clinical clues to the cause of Addison's disease, *Am J Med* 78:461-466, 1985.

Cross-Reference

Genitourinary Radiology: THE REQUISITES, pp 367-369.

Comment

In the United States, primary adrenal insufficiency presents most commonly in middle-aged women; idiopathic adrenal atrophy is the most common cause of Addison's disease. Immunohistochemical staining reveals the antibody and complement on the few remaining glandular cells. Primary ovarian failure caused by autoimmune oophoritis also may occur. Addison's disease also can be a part of an autoimmune endocrinopathy called *polyglandular syndrome* (PGS). This syndrome accounts for all of the cases of Addison's disease in juveniles and more than one third of all cases in adults. There are three types of PGS. Type 1 PGS usually begins in early childhood and is defined by mucocutaneous candidiasis and hypoparathyroidism. More than half of these patients develop Addison's disease; gonadal failure, chronic hepatitis, and alopecia also may occur. Addison's disease and either insulin-dependent diabetes or autoimmune thyroid disease defines PGS type 2 (Schmidt's syndrome). Addison's disease does not occur in type 3 PGS, which consists of autoimmune thyroid disease together with any two other autoimmune disorders, including insulin-dependent diabetes, pernicious anemia, or any nonendocrine autoimmune disorder (e.g., myasthenia gravis).

This case is unusual because the adrenal glands are slightly enlarged rather than atrophic; adrenal insufficiency was biochemical (as evidenced by abnormal results of a corticotropin-stimulation test), and the adrenal enlargement was incidentally discovered.

Notes

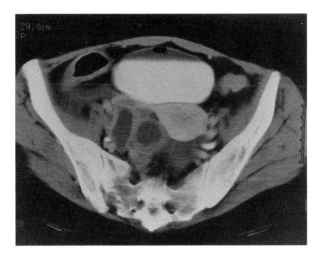 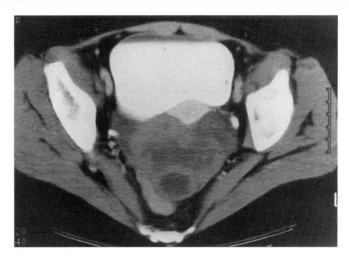

1. On the image on the left, what is the fluid-filled mass to the right of the uterus?

2. Name a cause of "massive ovarian edema."

3. What is the arterial supply of the ovary?

4. True or False: On Doppler sonography of the ovary, the presence of high resistance flow excludes malignancy and ovarian torsion.

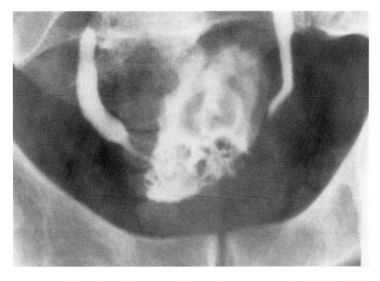 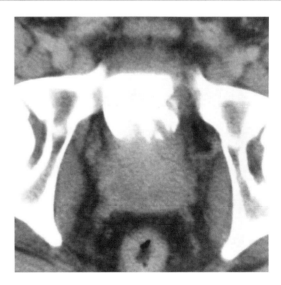

1. Given the clinical history of gross hematuria, what is the differential diagnosis for the bladder lesion or lesions?

2. Name three types of chronic proliferative cystitis that can mimic a papillary or invasive bladder neoplasm.

3. True or False: The majority of patients with malacoplakia are immunocompromised.

4. Cystitis cystica calcinosa, eosinophilic cystitis, and squamous cell carcinoma are associated with which bladder infection?

Ovarian Torsion

1. Dilated right fallopian tube with a thickened wall.

2. Partial or intermittent torsion of the ovary.

3. Ovarian artery (branch of the abdominal aorta) and uterine artery (branch of the anterior trunk of the internal iliac artery).

4. False.

References

Ghossain MA, Buy J-N, Sciot C, et al: CT findings before and after adnexal torsion: rotation of a focal solid element of a cystic mass as an adjunctive sign in diagnosis, *Am J Roentgenol* 169:1343-1346, 1997.

Kimura I, Togashi K, Kawakami S, et al: Ovarian torsion: CT and MR imaging appearances, *Radiology* 190:337-341, 1994.

Cross-Reference

Genitourinary Radiology: THE REQUISITES, pp 265, 266.

Comment

Ovarian torsion can be challenging to diagnose, particularly when the clinical presentation is atypical (e.g., the course is intermittent because of incomplete torsion or cycles of torsion and detorsion). In many cases an underlying ovarian mass predisposes to adnexal torsion, but torsion also occurs in patients with normal adnexa. In prepubertal girls, ovarian torsion should be suspected when there is a large unilateral pelvic mass with multiple peripheral "cysts" representing cortical follicles. An enlarged ovary bearing multiple enlarged follicles (8 to 12 mm in diameter) is unexpected in this age group. Kimura and co-workers found that deviation of the uterus to the twisted side, engorgement of blood vessels, ascites, and obliteration of pelvic fat planes identified on pelvic CT and MRI suggested ovarian torsion. Other reported signs include an ipsilateral, dilated fallopian tube with a thickened wall; this finding is illustrated in this case. In adnexal torsion associated with an ovarian tumor, a marked change in the position of an identifiable tumor marker (e.g., calcified vegetation or Rokitansky protuberance on a dermoid tumor) on CT scans obtained before and after the onset of adnexal torsion has been reported. An atypical presentation of partial or intermittent ovarian torsion is massive ovarian edema. Venous and lymphatic congestion result in marked edema in the stroma; the ovary may measure up to 35 cm in diameter!

Doppler sonography has limited usefulness for the diagnosis of adnexal torsion. Doppler flow may be absent in masses without torsion, and the identification of blood flow in a mass does not exclude this diagnosis. Arterial flow may be preserved in cases of torsion when only venous flow is compromised. Furthermore, the ovary is supplied by both the uterine artery and the ovarian artery, and therefore arterial flow to the adnexa may persist when arterial flow to the ovary is reduced.

Notes

Cystitis Glandularis

1. Bladder carcinoma, focal proliferative cystitis, and adherent blood clots.

2. Cystitis cystica, cystitis glandularis (CG), malacoplakia, bullous cystitis, follicular cystitis, Hunner's ulcer, and eosinophilic cystitis.

3. True.

4. Bilharziasis (*Schistosoma haematobium* bladder infection).

References

Hochberg DA, Motta J, Brodherson MS: Cystitis glandularis, *Urology* 51(1):112-113, 1998.

Young RH: Pseudoneoplastic lesions of the urinary bladder and urethra: a selective review with emphasis on recent information, *Semin Diagn Pathol* 14(2):133-146, 1997.

Cross-Reference

Genitourinary Radiology: THE REQUISITES, p 211.

Comment

A typical sequence of pathologic changes has been observed in one final common pathway of long-term bladder inflammation. The urothelium retains the potential to form numerous epithelial variants, such as mucus-producing glandular epithelium and squamous epithelium, because of its complex embryonal derivation. In the initial stages of bladder inflammation, Brunn's nests are found with increasing frequency in the lamina propria. These nests are nodular proliferations of urothelium that grow inward into the submucosa. If the centers of these urothelial cell nests degenerate, fluid-filled cysts (cystitis cystica) may result. Intestinal or vaginal glandular metaplasia of Brunn's nests in the lamina propria results in CG. Parenthetically, squamous metaplasia probably occurs with a different sequence of events because it is not preceded by the formation of Brunn's nests. Follicular cystitis is characterized by the presence of reactive lymphoid follicles in the lamina propria and is more common in children with chronic urinary tract infections.

The metaplastic submucosal glands of CG may enlarge such that they present as multiple discrete nodules, clusters of lobulated nodules, or a discrete papillary mass. Thus CG may mimic a papillary bladder carcinoma, bullous cystitis or edema, or a bladder-invasive prostate or cervical cancer. This process has a predilection for the bladder neck and trigone and has been associated with the passage of mucus.

Although adenocarcinoma presents in 10% to 42% of cases, it is not clear whether CG is a premalignant condition. The association with adenocarcinoma has been reported only in patients with the intestinal type of CG, not in patients with the much more common, typical variant of CG.

Notes

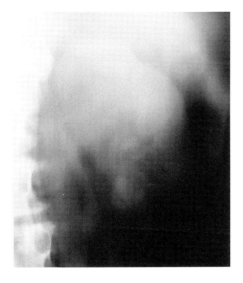
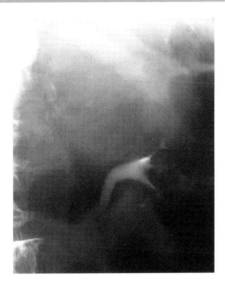
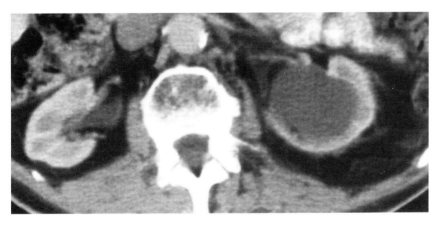

1. What lesion is likely in this 80-year-old patient with gross hematuria?

2. What is the fluid-containing structure filling the left renal sinus on the CT scan?

3. What term describes the opacified lower pole calyces in this and similar cases?

4. What associated congenital anomalies usually cause obstruction in this type of case?

Complete Duplication Anomaly

1. Duplication anomaly.

2. Obstructed upper pole pyelocalyceal system.

3. "Drooping lily" sign.

4. Ectopic ureterocele and extravesical ectopic insertion of the ureter.

Reference

Fernbach SK, Feinstein KA, Spencer K, Lindstrom CA: Ureteral dilatation and its complications, *Radiographics* 17:109-127, 1997.

Cross-Reference

Genitourinary Radiology: THE REQUISITES, pp 157, 158.

Comment

This patient has complete obstruction of the upper pole moiety of a duplicated system with resulting hydronephrosis, nonopacification of the upper pole calyces, and deviation of the lower pole calyces inferiorly. Otherwise the lower pole calyces appear normal. Upper pole obstruction is associated with complete duplication of the ureters. The two congenital causes of upper pole obstruction include ectopic ureterocele and extravesical ectopic insertion of the ureter. These anomalies are usually discovered during childhood. When the ureter inserts ectopically within the bladder, its abnormal course and position in the bladder wall may lead to formation of an obstructing ectopic ureterocele. Extravesical insertion of the ureter also may lead to ureteral obstruction. Because the upper moiety ureter is the ectopic ureter, it may insert inferior to the bladder. Its abnormal insertion may lead to obstruction because of limited outflow from its insertion site or fibrosis. If the ureter inserts in a site such as the female urethra or vagina, chronic infection can lead to stenosis of its orifice and resulting obstruction.

Duplication anomalies are commonly associated with other malformations. Approximately 30% of patients have other significant congenital urinary tract anomalies, such as renal agenesis or ureteropelvic junction stricture. Also, duplicated systems are susceptible to all of the pathologic problems that may occur in a single system. This 80-year-old patient with gross hematuria developed a transitional cell carcinoma of the ureter draining the upper pole moiety. This carcinoma was the cause of the hydronephrosis in this patient.

Notes

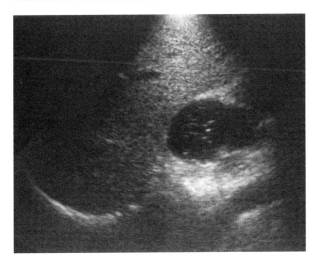
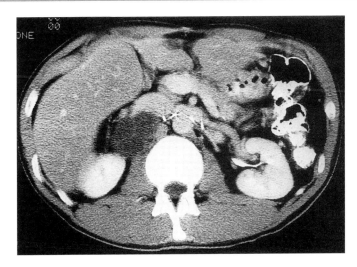

1. What surgical procedure has been performed on this patient?
2. What imaging test can be used to specifically diagnose lymphocele?
3. Nodal metastases from which primary malignancies may appear as a low density retroperitoneal mass?
4. Which infectious or inflammatory diseases may cause low density retroperitoneal lymph nodes?

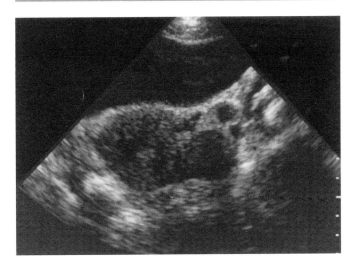
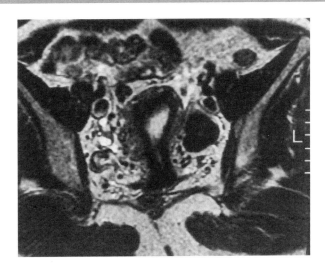

1. What is the differential diagnosis for the left adnexal mass?
2. On the T2W image, what feature of this adnexal mass is unusual for ovarian tumors?
3. What are potential histopathologic explanations for the appearance of this lesion on T2W MRI?
4. What two syndromes may be associated with this adnexal mass?

CASE 145

Recurrent Retroperitoneal Teratocarcinoma

1. Retroperitoneal lymph node dissection.

2. Lymphography.

3. Testicular cancer (particularly teratocarcinoma), epidermoid carcinoma of the genitourinary tract, lymphoma, and leiomyosarcoma.

4. Whipple's disease and *Mycobacterium avium*.

Reference

Hong WK, Wittes RE, Hajdu ST, et al: The evolution of mature teratoma from malignant testicular tumors, *Cancer* 40:553, 1977.

Cross-Reference

Genitourinary Radiology: THE REQUISITES, pp 316, 317.

Comment

The differential diagnosis of a predominantly cystic retroperitoneal mass includes lymphocele and low density lymph nodes; hypodense nodal conglomerates may result from infection, inflammation, or neoplasia. Surgical dissection of pelvic or retroperitoneal lymph nodes rarely may lead to a focal, cystlike accumulation of lymph from the transection of afferent lymphatics. These fluid-filled spaces are called *lymphoceles* or *lymphocysts* and most commonly occur in the pelvis after renal transplantation surgery. Lymphography may be used to show that contrast injected into the lymphatics opacifies these cysts.

This patient had a retroperitoneal lymph node dissection to treat teratocarcinoma of the testis and presented with a cystic recurrence 6 months later. The appearance of nodal metastases from a testicular tumor varies depending on the histologic characteristics of the primary tumor and whether or not treatment has been implemented. Before treatment, teratomas and mixed germ cell tumors containing teratomatous elements can be hypodense (measured attenuation value less than 30 HU), particularly when compared with metastases from seminomas and pure embryonal cell carcinomas. As a result of ischemic necrosis, large and bulky nodal masses caused by seminoma or embryonal cell carcinoma may be hypodense before treatment. After chemotherapy or radiation therapy, solid nodal masses may decrease in attenuation, and hypodense masses of lymph nodes may become cystic. This reduction in attenuation after treatment has been attributed to ischemic necrosis, appearance of lipid-laden macrophages surrounding areas of necrosis, or differentiation of an embryonal cell carcinoma or a mixed germ cell tumor to a more mature teratoma.

Notes

CASE 146

Fibrothecoma of the Ovary

1. Fibroma, fibrothecoma, subserosal leiomyoma, and broad ligament leiomyoma.

2. Signal intensity of the left adnexal mass is atypically low for an ovarian epithelial tumor.

3. Dense cellularity, abundant fibrosis or collagen content, calcification, and chronic hemorrhage.

4. Meigs' syndrome and basal cell nevus syndrome.

Reference

Troiano RN, Lazzarini KM, Scoutt LM, et al: Fibroma and fibrothecoma of the ovary: MR imaging findings, *Radiology* 204:795-798, 1997.

Cross-Reference

Genitourinary Radiology: THE REQUISITES, pp 272, 273.

Comment

Fibromas and fibrothecomas are tumors of the ovarian stroma and consist primarily of densely packed spindle cells, which produce relatively large amounts of collagen. Fibrothecomas also contain a smaller population of thecal cells, which have intracellular lipid and are often hormonally active. These stromal ovarian tumors are usually discovered incidentally or when they become very large and are almost always benign.

A fibroma can be associated with two unusual clinical syndromes. Meigs' syndrome complicates about 1% of all fibromas and is defined as ascites and pleural effusion that accompany a fibrous ovarian tumor and resolve after the removal of that tumor. Even in the absence of the complete syndrome, free intraperitoneal fluid is commonly associated with all but the smallest fibromas. When fibromas occur in basal cell nevus syndrome, they are typically bilateral, multinodular, and calcified.

The characteristic signal intensity of fibromas and fibrothecomas is homogeneously low on T1W images and predominantly low on T2W images. These tumors range in size from 3 to 18 cm; larger lesions (i.e., those greater than 5 cm in diameter) often show central or eccentric areas of cystic degeneration or edema.

Fibromas and fibrothecomas must be differentiated from pedunculated or broad ligament leiomyomas. On ultrasound, fibrous ovarian tumors are particularly difficult to distinguish from leiomyomas because both may be primarily hypoechoic with posterior wall attenuation. If a hypointense adnexal mass is demonstrated on pelvic MRI, the radiologist should try to identify either a pedicle to the uterine serosa or two normal ovaries. Either or both findings would support the diagnosis of a leiomyoma.

Notes

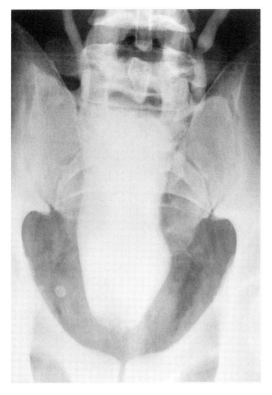 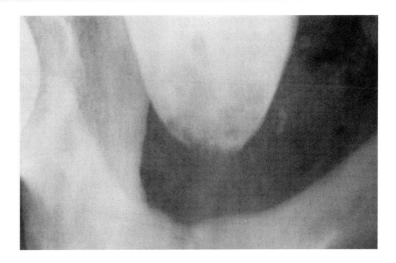

1. Two images of the bladder from an excretory urogram are shown. What is the differential diagnosis for the abnormal shape of the bladder?

2. On a barium enema examination (not shown), the rectosigmoid colon was elongated, straightened, and narrowed. What is the most likely diagnosis in this case?

3. What is the most likely cause of the lobulated filling defects in the urinary bladder?

4. True or False: In this disease, significant urinary obstruction is treated with excision of abnormal tissue around the bladder or ureters.

Pelvic Lipomatosis with Cystitis Glandularis

1. The differential diagnosis for a pear- or gourd-shaped bladder includes perivesical hematoma, urinoma, or abscess; iliopsoas hypertrophy; pelvic lipomatosis; lymphadenopathy (from lymphoma or carcinoma); and inferior vena cava obstruction.

2. Pelvic lipomatosis.

3. Proliferative cystitis.

4. False. The massive amount of fat, its adherence to the pelvic viscera, and the ill-defined fascial planes make surgery difficult. When treatment of urinary obstruction is necessary, supravesical urinary diversion or ureteroneocystostomy can be performed.

References

Heyns CF, de Kock MLS, Kirsten PH, van Velden DJJ: Pelvic lipomatosis associated with cystitis glandularis and adenocarcinoma of the bladder, *J Urol* 145:364-366, 1991.

Cross-Reference

Genitourinary Radiology: THE REQUISITES, pp 164, 224.

Comment

Pelvic lipomatosis is a rare and poorly understood disease typified by the proliferation of mature adipose tissue, fibrous tissue, and chronic inflammatory cells in the pelvis. There is a marked gender and racial predominance; 94% of patients are men, and two thirds of them are African-American. Many patients have systemic hypertension and are obese. As a result of displacement and compression of the pelvic viscera, obstruction of the urinary tract, rectum, iliac veins, and inferior vena cava may occur. Although usually confined to the pelvis, fibrofatty proliferation may extend cephalad to involve the perinephric space, omentum, and small bowel mesentery.

Urographic findings that suggest this diagnosis include anterosuperior elevation and symmetric compression of the urinary bladder (i.e., pear- or gourd-shaped bladder). The constriction is usually most marked inferiorly. The lower third of the ureters may be deviated medially, and there can be distal ureterectasia to severe hydroureteronephrosis.

Heyns and co-workers reported proliferative cystitis (i.e., cystitis cystica or cystitis glandularis) in 78% of patients with pelvic lipomatosis. Several other diseases have been associated with pelvic lipomatosis, including chronic urinary tract infection, superficial thrombophlebitis, retroperitoneal fibrosis, nontropical chyluria, and the Proteus syndrome (lipomatosis, cutaneous and visceral vascular malformations, hemihypertrophy, and exostoses).

Notes

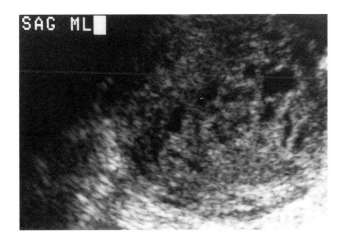

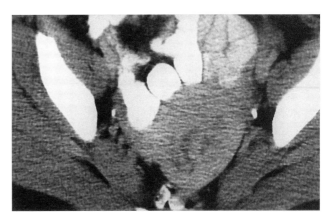

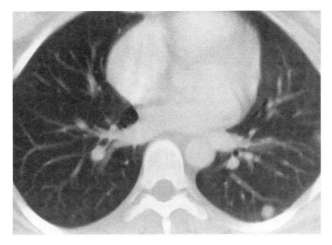

1. A sagittal transvaginal sonogram of the uterus and CT images of the upper pelvis and lower chest are shown. What is the most likely diagnosis?

2. What is the differential diagnosis based on the findings in the images of the uterus?

3. What are the clinical indications for staging this disease?

4. What is the abnormal karyotype of the diseased tissue?

Gestational Trophoblastic Disease

1. Molar pregnancy.

2. Degenerated uterine leiomyoma, hydropic degeneration of the placenta, and endometrial proliferative disease, including carcinoma.

3. Sonographic evaluation is warranted when the uterus is too large for the fetus' gestational age, human chorionic gonadotropin (hCG) titers are disproportionate to the gestational age, there is severe pregnancy-induced hypertension before 24 weeks gestation, and there is vaginal bleeding. CT examination is performed when malignancy is suspected.

4. A complete mole has a 46XX karyotype and likely develops when an egg with an absent nucleus is fertilized by a haploid sperm. Incomplete moles usually (80%) have a karyotype of XXY and present with a triploid dysmorphic fetus.

Reference

Jauniaux E: Ultrasound diagnosis and follow-up of gestational trophoblastic disease, *Ultrasound Obstet Gynecol* 11(5):367-377, 1998.

Cross-Reference

Genitourinary Radiology: THE REQUISITES, pp 294-298.

Comment

The term *gestational trophoblastic disease* (GTD) refers to a spectrum of gestational disease, ranging from the benign (complete [hydatidiform] or partial mole) to the overtly malignant (chorioadenoma destruens and choriocarcinoma). All of these diseases can produce hCG. Affected patients usually have painless vaginal bleeding in the first trimester of pregnancy. Less commonly, patients have severe pregnancy-induced hypertension or hyperemesis gravidarum. Treatment for a molar pregnancy is suction curettage of the endometrial cavity. Successful treatment is heralded by the return of serum hCG levels to normal in 12 weeks.

The sonographic appearance of molar pregnancy is characteristic. The uterus is enlarged, and hydropic degeneration of molar villi produces multiple small (3 to 10 mm in diameter) anechoic structures; this finding has been termed the *cluster of grapes appearance.* The myometrium appears normal. Frequently, accompanying areas of hemorrhage or necrosis present as irregular hypoechoic or anechoic areas. The presence of fetal membranes and parts suggests a partial molar pregnancy. This characteristic appearance may not be present in the first trimester, when the molar tissue may appear as a homogeneous echogenic endometrial mass. Myometrial invasion or abdominal metastatic disease confirms the diagnosis of the malignant form of GTD.

Notes

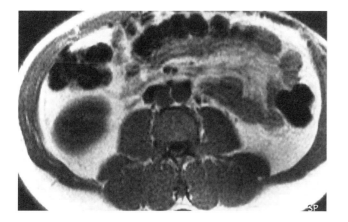
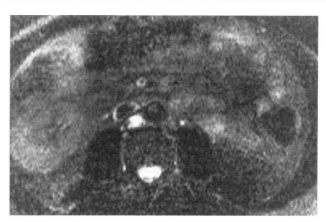

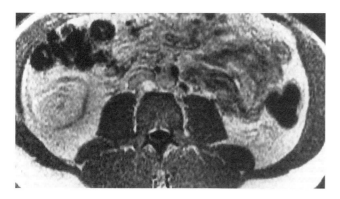

1. Describe the MR images shown.
2. Identify the location of the abnormal tissue on these images.
3. What are the organs of Zuckerkandl? Where are they found?
4. Why is pheochromocytoma sometimes referred to as the *10% tumor?*

Recurrent Extraadrenal Pheochromocytoma

1. The image on the upper left is a transaxial T1W image, the image on the right is a T2W image with fat saturation, and the image on the bottom is an enhanced T1W image.

2. There is a small mass located between and posterior to the aorta and the inferior vena cava.

3. A collection of sympathetic ganglia found at the aortic bifurcation.

4. Approximately 10% are extraadrenal, 10% are found in both adrenal glands, and 10% are malignant. About 10% of patients with von Hippel-Lindau disease have pheochromocytomas, and 10% of pheochromocytomas are inherited (majority as autosomal dominant).

Reference

Francis IR, Korobkin M: Pheochromocytoma, *Radiol Clin North Am* 34(6):1101-1112, 1996.

Cross-Reference

Genitourinary Radiology: THE REQUISITES, pp 351-355.

Comment

Arising from chromaffin cells of the sympathetic nervous system, pheochromocytomas may retain the capacity to produce and secrete catecholamines. Release of norepinephrine and epinephrine may lead to classic symptoms of a "crisis," or the five *p*'s—*p*ain (head, chest, or abdomen), high blood *p*ressure, *p*alpitations, *p*erspiration, and *p*anic. Measurement of unconjugated catecholamines (norepinephrine is more sensitive than epinephrine) or their metabolites (vanillylmandelic acid) in 24-hour urine samples is the most common screening test. A general rule of thumb is that an adrenal pheochromocytoma is more likely when the urine or plasma epinephrine represents 20% or more of the total catecholamines, whereas an extraadrenal pheochromocytoma is found in about one third of cases in which the norepinephrine level alone is elevated.

Pheochromocytomas can arise in sympathetic paraganglia cells from the skull base to the urinary bladder, but 98% are discovered in the abdomen or pelvis. CT is the modality most commonly used for localizing these tumors. On CT, pheochromocytomas are most often single, solid adrenal masses that are more than 2 cm in diameter. However, adrenal pheochromocytomas can be predominantly cystic or complicated by hemorrhage. MRI can be used to confirm a suspected pheochromocytoma; on high-field MRI a pheochromocytoma is isointense to hypointense on T1W images, and 90% are hyperintense on T2W images. Because pheochromocytomas are hypervascular tumors, rapid and prolonged contrast enhancement is typical on MRI. Scintigraphy with either or both metaiodobenzylguanidine I 123 (a guanethidine derivative) and octreotide In 111 (a somatostatin receptor agonist) has been used successfully to localize the tumor.

Notes

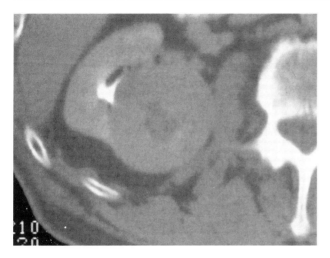

1. What are the two main differential diagnoses for this right renal mass?
2. What feature suggests that this mass may be benign?
3. What angiographic feature helps support the diagnosis of a benign mass?
4. Whether this mass is benign or malignant, what is the conventional management?

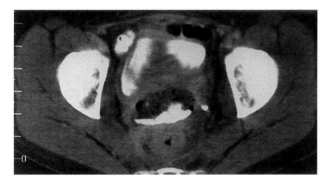 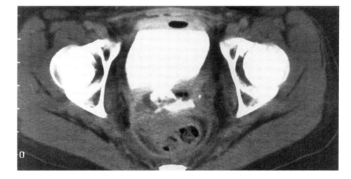

1. What is the most likely diagnosis in this case? What is the most common cause of this lesion in the United States?
2. What is the most common cause of this lesion worldwide?
3. What technical modifications of the CT protocol may improve detection of this lesion?
4. True or False: When this lesion is identified in the patient with cancer, viable tumor is always present.

CASE 150

Renal Oncocytoma

1. Oncocytoma and renal cell carcinoma (RCC).

2. Central stellate low attenuation area.

3. "Spoke wheel" pattern of feeding arteries.

4. Nephrectomy, radical or partial. If the mass is benign, partial nephrectomy is probably favorable.

Reference

Harrison RB, Dyer RB: Benign space-occupying conditions of the kidneys, *Semin Roentgenol* 22:275-283, 1987.

Cross-Reference

Genitourinary Radiology: THE REQUISITES, pp 99-101.

Comment

Of solitary solid, ball-shaped renal masses with no visible fat, 90% are RCCs. However, certain features may suggest alternative diagnoses. One of these features is a central stellate scar in an otherwise homogeneous solid renal mass. This feature is suggestive but not diagnostic of oncocytoma. There are no absolute diagnostic imaging features of oncocytoma. It is best to consider this a surgical renal mass, and if there is no evidence of spread beyond the kidney and if the mass has a favorable location, the surgeon may attempt partial nephrectomy. RCCs may contain oncocytic components, and therefore preoperative percutaneous biopsy does not help the physician make management decisions. Up to 30% of tumors that are predominantly oncocytomas contain foci of RCC. If partial nephrectomy is being contemplated, renal arteriography may help to delineate the number and distribution of renal arteries supplying the kidney and the tumor. Oncocytomas typically have a characteristic angiographic pattern—the "spoke wheel" arteriogram. Unfortunately, this appearance is not diagnostic of oncocytoma and may be seen with RCCs.

Therefore a solitary renal mass containing a central stellate scar should be considered a surgical renal mass. The surgeon should be alerted that the tumor may be benign, and he or she may elect to attempt renal-sparing surgery if the mass' location is amenable.

Notes

CASE 151

Vesicovaginal Fistula After Radiation Therapy for Cervical Cancer

1. Fistula from vagina to bladder. Radiation therapy for cervical carcinoma.

2. Obstetric trauma.

3. Administration of intravenous contrast only, thin-section imaging through the bladder and vagina, and delayed imaging.

4. False.

Reference

Kuhlman JE, Fishman EK: CT evaluation of enterovaginal and vesicovaginal fistulas, *J Comput Assist Tomogr* 14(3):390-394, 1990.

Cross-Reference

Genitourinary Radiology: THE REQUISITES, pp 215, 219.

Comment

Vaginal fistulas to the urinary or gastrointestinal tract reportedly occur in 1% to 10% of patients with cervical cancer who are treated with radiation therapy. Although vesicovaginal or ureterovaginal fistulas occur in patients who have not received radiation treatment, this presentation is uncommon. Some of the risk factors for the development of vaginal fistulas include extensive disease, the addition of hysterectomy to irradiation, and a high cumulative dose of radiation.

Many patients with vesicovaginal fistulas experience the classic symptom of passing urine via the vagina. Urography, cystography, vaginography, cystoscopy, and vaginoscopy have been used to evaluate vaginal fistulas to the urinary tract with variable results. Contrast radiologic studies may not demonstrate the fistula tract, particularly if the fistula is small or if its course is oblique or tortuous. Kuhlman and Fishman report that carefully performed enhanced CT detected 60% of vaginal fistulas to the bladder and bowel, whereas other radiologic and endoscopic studies provided false negative results in 72% of cases. To detect vesicovaginal fistulas, their recommendations for optimal CT technique include (1) administration of intravenous contrast medium but no oral or rectal contrast and (2) additional delayed imaging 5 to 15 minutes later if the initial images show intravesical contrast but no contrast in the vagina. Thin-section (3 to 5 mm) images through the bladder and vagina may detect a small fistula. An additional advantage of CT is that it can provide insight regarding the cause of a vaginal fistula. For instance, in this case note the thickened rectal wall and the stranding of the perirectal fat resulting from radiotherapy.

Notes

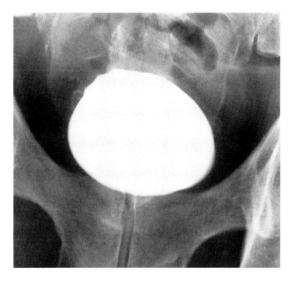 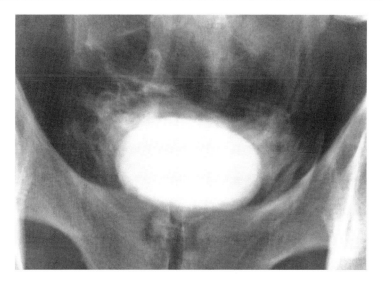

1. What are the different types of blunt traumatic bladder injury?

2. In what percentage of traumatic injuries of the anterior pelvic ring does bladder injury occur?

3. What are some causes of spontaneous bladder rupture?

4. This patient has chronic renal failure and is being evaluated for renal transplantation. What is the diagnosis?

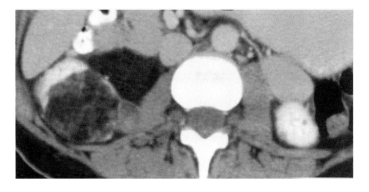 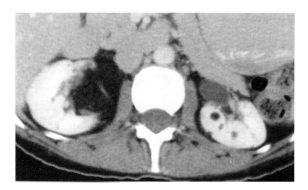

1. What is the diagnosis of the mass in the upper pole of the right kidney?

2. What syndrome does this patient probably have?

3. Besides the mass in the right kidney, what is another common renal manifestation of this syndrome?

4. What are some of the common extrarenal manifestations of this syndrome?

CASE 152

Extravasation in an Unused Urinary Bladder

1. Mural contusion, partial-thickness laceration, and full-thickness bladder laceration.

2. 7% to 10%.

3. Lesions that thin or weaken the bladder wall, bladder outlet obstruction, neurogenic bladder, cystitis, radiation treatment, tumor, and perivesical inflammation.

4. Extraperitoneal rupture of an unused bladder.

References

Caroline DF, Pollack HM, Banner MP, Schneck C: Self-limiting extravasation in the unused urinary bladder, *Radiology* 155(2):311-313, 1985.

Matsumoto AH, Clark RL, Cuttino JT Jr: Bladder mucosal tears during voiding cystourethrography in chronic renal failure, *Urol Radiol* 8:81-84, 1986.

Cross-Reference

Genitourinary Radiology: THE REQUISITES, pp 224-229.

Comment

Full-thickness rupture of the bladder most often occurs after pelvic trauma and is generally accompanied by local (pain, tenderness, and guarding) and systemic (fever and malaise) symptoms. However, bladder rupture can be spontaneous or iatrogenic (e.g., occurring after cesarean section or transurethral bladder resection). Isolated extraperitoneal rupture (prevalence, 50% to 85%) is more common than either isolated intraperitoneal rupture (prevalence, 15% to 45%) or combined intraperitoneal and extraperitoneal rupture (prevalence, 5% to 10%). Although intraperitoneal bladder lacerations are less commonly associated with traumatic osseous pelvic injury, between 80% and 95% of traumatic extraperitoneal ruptures are associated with fractures of the anterior pubic ring or diastasis of the pubic symphysis.

Although complications are rare, mucosal tears and self-limited contrast extravasation have been reported in unused urinary bladders during cystourethrography. Over time, the nonfunctioning bladder becomes hypertonic and less compliant. These changes are likely to be intrinsic properties of the unused detrusor muscle because they develop independent of infection, inflammation, denervation, or fibrosis. Unused bladders are studied to evaluate bladder capacity, vesicoureteral reflux, or urethral anatomy. Acute distention of the bladder beyond its normal capacity during cystourethrography may cause small rents in the mucosa. Contrast gradually dissects within the bladder wall, and extravasation may be visible at the lateral border of the bladder trigone near the ureteral orifices. However, it never extends much further than the immediate perivesical space.

Notes

CASE 153

Tuberous Sclerosis

1. Angiomyolipoma (AML).

2. Tuberous sclerosis.

3. Renal cysts.

4. Central nervous system hamartomas, facial adenoma sebaceum, pulmonary lymphangioleiomyomatosis, cardiac rhabdomyomas, and cutaneous shagreen patches.

Reference

Wagner BJ, Won-You-Cheong JJ, Davis CJ: Adult renal hamartomas, *Radiographics* 17:155-169, 1997.

Cross-Reference

Genitourinary Radiology: THE REQUISITES, pp 111, 112, 142.

Comment

Renal tumors that contain fat can be diagnosed as AMLs with near certainty. These tumors usually are isolated findings in middle-aged or older adults. Of patients with tuberous sclerosis, 80% develop AMLs. Patients with tuberous sclerosis usually develop AMLs earlier in life and develop larger and more numerous masses than patients who do not have this syndrome. This patient demonstrates multiple bilateral AMLs, with two large AMLs in the right kidney, one of which extends into the renal sinus and perirenal space. Tuberous sclerosis is an autosomal dominant hereditary disorder characterized by the triad of facial adenoma sebaceum, periventricular hamartomas in the brain, and mental retardation. The extent of penetrance of each of these symptoms varies among patients with tuberous sclerosis. Approximately 20% of patients with tuberous sclerosis also develop renal cysts.

Notes

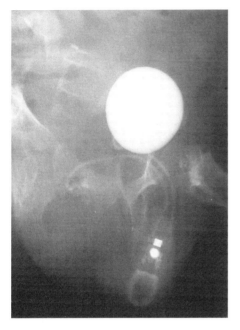 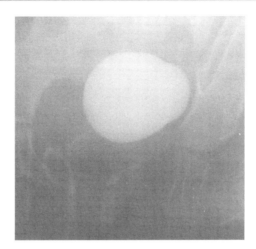

1. What device is shown on the radiograph to the left?

2. The radiograph on the right was taken 2 years later. What is the diagnosis?

3. What is the most common indication for the implantation of this device in children?

4. True or False: A normal upper urinary tract is considered a prerequisite for implanting this device.

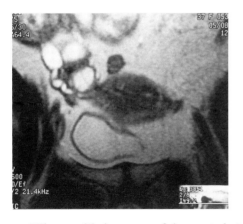 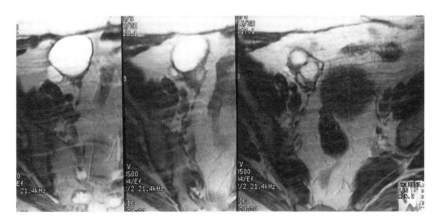

1. What are likely causes of the cystic lesion demonstrated on these T2W images?

2. Stenosis or occlusion is most likely to occur in which segment of the fallopian tube?

3. What are some of the common causes of hydrosalpinx?

4. Is hydrosalpinx often caused by primary or metastatic tumors of the fallopian tube?

Artificial Urinary Sphincter

1. Artificial urinary sphincter (AUS).

2. Deformity suggests mechanical failure of the reservoir.

3. Incontinence as a result of spinal dysraphism.

4. True.

Reference

Simeoni J, Guys JM, Mollard P, et al: Artificial urinary sphincter implantation for neurogenic bladder: a multi-institutional study in 107 children, *Br J Urol* 78:287-293, 1996.

Cross-Reference

Genitourinary Radiology: THE REQUISITES, pp 229-233.

Comment

The AUS was introduced in 1972 and has been used in the management of stress incontinence and postprostatectomy sphincter weakness and as a part of complex reconstructive surgery of the lower urinary tract. In the large series referenced above, the most common indication for implantation of the AUS in children was incontinence caused by spinal dysraphism.

The AUS consists of the following three tube-connected components: (1) a pressure-regulated reservoir in the abdomen, (2) a pump (in this case placed in the scrotum), and (3) a peri-urethral cuff. The reservoir, filled with dilute iodinated contrast, maintains a constant and predetermined pressure in the peri-urethral cuff, which can be placed around the bladder neck or bulbar urethra. When squeezed, the scrotal pump shifts fluid out of the cuff and into the reservoir. This action decreases the urethral pressure to permit bladder emptying. Fluid then is automatically returned to the cuff by a resistor that is incorporated in the pump.

Despite achieving urinary continence in 77% of children, the AUS has a reported long-term complication rate of 59%. Complications include mechanical problems with the AUS, surgical complications, and long-term bladder adaptations. The most common mechanical problem is pump malfunction. A common surgical complication is erosion of the bulbous urethra or bladder neck caused by an improperly fitted cuff. Detrusor hyperreflexia and low bladder compliance are the most common changes in bladder function that occur with long-term use. There is a high incidence of secondary reflux in patients with neurogenic bladder that might be exacerbated by the AUS. Hence a normal upper urinary tract and, if necessary, surgical treatment of vesicoureteral reflux are necessary before implantation of the AUS.

Notes

Hydrosalpinx on MRI

1. Ovarian cyst, paraovarian cyst, hydrosalpinx, and endometrial cyst.

2. Fimbria.

3. Salpingitis, tubal surgery, pelvic endometriosis, and tubal adenomyosis.

4. No.

Reference

Outwater EK, Siegelman ES, Chiowanich P, Kilger AM, Dunton CJ, Talerman A: Dilated fallopian tubes: MR imaging characteristics, *Radiology* 208:463-469, 1998.

Cross-Reference

Genitourinary Radiology: THE REQUISITES, pp 277, 278, 283-289.

Comment

Tubal occlusion may occur at the fimbrial end, at the middle segment, or at the isthmus-cornua junction of the fallopian tube. Causes of fimbrial occlusion include prior salpingitis and use of an intrauterine device. Tubal sterilization is the most common cause of middle segment occlusion; in countries where the disease is endemic, tuberculosis also may cause ampullary tubal stenosis. Occlusion of the tube at the isthmus near the cornu may be congenital or may be caused by endometriosis, tubal adenomyosis, or infection.

The diagnosis of hydrosalpinx is relatively simple to make on hysterosalpingography but is often more difficult on ultrasound and MRI. A dilated fallopian tube can mimic a complex cystic ovarian or adnexal mass, but there are several clues to its diagnosis. Dilated uterine tubes may appear as fluid-filled tubular structures folded into partial C or S shapes. Within the dilated fallopian tube, longitudinal mucosal folds, called *plicae,* may be visible. Pathologic correlation shows that these longitudinal folds result from effacement of the mucosa and submucosa by the dilated lumen. Alternatively, plicae may be visible because normal mucosal folds are blunted by chronic salpingitis. The signal intensity of the fluid within the dilated tube on MRI may suggest a cause of the hydrosalpinx. For example, Outwater and colleagues reported that fluid of high signal intensity on T1W images was significantly correlated with endometriosis in the tubes and pelvis. On T2W images the signal intensity of fluid within the dilated tube also was high, in contrast to the signal intensity of a typical endometrial cyst (i.e., moderate or marked T2 shortening caused by "shading").

Notes

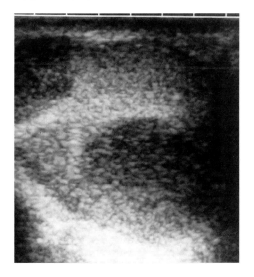 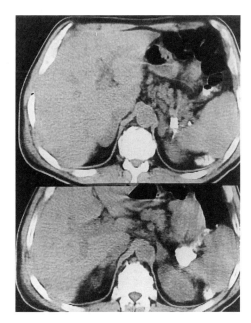

1. A sagittal sonogram of the testis and images from an abdominal CT scan in a 57-year-old man are shown. What is the most likely diagnosis?

2. What is the differential diagnosis for bilateral adrenal masses?

3. Given the clinical history of a bronchogenic carcinoma, what is the most likely cause of bilateral adrenal masses?

4. True or False: Adrenal insufficiency is a common presentation of this disease.

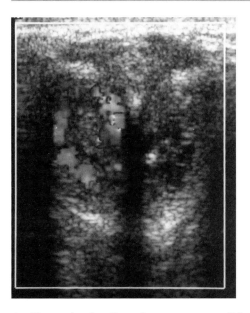 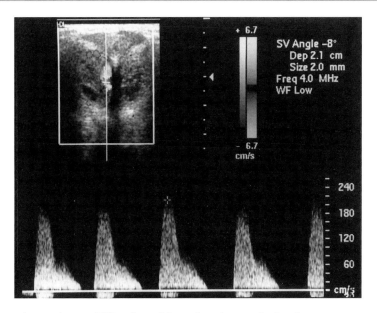

1. Coronal color Doppler sonograms of the penis are shown. Why does this patient have priapism?

2. What is the differential diagnosis for a vascular penoscrotal mass?

3. What clinical sign or signs may be helpful in differentiating this lesion from other scrotal vascular lesions?

4. How is this lesion treated?

Adrenal Lymphoma

1. Adrenal lymphoma or leukemia.

2. Benign tumors (adenomas, nonsporadic pheochromocytomas, and macronodular hyperplasia), malignancies (metastases and lymphoma), hemorrhage, and granulomatous adrenalitis (tuberculosis and histoplasmosis).

3. Bilateral adenomas.

4. True.

Reference

Wang J, Sun NCJ, Rensio R, et al: Clinically silent primary adrenal lymphoma: a case report and review of the literature, *Am J Hematol* 58:130-136, 1998.

Cross-Reference

Genitourinary Radiology: THE REQUISITES, pp 359, 360.

Comment

Primary lymphoma of the adrenal gland (PLA) is thought to arise from intrinsic hematopoietic tissue and is extremely uncommon; only about 65 cases have been reported. PLA tends to affect older men (median age, 68 years; male/female ratio, 2.2:1). Half of the cases manifested adrenocortical insufficiency even when the tumors were small. There also was a high incidence of immunodeficiency in patients with PLA; concurrent cancer or a medical history of cancer, HIV infection, or other autoimmune diseases were reported in 15% of patients. Diffuse large cell non-Hodgkin's lymphoma is the most common morphologic type, and the majority are B cells. The prognosis for patients with PLA is decidedly grim; of the case reports and series that reported follow up, most patients died as a result of tumor, intercurrent diseases, or infection within 1 year.

On CT, adrenal lymphoma presents as a complex mass with variable density, although some lymphomas are homogeneous, as in the case presented here. Cystic and necrotic adrenal masses also have been reported. Masses ranged in size from 3 to 17 cm in diameter, and bilateral masses were reported in 72% of cases. Because there is no pathognomonic appearance of adrenal lymphoma, percutaneous needle biopsy has been an effective means of establishing the diagnosis. Percutaneous aspiration is less reliable because PLA may be misdiagnosed as poorly differentiated carcinoma.

Notes

Posttraumatic Scrotal Arteriovenous Fistula

1. Markedly increased arterial inflow.

2. Varicocele, hemangioma, lymphangioma, and arteriovenous (AV) malformation.

3. Bruit may be audible in cases of penoscrotal AV malformation.

4. Surgical excision; successful endovascular treatment has not been reported.

References

Forstner R, Hricak H, Kalbhen CL, Kogan BA, McAninch JW: Magnetic resonance imaging of vascular lesions of the scrotum and penis, *J Urol* 46(4):581-583, 1995.

Sule JD, Lemmers MJ, Barry JM: Scrotal arteriovenous malformation: case report and literature review, *J Urol* 150:1917-1919, 1993.

Cross-Reference

Genitourinary Radiology: THE REQUISITES, pp 337-341.

Comment

The differential diagnosis of a scrotal vascular mass includes varicocele, vascular tumor (hemangioma and lymphangioma), and AV malformation. Varicocele is by far the most common and is diagnosed by the presence of multiple, dilated (≥ 2 mm in diameter) veins in the pampiniform plexus of the spermatic cord. Hemangioma and lymphangioma are benign congenital vascular tumors that usually manifest in the third to fifth decades of life as scrotal swelling, bleeding, or severe pain. Scrotal AV malformations are rare; only five cases have been reported. These vascular malformations may be congenital or may slowly develop after traumatic injury; patients have bloody meatal discharge, a palpable mass, or priapism. A bruit at auscultation may allow differentiation of AV malformation from the varicocele and vascular tumor. Angiographic embolization has been used to reduce flow before surgery but has not been successful as definitive treatment of AV malformations.

Noninvasive investigation of scrotal vascular masses has included sonography and MRI. Duplex sonography may demonstrate a venous flow pattern in varicoceles and high velocity arterial flow in the more extensive AV malformation. MRI of the AV malformation may demonstrate multiple serpentine vessels in the subcutaneous tissues of the scrotum and penis; involvement of the testes and urethra by the malformation also can be evaluated. In contrast, a lymphohemangioma appears as a focal hyperintense mass on T2W MRI.

Notes

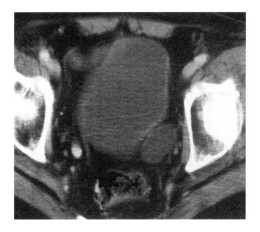 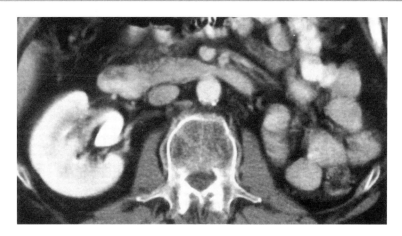

1. What is the differential diagnosis for a paraprostatic cyst?
2. What prostatic cysts are associated with renal agenesis?
3. What renal and ureteral anomalies are associated with seminal vesicle cysts?
4. Are seminal vesicle cysts congenital or acquired?

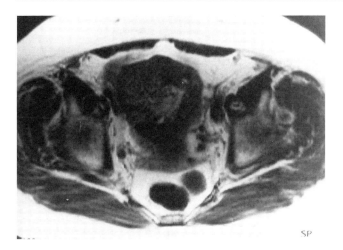 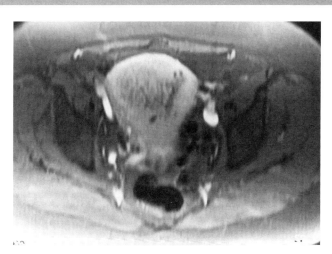

1. Describe the type of MR images (i.e., T1W or T2W, with or without contrast administration, with or without fat saturation) shown.
2. Given a history of postmenopausal bleeding, what is the most likely diagnosis?
3. What are the major prognostic factors for this disease?
4. True or False: MRI is routinely used to stage this disease before surgery.

Zinner Syndrome (Seminal Vesicle Cyst with Renal Agenesis)

1. Lateral paraprostatic cysts include seminal vesicle and vas deferens cysts; müllerian duct cysts tend to be midline. Bladder diverticula may be either lateral or midline.

2. Cysts of Wolffian duct derivation; rarely renal agenesis is associated with utricular and müllerian duct cysts.

3. Ipsilateral renal agenesis, renal ectopia, adult polycystic kidney disease, collecting system duplication, and ectopic ureteral insertion.

4. Either.

Reference

King BF, Hattery RR, Lieber MM, et al: Congenital cystic disease of the seminal vesicle, *Radiology* 178:207-211, 1991.

Cross-Reference

Genitourinary Radiology: THE REQUISITES, pp 326, 327.

Comment

The duct of the seminal vesicle joins the ampulla of the vas deferens to form the ejaculatory duct. Cysts of the seminal vesicle may form after either congenital (atresia) or acquired obstruction of the ejaculatory duct. Some examples of acquired causes include chronic prostatitis and benign prostatic hyperplasia. Patients with seminal vesicle cysts may have an asymptomatic pelvic mass, infertility, hematuria, hemospermia, postejaculatory perineal pain, or epididymitis. Fluid aspirated from a seminal vesicle cyst is often hemorrhagic and contains inactive sperm.

Zinner syndrome, or the coexistence of renal dysgenesis or agenesis and ipsilateral seminal vesicle cysts, was first described in 1914. Approximately two thirds of patients with seminal vesicle cysts have ipsilateral renal agenesis. The association is explained by the common embryologic origin of the male internal genital system and the ureters. At about the fifth fetal week, the ureteric buds (metanephric ducts) branch from the mesonephric (Wolffian) ducts and extend to the metanephric blastema; the ureteric bud eventually induces the formation of the permanent kidney. Later in normal development, the Wolffian duct separates from the metanephric duct and persists in the male as the appendix of the epididymis, paradidymis, epididymis, vas deferens, ejaculatory duct, seminal vesicle, and hemitrigone of the bladder. Early dysgenesis of the mesonephric duct may explain the association of unilateral renal agenesis (which affects about 0.1% of the population) and ipsilateral genital tract anomalies.

Seminal vesicle cysts also are associated with cystic renal disease. Even in the absence of a family history, an evaluation of the kidneys for adult-type polycystic renal disease is warranted in patients with seminal vesicle cysts, particularly when bilateral.

Notes

Endometrial Carcinoma: Depth of Myometrial Invasion

1. Spin-echo T1W image through the uterus (on the left) and enhanced T1W image with frequency-selective fat saturation (on the right).

2. Endometrial carcinoma with deep myometrial invasion.

3. Histologic type and differentiation (grade) and stage of disease.

4. False.

References

Rose PG: Endometrial carcinoma, *N Engl J Med* 335(9):640-649, 1996.

Takahashi S, Murakami T, Narumi Y, et al: Preoperative staging of endometrial carcinoma: diagnostic effect of T2-weighted fast spin-echo MR imaging, *Radiology* 206:539-547, 1998.

Cross-Reference

Genitourinary Radiology: THE REQUISITES, pp 290-294.

Comment

The depth of myometrial invasion is a consistent indicator of the virulence of endometrial carcinoma. Patients with deeper myometrial invasion, defined as invasion of the outer half of the myometrium, are more likely to have local recurrence and have lower survival rates.

Because surgery is the initial treatment in most patients with uterine cancer, the comprehensive evaluation of disease extent at the time of surgery has supplanted routine abdominopelvic imaging for the initial staging of this disease. Preoperative staging of myometrial invasion by transvaginal sonography or enhanced MRI may be necessary if the gynecologist does not perform routine nodal dissection or if the patient is premenopausal and wishes to preserve fertility. If the myometrium is not invaded, nodal metastases are present in about 3% of patients, but if myometrial invasion is deep (stage Ic), the prevalence of nodal metastases increases to about 40%. The reported concordance of MRI with the histologic examination for distinguishing superficial from deep myometrial invasion is about 80%. Myometrial invasion is staged by comparing the maximal depth of tumor relative to the absolute thickness of the myometrial wall; if more than half of the wall is occupied by tumor, deep myometrial invasion is diagnosed. Assessing the integrity of the junctional zone (inner third of the myometrium) is crucial because myometrial invasion is superficial if the T2 hypointense junctional zone is intact.

Notes

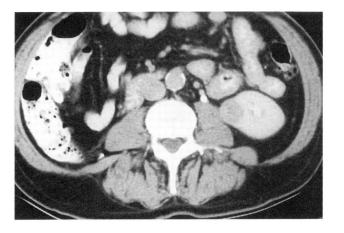

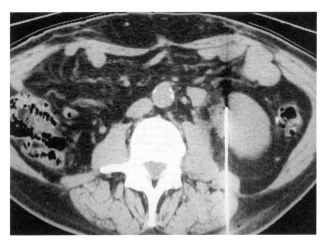

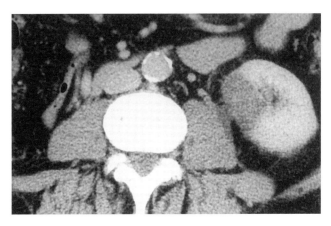

1. What are the important findings on the upper-left image?

2. The patient had a right total nephrectomy to treat renal cell carcinoma. How does this impact treatment options?

3. Name two treatment options for this patient.

4. What is the mechanism of action of radiofrequency ablation?

Radiofrequency Ablation of a Renal Cell Carcinoma

1. Solid mass in the left kidney and right nephrectomy.

2. Left nephrectomy would necessitate long-term dialysis because patients with a history of cancer are not usually considered for renal transplantation.

3. Partial nephrectomy and percutaneous tumor ablation using cryotherapy or radiofrequency (RF) therapy.

4. Deposition of RF energy into a tissue causes local heating of the tissue and cell death.

References

Lewin JS, Connell CF, Duerk JL, et al: Interactive MR imaging-guided radiofrequency interstitial thermal ablation of abdominal tumors: clinical trial for evaluation of safety and feasibility, *J Magn Reson Imaging* 8:40-47, 1998.

Zlotta AR, Wildschutz T, Raviv G, et al: Radiofrequency interstitial tumor ablation (RITA) is a possible new modality for treatment of renal cancer: ex vivo and in vivo experience, *J Endourol* 11:251-258, 1997.

Cross-Reference

Genitourinary Radiology: THE REQUISITES, pp 89-100, 390, 391.

Comment

The image on the right shows an RF probe positioned in a small, solid left renal tumor. The bottom image, obtained weeks later, shows local tissue necrosis and normal enhancement of untreated renal parenchyma.

Nephrectomy is the first-line treatment for patients with localized renal cell carcinoma (RCC). More recently, partial nephrectomy or nephron-sparing surgery has been advocated. However, these operations are technically difficult and when compared with total nephrectomy are associated with higher rates of complications from bleeding and postoperative collections.

New percutaneous techniques have been developed to treat patients with either primary or metastatic abdominal neoplastic disease. These techniques include cryoablation and RF ablation. The advantage of RF ablation therapy is that a smaller electrode can be used, the equipment is less complicated, and the area of tumor "kill" is easier to control. Alternating current in the RF range causes local ionic agitation and frictional heat. As a result, interstitial temperatures in excess of 50° C produce coagulative necrosis. Shielded probes and electrodes of various sizes have been designed to concentrate the RF energy in different tissue volumes. The largest volume of tumor necrosis per ablation is a 3-cm-diameter sphere.

Notes

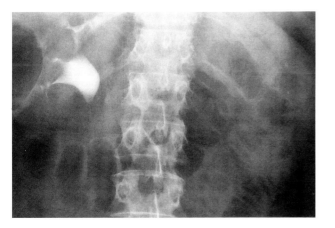
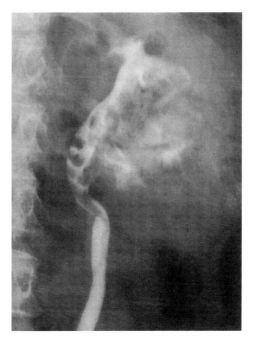

1. An intravenous urogram and a retrograde pyelogram are shown. What is the most likely cause of the ureteral obstruction in this patient?

2. In this patient with gross hematuria, what are likely underlying causes of the bleeding?

3. What are the most common causes of radiolucent filling defects that are visible on contrast studies of the pyelocalyceal system?

4. What enzyme in urine leads to rapid change of pyelocalyceal blood clots?

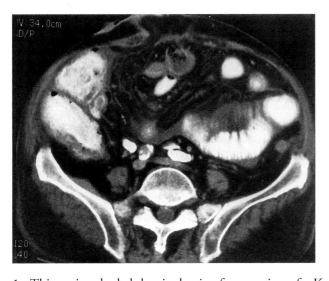
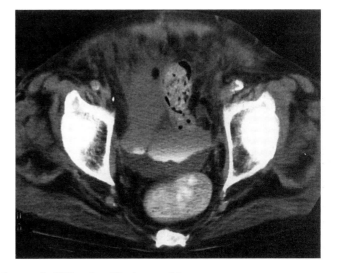

1. This patient had abdominal pain after creation of a Kock pouch. What is a Kock pouch?

2. What complication should be diagnosed in this case?

3. Name late complications of the Kock pouch.

4. Why do some patients with a Kock pouch develop megaloblastic anemia?

Pyelocalyceal Blood Clot

1. Blood clot, infectious debris, or fungal material.

2. Transitional cell carcinoma, renal cell carcinoma, or vascular malformation.

3. In order of descending frequency, radiolucent stones, urothelial neoplasms, blood clots, infectious debris, sloughed papilla, and fungal material.

4. Urokinase.

References

Fein AB, McClennan BL: Solitary filling defects of the ureter, *Semin Roentgenol* 21:201-213, 1986.

Williamson J Jr, Hartman GW, Hattery RR: Multiple and diffuse ureteral filling defects, *Semin Roentgenol* 21:214-223, 1986.

Cross-Reference

Genitourinary Radiology: THE REQUISITES, pp 185, 186.

Comment

There are numerous causes of radiolucent filling defects in the urinary tract. The most common of these causes are solid lesions, including uric acid stones and neoplasms, which are noncompliant. Alternatively, other causes of radiolucent filling defects, such as blood clot, infectious debris, and fungal material, are compliant and tend to conform to the shape of their container, in this case the pyelocalyceal system. In this case the intravenous urogram demonstrates unilateral nephromegaly and evidence of ureteral obstruction with delayed pyelogram. The retrograde study shows a large amount of radiolucent material, some of which is linear, that conforms to the shape of the ureter. This finding indicates a liquid or semisolid material in the pyelocalyceal system, making the diagnosis of blood clot the most likely in this patient with gross hematuria. Unfortunately, blood clots obscure the pyelocalyceal system, making diagnosis of an underlying lesion difficult. When gross hematuria is present, a search for the source of the bleeding is relevant. Sometimes the cause of intermittent gross hematuria remains occult, but common causes include urothelial neoplasm, renal cell carcinoma, vascular malformation, and traumatic injury.

In this case a follow-up retrograde study performed 1 week later demonstrated complete resolution of the filling defect and a normal-appearing pyelocalyceal system with no evidence of urothelial neoplasm. As is typical of clots in the urinary tract, it evolved and changed rapidly because of urokinase in the urine. Large clots can be completely lysed within a few days. This rapid change, when seen on sequential studies, helps to confirm the diagnosis of blood clot as the cause of radiolucent filling defects.

Notes

Urinary Leak from Kock Pouch

1. Continent cutaneous urinary diversion created from detubularized ileum.

2. Urinary leak.

3. Pouch stones, afferent nipple stenosis, ureteral reflux, incisional hernia, and anterior urethral stricture (in patients with hemi-Kock neobladder).

4. If more than 50 cm of terminal ileum is used to create this reservoir, diminished absorption of vitamin B_{12} may occur.

Reference

Nieh PT: The Kock pouch urinary reservoir, *Urol Clin North Am* 24(4):755-772, 1997.

Cross-Reference

Genitourinary Radiology: THE REQUISITES, pp 233-235.

Comment

The Kock pouch is a continent cutaneous urinary reservoir created from an 80-cm segment of ileum that has been detubularized (split longitudinally). The proximal end of ileum is intussuscepted to create a long, nonrefluxing nipple valve, and spatulated distal ureters are attached to this afferent limb. An efferent continence nipple valve is formed for the stoma, sited on the lower abdominal wall. Over time, long-term exposure of the ileal mucosa to urine results in diminished prominence of the villi and production of mucus. A modification of this procedure is the hemi-Kock neobladder in which the most dependent portion of the pouch is anastomosed to the urethra.

Kock reservoirs are most often created for patients undergoing total cystectomy to treat bladder cancer; other situations in which these reservoirs are used include salvage prostatectomy to treat prostate cancer, refractory interstitial cystitis, neurogenic bladder, radiation cystitis, and conversion from other types of urinary diversions.

Early and late complications occur in approximately 15% of patients. The major early complications related to the pouch include anastomotic urine leak (2.5%), dehydration (2%), and urosepsis (1.7%). In this case urinary leak was suspected when a large amount of "free fluid" was noted on noncontrast CT. Anastomotic leak was confirmed on enhanced CT that demonstrated extravasated contrast pooling in the pelvis. Major late complications include struvite pouch stones (4%), afferent nipple stenosis (3%), and reflux (2%). Tumor may recur in the reservoir or upper urinary tracts.

Notes

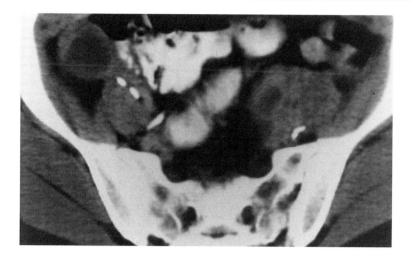

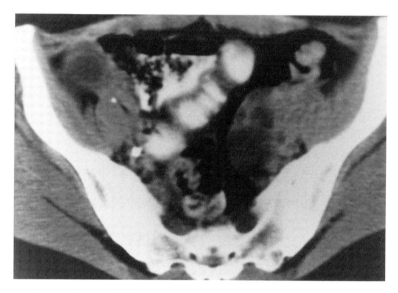

1. Images from a CT scan through the upper pelvis are shown. What are the bilateral low density masses?

2. The patient underwent an operative procedure to move the gonads out of the lower pelvis. What is the name of this procedure?

3. Why was this operation performed?

4. What imaging procedure could be performed to confirm this anatomic finding?

Ovarian Pexy

1. Ovaries.

2. Ovarian pexy.

3. To remove gonadal tissue from the therapeutic radiation field.

4. Transabdominal sonography or MRI.

Reference

Hricak H, Yu KK: Radiology in invasive cervical cancer, *Am J Roentgenol* 167:1101-1108, 1996.

Cross-Reference

Genitourinary Radiology: THE REQUISITES, pp 295-301.

Comment

This young woman with cervical carcinoma was treated with hysterectomy and postoperative radiation therapy. The ovaries were moved out of the pelvis and "pexed" along the superior pelvic sidewall so that they would not be included in the radiation field. Knowledge of this procedure is important so that the pexed ovary is not confused with adenopathy, particularly if one ovary has been removed. If necessary, appropriate imaging modalities, including transabdominal ultrasound (the ovaries are usually too high to be seen with transvaginal sonography) or MRI, can confirm the location of a pexed ovary.

Patients with early invasive carcinoma (stages Ib and IIa) have a 10% to 15% risk of pelvic nodal spread of disease and a 5% risk of periaortic lymph node involvement. These patients usually require radical hysterectomy with lymphadenectomy, with or without radiation therapy. Because early cervical carcinoma rarely spreads to the ovaries, oophorectomy usually is not performed. Patients retain ovarian function; do not suffer from secondary complications of oophorectomy, such as osteoporosis; and do not require exogenous hormone supplementation. Pelvic radiation to the ovaries results in loss of ovarian function. This disadvantage favors surgical treatment of early cervical cancer over radiation and explains why ovarian pexy is performed in patients who may subsequently undergo radiation therapy.

Notes

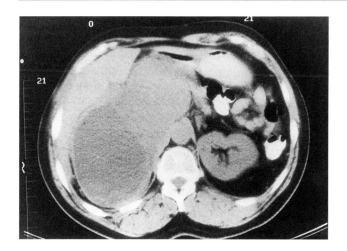 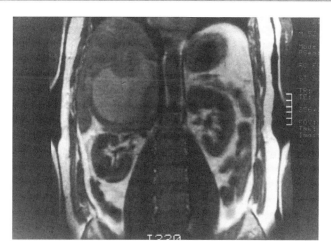

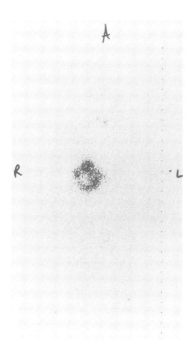

1. What is the differential diagnosis for this right adrenal mass?

2. What is the finding on the nuclear medicine study? What type of radiopharmaceutical was administered?

3. True or False: Aspiration of cyst fluid should be recommended next.

4. True or False: The majority of adrenocortical carcinomas are larger than 6 cm in diameter, contain areas of cystic necrosis, and may have foci of calcification.

Cystic Pheochromocytoma

1. Chronic hematoma (pseudocyst), necrotic metastasis, "cystic" pheochromocytoma, adrenocortical carcinoma, adrenal cyst, and parasitic cyst.

2. Metaiodobenzylguanidine (MIBG) I-123 scan shows increased uptake in right adrenal mass.

3. False.

4. True.

References

Belden CJ, Powers C, Ros PR: MR demonstration of a cystic pheochromocytoma, *J Magn Reson Imaging* 5:778-780, 1995.

McCorkell SJ, Niles NL: Fine-needle aspiration of catecholamine-producing adrenal masses: a possibly fatal mistake, *Am J Roentgenol* 145:113-114, 1985.

Cross-Reference

Genitourinary Radiology: THE REQUISITES, pp 351-355.

Comment

Rarely, pheochromocytoma may present as a large cystic adrenal mass because of central necrosis. Biochemical screening (measurement of unconjugated catecholamines and vanillylmandelic acid levels in a 24-hour urine collection) or nuclear medicine tests (MIBG I 123 or octreotide In 111) to exclude a pheochromocytoma should precede aspiration or biopsy of an adrenal mass. However, normal or only minimally abnormal results of biochemical screening tests for catecholamine production have been reported in some cases of cystic pheochromocytoma.

Percutaneous needle aspiration or biopsy (PNAB) of a pheochromocytoma may result in potentially fatal complications. During adrenal angiography, catecholamine storm leading to hypertensive crisis has been reported in up to half of patients with unsuspected pheochromocytomas, and a similar risk has been postulated for PNAB. Because pheochromocytoma is a hypervascular neoplasm, catastrophic retroperitoneal hemorrhage is another potential complication.

Sympathomedullary imaging has been made possible with MIBG, an analog of norepinephrine. MIBG I 123 is particularly useful for detecting extraadrenal and metastatic pheochromocytomas because the whole body can be evaluated. It is also useful in the patient who has a suspected recurrence of pheochromocytoma after adrenalectomy because surgical clips or distorted anatomy may reduce the accuracy of CT or MRI. A significant number of medications may interfere with the accumulation of MIBG. Tricyclic antidepressants, labetalol, and cocaine are just a few of the medications that can decrease MIBG uptake by sympathomedullary tissues.

Notes

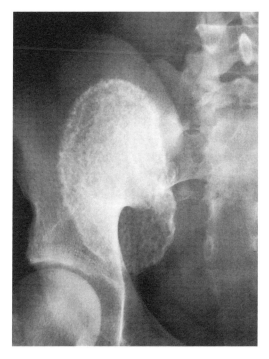

1. What part of the renal parenchyma is calcified in this kidney?
2. What are the major causes of this pattern of renal calcification?
3. What are the common causes of medullary nephrocalcinosis?
4. What causes calcification in patients with this pattern of nephrocalcinosis?

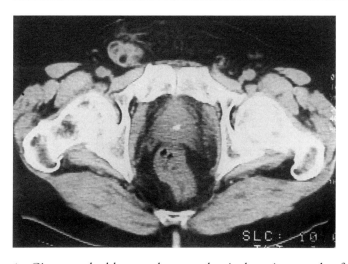 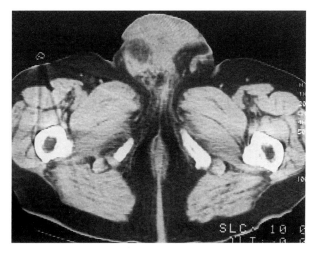

1. Given a palpable scrotal mass, what is the primary role of scrotal sonography? Why is this distinction important?
2. What is the most common tumor of the epididymis?
3. True or False: The most common extratesticular malignant tumor is a peritoneal metastasis.
4. What is the most common tumor that arises from an undescended testicle?

Cortical Nephrocalcinosis

1. Cortex.

2. Chronic renal failure, acute cortical necrosis, oxalosis, Alport's syndrome, and chronic transplant rejection.

3. Hypercalcemia, medullary sponge kidney, and renal tubular acidosis.

4. Dystrophic calcification of necrotic renal cortex.

Reference

Davidson AJ, Hartman DS, editors: *Radiology of the kidney and urinary tract,* ed 2, Philadelphia, 1994, Saunders, pp 177-189.

Cross-Reference

Genitourinary Radiology: THE REQUISITES, pp 146, 147.

Comment

Unlike medullary nephrocalcinosis, which usually results from precipitation of calcium products within tubules or in normal renal tissue, cortical nephrocalcinosis results from dystrophic calcification secondary to a prior insult, usually ischemia. The major causes of this pattern of renal calcification have in common cortical necrosis caused by either ischemia or inflammation.

Cortical nephrocalcinosis is easily recognized by its eggshell pattern of calcification. At the edges of the kidney, where it is seen in profile, the calcification tends to have a "tram track" pattern, as seen in this image of a transplant kidney. As is also illustrated by this patient with chronic transplant rejection, most patients with cortical nephrocalcinosis have global atrophy of the kidney, causing small, smooth kidneys and chronic renal insufficiency.

Notes

Liposarcoma of the Spermatic Cord

1. To distinguish an intratesticular mass from an extratesticular one. Solid intratesticular masses are often malignant neoplasms; solid extratesticular masses are rarely malignant.

2. Adenomatoid tumor.

3. False.

4. Seminoma.

References

Cardenosa G, Papanicolaou N, Fung CY, et al: Spermatic cord sarcomas: sonographic and CT features, *Urol Radiol* 12:163-167, 1990.

Frates MC, Benson CB, DiSalvo DN, et al: Solid extratesticular masses evaluated with sonography: pathologic correlation, *Radiology* 204:43-46, 1997.

Cross-Reference

Genitourinary Radiology: THE REQUISITES, p 310.

Comment

Malignant tumors account for only 3% of all solid extratesticular lesions, whereas 90% to 95% of solid intratesticular lesions are malignant. Ultrasound accurately distinguishes intratesticular from extratesticular solid masses in 95% to 100% of cases and therefore is usually performed early in the evaluation of a palpable scrotal mass. However, no sonographic features reliably permit the distinction between a benign and malignant extratesticular mass. In the series of 19 solid extratesticular masses reported by Frates and colleagues, 16 were benign and included adenomatoid tumor of the epididymis, lipoma, sarcoidosis (bilateral), sperm granuloma, leiomyoma, benign inflammatory nodule, and fibroma; two of the three malignant tumors arose from the spermatic cord.

The spermatic cord originates at the internal inguinal ring and descends to the testis through the inguinal canal. It contains the testicular artery and vein, the cremasteric and deferential vessels, and the lymphatics. In addition, components of the ventral abdominal wall are incorporated in the spermatic cord and include the internal and external spermatic fascia and cremasteric layer. The predominance of mesodermal elements explains the prevalence of sarcomas amongst malignant tumors that arise from the spermatic cord.

Spermatic cord sarcoma is a rare cause of a solid extratesticular mass. In adults, liposarcoma, leiomyosarcoma, and malignant fibrous histiocytoma have been reported, and in infants and children, rhabdomyosarcoma is the most common type of tumor. Lymphatic spread (paraaortic lymphadenopathy) has been reported in up to one third of patients with poorly differentiated tumors.

Notes

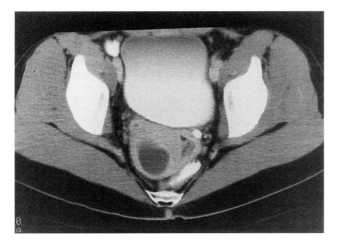
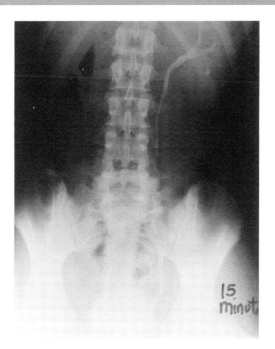

1. What is the differential diagnosis for this fluid-filled pelvic mass?
2. How does the urogram help with the diagnosis in this case?
3. What is the most common structural cause of primary amenorrhea in the genitourinary tract?
4. How can a transverse vaginal septum be differentiated from an imperforate hymen?

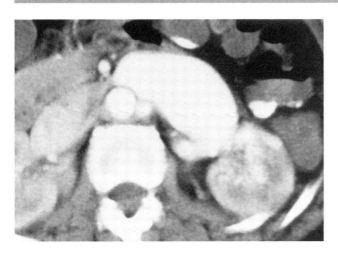
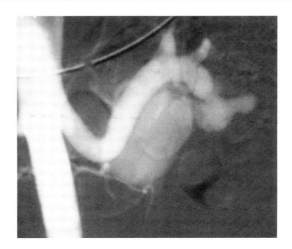

1. In this patient with gross hematuria, what is the most likely diagnosis?
2. What features on the CT scan indicate an abnormal connection between the arterial and venous systems?
3. What symptoms may result from this type of abnormality?
4. What are the common causes of this type of abnormality?

CASE 167

Obstructed Didelphys Uterus Resulting from Vaginal Septum

1. Cystic ovarian mass, hematometra or hematocolpos, enteric duplication cyst, and long-standing hematoma or lymphocele.

2. Ipsilateral renal anomalies often coexist with genital tract anomalies.

3. Congenital agenesis of the vagina.

4. Most transverse septa are located in the upper third of the vagina, whereas an imperforate hymen obstructs at the introitus.

Reference

Golan A, Langer R, Bukovsky I, Caspi E: Congenital anomalies of the müllerian system, *Fertil Steril* 51:747-755, 1989.

Cross-Reference

Genitourinary Radiology: THE REQUISITES, pp 253-257.

Comment

Notwithstanding vaginal agenesis, obstructed drainage of the uterus occurs in only two types of müllerian duct anomalies. One of these anomalies is a type of unicornuate uterus (class II anomaly). Unicornuate uterus results from either agenesis or incomplete development of one müllerian duct. If a unicornuate uterus occurs with a coexistent rudimentary horn containing functional endometrial tissue, hematometra of the rudimentary horn may develop if that horn does not connect with the unicornuate uterus. The diagnosis in this case is the other müllerian anomaly that can be associated with obstructed drainage—uterus didelphys with an obstructing transverse vaginal septum. Both of these müllerian anomalies may be associated with hematometra. In this case a clue to the diagnosis is the thin rim of contrast-enhancing endometrium surrounding the obstructed, fluid-filled endometrial cavity. Uterus didelphys (class III anomaly) is diagnosed when complete duplication of separate uteri, cervices, and upper vaginas is demonstrated. Between unicornuate uterus and uterus didelphys with transverse vaginal septum, only the latter is associated with hematocolpos, a double cervix, and a double upper vagina. Based on imaging findings, differentiation between a vaginal septum and a short atretic segment of the vagina may be difficult. However, in this case the small and nonobstructed left uterine cornua can be identified separate from the obstructed right horn.

In virtually all reported cases of uterus didelphys with atresia of one vagina, ipsilateral renal agenesis coexists. Conversely, about 50% of women with unilateral renal agenesis have associated anomalies of the lower genital tract.

Notes

CASE 168

Renal Arteriovenous Malformation

1. Arteriovenous malformation (AVM).

2. Marked left renal vein enlargement and renal vein opacification to the same degree as in the aorta and superior mesenteric artery.

3. Gross hematuria and high output heart failure.

4. Congenital malformation and AVM in association with other syndromes, such as congenital telangiectasias (Osler-Weber-Rendu syndrome).

Reference

Tarkington MA, Matsumoto AH, Dejter SW, Regan JB: Spectrum of renal vascular malformation, *Urology* 4:297-300, 1991.

Cross-Reference

Genitourinary Radiology: THE REQUISITES, p 397.

Comment

Most AVMs of the kidney are congenital. They usually come to light as a result of gross hematuria, but when there is massive shunting of blood, evidence of heart failure may develop. These abnormalities are usually diagnosed in young patients. Because of the low-resistance pathway of the AVM, the normal kidney may be underperfused, as in this case. Massive enlargement of the draining left renal vein was detected by CT scanning and led to the diagnosis of renal AVM. Selective embolization of the malformation is possible in some cases. However, when the arteriovenous connection is of large caliber with very high flow, embolic occlusion of the AVM, with maintenance of perfusion to the kidney, may be impossible.

Notes

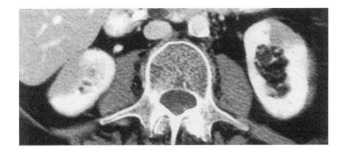 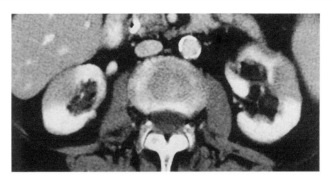

1. Which abnormalities commonly cause bilateral renal lesions with this radiologic pattern?

2. What lesions typically cause bilateral exophytic renal masses?

3. What nephrographic pattern would be diagnostic of infarction, if present?

4. What is the most common pattern of renal involvement with lymphoma?

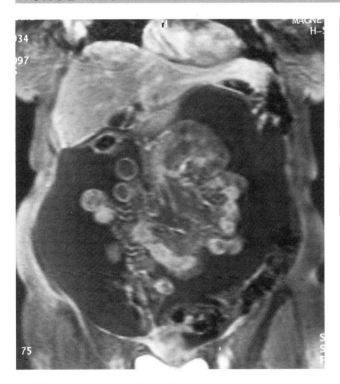 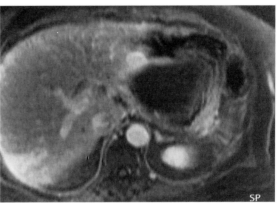

1. What is the most likely diagnosis?

2. What are the most common sites of peritoneal tumor implantation?

3. What technical options for MRI may improve detection of this disease?

4. What is pseudomyxoma peritonei?

Renal Lymphoma

1. Renal infarcts; infiltrative renal neoplasms, including lymphoma; and renal infections.

2. Renal cysts, bilateral renal cell carcinoma, angiomyolipomas, Wilms' tumors, and renal metastases.

3. Rim nephrogram, which is absent in this case.

4. Multiple renal parenchymal masses.

Reference
Gash JR, Zagoria RJ, Dyer RB: Imaging features of infiltrating renal lesions, *Crit Rev Diagn Imaging* 33:293-310, 1992.

Cross-Reference
Genitourinary Radiology: THE REQUISITES, pp 115, 116.

Comment
This patient has bilateral, homogeneous renal masses with an infiltrative growth pattern. The cortical rim sign is absent. The cause of bilateral infiltrative renal lesions is usually renal metastases, including lymphoma, renal infarcts, or bilateral pyelonephritis. The lack of the nephrographic rim sign and the homogeneous, nonstriated nature of the lesions make renal infarcts and pyelonephritis less likely. The homogeneous appearance of these infiltrative lesions suggests lymphoma. Renal lymphoma is usually a late finding in the course of systemic lymphoma. As in this patient, non-Hodgkin's lymphoma is the usual cell type when the kidneys are involved.

Renal lymphoma can occur with several different patterns. The most common pattern, which is illustrated in this case, is multifocal renal parenchymal lesions. These lesions usually have an infiltrative growth pattern and are homogeneous, with some contrast enhancement. On sonography, lymphoma typically has a homogeneous hypoechoic pattern. Other patterns of renal involvement with lymphoma include diffuse infiltration of one or both of the kidneys and a solitary renal mass. Additionally, renal lymphoma may result from direct spread of lymphoma from the retroperitoneal lymphatics to the renal sinus and perinephric space, with subsequent parenchymal invasion.

Notes

Peritoneal Carcinomatosis on MRI

1. Peritoneal carcinomatosis caused by epithelial carcinoma of the ovary.

2. Pouch of Douglas, ileocecal region, and right paracolic gutter.

3. Gadolinium enhancement, air distention of the bowel, and glucagon administration.

4. Accumulation of large amounts of gelatinous material in the peritoneal cavity caused by the transformation of peritoneal mesothelium to a mucin-secreting epithelium after perforation of a mucinous cystadenoma or cystadenocarcinoma.

Reference
Chou CK, Liu GC, Su JH, Chen LT, Sheu RS, Jaw TS: MRI demonstration of peritoneal implants, *Abdom Imaging* 19:95-101, 1994.

Cross-Reference
Genitourinary Radiology: THE REQUISITES, pp 288, 289.

Comment
Epithelial carcinoma of the ovary is one of the classic neoplasms that can present with extensive peritoneal disease. There are two theories for this observed disease pattern. One theory is that cells exfoliate into the peritoneal cavity only after the tumor has grown locally and invaded the ovarian capsule and mesovarium. Another theory is that the entire coelomic epithelium of the peritoneum undergoes malignant transformation. This theory may explain primary peritoneal or surface papillary adenocarcinoma in which multifocal or diffuse peritoneal carcinoma occurs with minimal or no ovarian involvement. In the International Federation of Gynecology and Obstetrics (FIGO) staging system of ovarian carcinoma, histologically confirmed abdominopelvic peritoneal implants less than 2 cm in diameter are designated as stage IIIb disease, and those that exceed 2 cm in diameter are considered stage IIIc ovarian cancer. Retrospective studies have suggested that survival in patients with stage III disease is related to residual tumor after surgery, and therefore detection and surgical debulking of peritoneal carcinomatosis are essential.

Although enhanced CT remains the imaging test of choice for the detection of peritoneal carcinomatosis, MRI also has been used to stage ovarian carcinoma. Although most implants have higher signal intensity than ascites on T1W images, differentiation of implants from ascites is facilitated by intravenous administration of gadolinium contrast. In this case nodular implants can be identified along the surface of the liver and in the gastrosplenic ligament.

Notes

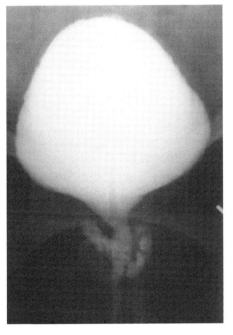
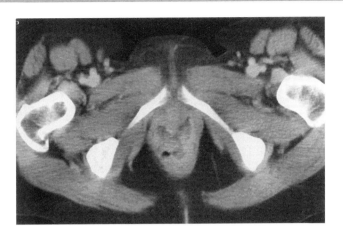

1. What imaging studies were performed?

2. What is the differential diagnosis for the abnormal urethra?

3. What should be recommended next to further evaluate this finding?

4. Name three complications of urethral diverticula.

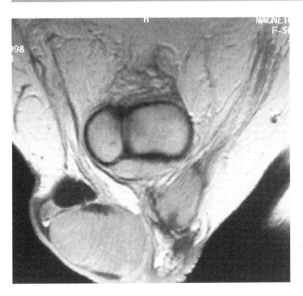
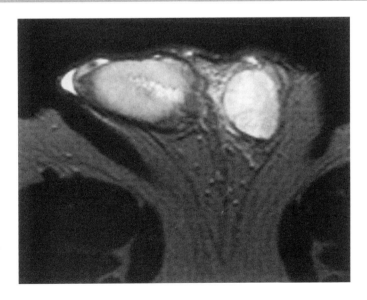

1. What are the findings on MRI in this case?

2. Name three complications of cryptorchidism.

3. In cases of "impalpable" testis, where are true cryptorchid and ectopic testes eventually located?

4. Why is the clinical diagnosis of cryptorchidism unreliable in patients younger than 3 months of age?

Adenocarcinoma Arising from a Urethral Diverticulum

1. Voiding cystourethrography and CT.

2. Neoplasm, abscess, and ureteral tear with contrast extravasation.

3. Depends on the clinical history. If a mass is palpable, aspiration or biopsy could be performed.

4. Infection, stone formation, and neoplasia.

References

Rajan N, Tucci P, Mallouh C, Choudhury M: Carcinoma in female urethral diverticulum: case reports and review of management, *J Urol* 150:1911-1914, 1993.

Seballos RM, Rich RR: Clear cell adenocarcinoma arising from a urethral diverticulum, *J Urol* 153:1914-1915, 1995.

Cross-Reference

Genitourinary Radiology: THE REQUISITES, pp 244, 245.

Comment

Urethral diverticula may be complicated by infection and calculus formation, and an association with benign and malignant neoplasms has been reported. The development of malignancy in a urethral diverticulum is rare; fewer than 100 cases have been reported. The average age at diagnosis is 40 years, and the development of hematuria and irritative voiding symptoms usually brings the patient to medical attention. Dyspareunia is reported in only 5% of patients, although it is a common symptom in women with uncomplicated urethral diverticula. On physical examination a tender, suburethral mass may be palpable. Further evaluation may include urethroscopy, cystourethrography, or double balloon urethrography. Urethrography may demonstrate a paraurethral mass displacing the urethra or an irregular filling defect within a diverticulum, as in this case.

Although the most common primary urethral malignancy is a squamous cell carcinoma, adenocarcinoma and transitional cell carcinoma account for two thirds of the malignancies that arise from within a urethral diverticulum. This finding is consistent with the theory that diverticula result from inflammation of obstructed paraurethral glands. Transitional cell carcinoma is more common in the proximal third of the urethra.

The prognosis for these carcinomas is poor, and failures can be both local and systemic. Diverticulectomy alone is inadequate; anterior exenteration with total urethrectomy, wide excision of the vaginal wall, and postoperative radiation are recommended.

Notes

Testicular Atrophy on MRI After Orchiopexy to Treat Cryptorchidism

1. Left testicular atrophy after orchiopexy, normal right testis, and right epididymal cyst.

2. Infertility, neoplasia, torsion, and trauma.

3. 50% are inguinal; 25% are abdominal; 15% are below external inguinal ring; 10% are absent (anorchia).

4. Because the testis may descend into the scrotal sac between the ages of 3 and 6 months.

Reference

Gill B, Kogan S: Cryptorchidism: current concepts, *Pediatr Clin North Am* 44(5):1211-1227, 1997.

Cross-Reference

Genitourinary Radiology: THE REQUISITES, pp 319-320.

Comment

This patient underwent orchiopexy for an undescended left testis and years later has a palpable right testicular mass. MRI demonstrates left testicular atrophy; the asymmetric scrotal examination was the result of a normal right testicle and the epididymal cyst. There is a 22-fold increased risk of testicular cancer in patients with undescended testis, and approximately one fourth of all cancers occur in the contralateral, descended testicle.

The objectives of orchiopexy are to improve fertility, reduce the risk of malignancy (in both the undescended and contralateral testicle), and restore the normal appearance of the scrotum. Although descended and cryptorchid testes have identical histologic findings during the first year of development, soon thereafter, progressive deterioration in the cryptorchid testis appears. An extrascrotal location caused by untreated cryptorchidism results in decreased testicular volume and histologic change, including loss of germ cells, appearance of abnormal Leydig cells, diminished seminiferous tubule diameter, and peritubular fibrosis. In addition, when cryptorchidism is not corrected, 40% of contralateral testes show decreased germ cell count. Abnormalities of the male genital ductal system (abnormal epididymal attachment to the testes and vasal atresia) also occur more frequently when cryptorchidism is not corrected.

The Action Committee of the American Academy of Pediatrics recommends that orchiopexy be performed when the patient is 1 year old. Some data suggest that when orchiopexy is performed at this age the result is higher fertility rates than when it is performed at an older age. Another study reported an increase in the likelihood of testicular carcinoma as the age at orchiopexy increases.

Notes

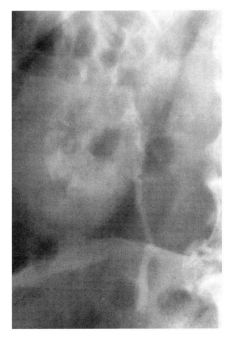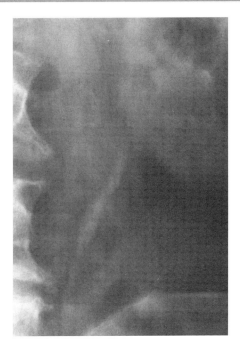

1. In this elderly patient with recurrent urinary tract infections, what is the most likely diagnosis for the abnormality shown?

2. In what percentage of patients does transitional cell carcinoma involve the upper tracts bilaterally?

3. What multifocal ureteral lesions are closely associated with recurrent urinary tract infections?

4. Between cystitis cystica and cystitis glandularis, which inflammatory bladder lesion is believed to be premalignant?

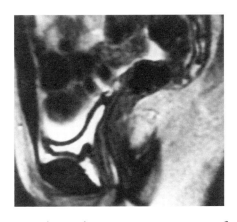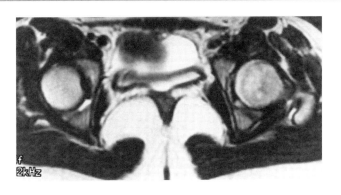

1. What is the most common cause of primary amenorrhea?

2. What is the role of imaging with regard to the selection of appropriate surgery for the lesion shown?

3. What renal anomalies have been reported in patients with Mayer-Rokitansky-Kuster-Hauser syndrome?

4. True or False: Patients with Mayer-Rokitansky-Kuster-Hauser syndrome have ovaries.

Pyeloureteritis Cystica

1. Pyeloureteritis cystica.

2. 1% to 2%.

3. Pyeloureteritis cystica and malakoplakia.

4. Cystitis glandularis.

Reference

Banner MP: Genitourinary complications of inflammatory bowel disease, *Radiol Clin North Am* 25:199-209, 1987.

Cross-Reference

Genitourinary Radiology: THE REQUISITES, p 188.

Comment

This case demonstrates poor excretion of contrast material from both kidneys and numerous filling defects within the ureter and marginal irregularity of the ureter and renal pelvis. There are numerous causes of multifocal radiolucent filling defects, most of which are unilateral. In addition, the history of recurrent urinary tract infections suggests the diagnosis of pyeloureteritis cystica. Malakoplakia is extremely rare but is associated with recurrent urinary tract infections. This condition could have a similar appearance, but its rarity in comparison with pyeloureteritis cystica makes it much less likely.

Pyeloureteritis cystica is analogous to cystitis cystica, which occurs in the bladder. Both result from chronic or recurrent urinary tract infections that cause encystment of submucosal glands. These cysts are usually multifocal and small. Rarely they can be unifocal and may be several centimeters in diameter. These filling defects can persist for months after resolution of the infection, but they have no known malignant potential. A similar-appearing abnormality in the bladder is cystitis glandularis. Unlike cystitis cystica, which is always associated with urinary tract infections, cystitis glandularis often occurs without bacterial infection. In addition, cystitis glandularis is believed to be premalignant. Multifocal, bilateral transitional cell carcinoma can have a similar appearance, but it is quite rare and is unrelated to recurrent urinary tract infections.

Notes

Vaginal Atresia

1. Vaginal agenesis.

2. To determine whether there is a normal, patent cervix and an endometrial canal.

3. Pelvic kidney and renal agenesis.

4. True.

Reference

Reinhold C, Hricak H, Forstner R, et al: Primary amenorrhea: evaluation with MR imaging, *Radiology* 203:383-390, 1997.

Cross-Reference

Genitourinary Radiology: THE REQUISITES, pp 253-257.

Comment

Primary amenorrhea is defined as the absence of menarche by the age of 16 years. The most common cause is congenital absence of the vagina, which occurs in approximately 1 in every 4000 to 5000 women; other causes of primary amenorrhea include müllerian duct anomalies, congenital disorders of sexual differentiation, ovarian dysfunction or failure, and hormonal abnormalities caused by hypothalamic or pituitary disorders. Patients with Mayer-Rokitansky-Kuster-Hauser syndrome have vaginal hypoplasia or agenesis and normal fallopian tubes and ovaries. There are variable associated anomalies of the uterus, urinary tract, and musculoskeletal system, but these patients are endocrinologically normal, are phenotypically female, and have complete gonadal development.

Transperineal sonography and MRI are effective in the evaluation of patients with vaginal agenesis. The primary role of imaging in these patients is to evaluate the length of the atretic segment and the patency of the endometrial canal and cervix. Vaginal agenesis with a functioning uterus and cervix can be treated with vaginoplasty. The distance between the agenetic vaginal segment and the introitus has implications for the particular type of vaginoplasty (primary anastomosis versus skin grafting). If the cervix is absent but there is functioning endometrial tissue, hysterectomy usually is performed because a surgically formed uterovaginal fistula or an artificial cervix often closes and cannot sustain a pregnancy. Closure of the uterovaginal fistula results in endometriosis.

Notes

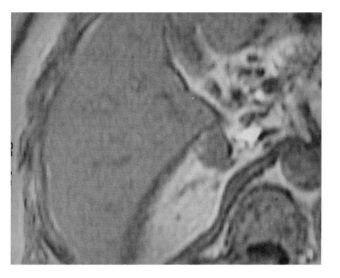 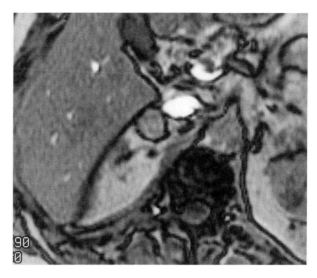

1. Identify the type (pulse sequence and weighting) of MR images shown.
2. What is the typical appearance of an adrenal metastasis on T1W and T2W images?
3. With regard to chemical shift MRI of adrenal adenomas, what is the explanation for false negative cases?
4. What is the explanation for false positive cases?

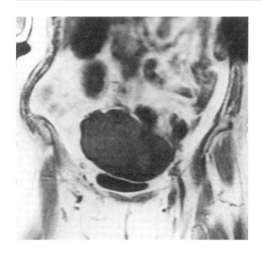 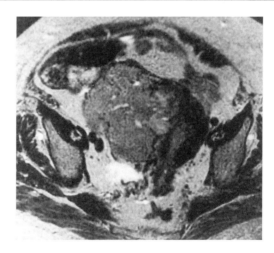

1. What is the differential diagnosis for this pelvic mass?
2. True or False: On MRI, degenerating leiomyomas enhance.
3. Of submucosal, intramural, and subserosal, which location is the least common for uterine leiomyosarcomas?
4. Name two prognostic factors for endometrial carcinoma.

Adrenal Chemical Shift Imaging: False Negatives and False Positives

1. In-phase and out-of-phase T1W gradient echo MR images of a right adrenal mass.

2. On T1W images, hypointense compared with liver and retroperitoneal fat; on T2W images hyperintense compared with liver.

3. Histologic variability. Some adenomas have a large proportion of fat-poor cells.

4. Metastases that contain fat or envelop periadrenal fat.

References

Mitchell DG, Crovello M, Matteucci T, Petersen RO, Miettinen MM: Benign adrenocortical masses: diagnosis with chemical shift MR imaging, *Radiology* 185:345-351, 1991.

Reinig JW: MR imaging differentiation of adrenal masses: has the time finally come? *Radiology* 185:339-340, 1992.

Cross-Reference

Genitourinary Radiology: THE REQUISITES, pp 29-30, 346-351.

Comment

The now classic paper by Mitchell and colleagues established chemical shift imaging as the method of choice for characterizing adrenal mass lesions on MRI. However, like many noninvasive imaging tests, chemical shift imaging is imperfect. The chemical shift MR images presented show a false negative case of a biopsy-proven right adrenal adenoma.

For the diagnosis of adrenal adenoma, the sensitivity of chemical shift imaging is lower than its specificity. The rate of false negatives (i.e., no loss of signal in the mass on an opposed-phase T1W gradient echo image compared with an in-phase image) may be as high as 20% in some series. The explanation is that adenomas contain variable amounts of cytoplasmic fat. Most benign, nonhyperfunctional adenomas consist of "clear" cells with abundant intracytoplasmic cholesterol, fatty acids, and neutral fat. However, other adenomas are composed of relatively lipid-poor "compact" cells.

Conversely, in most reported series the specificity of chemical shift imaging for characterizing an adrenal adenoma is close to 100%, and false positive cases are largely theoretical. Some malignant tumors may contain cytoplasmic lipid (e.g., renal cell carcinoma, hepatoma, liposarcoma, and well-differentiated adrenocortical carcinoma).

Notes

Leiomyosarcoma of the Uterus

1. Endometrial carcinoma, degenerating fibroid, and uterine sarcoma.

2. True.

3. Subserosal.

4. Surgical stage, tumor grade, presence of malignant peritoneal cytology, invasion of the vascular space in the hysterectomy specimen, and tumor size.

References

Pattani SJ, Kier R, Deal R, Luchansky E: MRI of uterine leiomyosarcoma, *Magn Reson Imaging* 13(2):331-333, 1995.

Schwartz LB, Diamond MP, Schwartz PE: Leiomyosarcomas: clinical presentation, *Am J Obstet Gynecol* 168:180-183, 1993.

Cross-Reference

Genitourinary Radiology: THE REQUISITES, pp 290-294.

Comment

Approximately 1 of every 800 uterine smooth muscle neoplasms is a leiomyosarcoma (LMSA), and they comprise 25% of all uterine sarcomas. The mean age of patients at diagnosis is 52 years, which is about 10 years older than the mean age of patients with leiomyoma.

There are some clinical clues to suggest that a uterine mass is an LMSA. In 19 of 20 subjects reported in the article by Schwartz and colleagues, the LMSA was either the largest or the only uterine mass. In this study, benign myomas ranged in size from microscopic to approximately 5 cm in diameter, whereas LMSAs ranged in diameter from 5 to 18 cm. A rapid increase in the size of any fibroid after menopause should raise concern. Similarly, others have reported that LMSAs may not shrink or may continue to grow when leiomyomas and nonmyomatous myometrial tissue decrease in size during gonadotropin-releasing hormone agonist treatment. Most LMSAs are intramural or submucosal in location; a subserosal location is unusual. A high proportion of LMSAs involve the cervix.

Notes

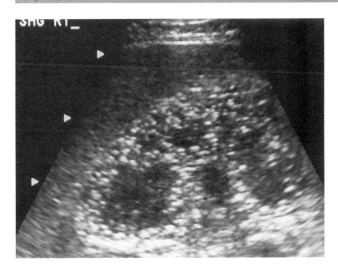
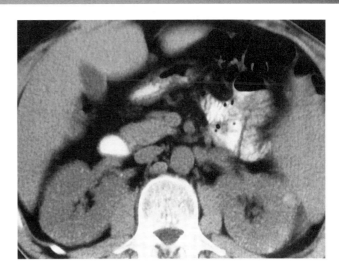

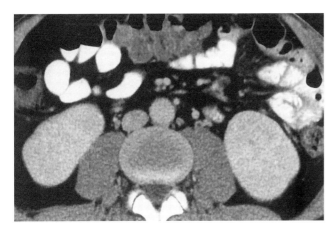

1. In an immunocompromised host, infection with what organisms may manifest as punctate calcifications in the kidneys?

2. Why has the incidence of renal infection with this organism increased recently?

3. Infection in what other organs is commonly caused by this organism? How can the diagnosis be made?

4. Do calcifications imply healed inactive disease?

Pneumocystis Carinii Infection of the Kidney

1. *Pneumocystis carinii, Mycobacterium avium-intracellulare,* and cytomegalovirus (CMV).

2. Increased use of aerosolized pentamidine.

3. Lung, liver, spleen, lymph nodes, and bone marrow. By percutaneous biopsy of involved organ.

4. No.

Reference
Miller, FH, Parikh S, Gore RM, et al: Renal manifestations of AIDS, *Radiographics* 13:587, 1993.

Cross-Reference
Genitourinary Radiology: THE REQUISITES, p 148.

Comment
A wide variety of renal abnormalities are described in patients with acquired immunodeficiency syndrome (AIDS). The most common renal abnormality in this patient population is human immunodeficiency virus (HIV) nephropathy, which is diagnosed when there is renal insufficiency, nephrotic syndrome, and glomerulopathy.

Patients with AIDS have an increased incidence of opportunistic infections with agents such as *Pneumocystis carinii, Mycobacterium avium-intracellulare, Mycobacterium tuberculosis,* CMV, and others. When the CD4 count is low, prophylaxis against *P. carinii* infection is recommended, and oral Bactrim or aerosolized pentamidine is administered. Aerosolized pentamidine provides therapeutic levels of pentamidine to the lung (the most commonly affected organ) and does not cause systemic side effects. An adverse consequence of the use of aerosolized pentamidine is more frequent infection of other organs, such as the liver, spleen, lymph nodes, and bone marrow, because of subtherapeutic systemic levels of the drug. The imaging findings of renal pneumocystosis include echogenic foci in the renal cortex on ultrasound and small punctate calcifications on noncontrast CT. Calcifications are evident in both active and inactive forms of renal pneumocystic infection. Although most commonly associated with pneumocystic infections, these calcifications also may occur with *M. avium-intracellulare* and CMV infection. Diagnosis can be made by percutaneous biopsy. In the case presented, a splenic biopsy demonstrated multiple *Pneumocystis* organisms.

Notes

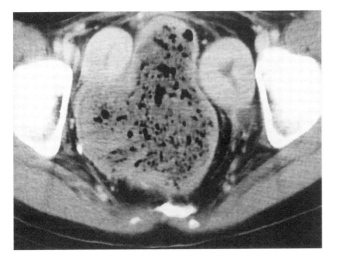

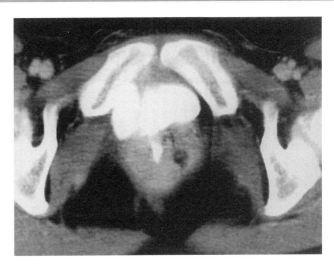

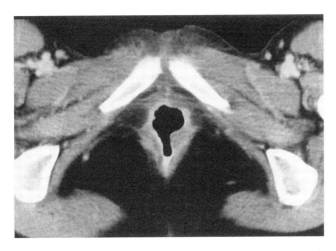

1. What are the abnormal findings on these images? What is the most likely diagnosis?
2. What is the most common cause of morbidity in these patients?
3. Which radiologic test usually is performed initially?
4. What is the meaning of the word *cloaca?*

Cloaca

1. Duplicated uterus, dilated rectum, and common cavity for urethra, vagina, and rectum are the abnormal findings. Cloacal malformation is the most likely diagnosis.

2. Renal failure resulting from obstruction, vesicoureteral reflux, or chronic infection.

3. Instillation of water-soluble contrast through the perineal orifice under fluoroscopy. This test is useful to determine the anatomic relationship between the bladder, urethra, vagina, and rectum. Cross-sectional imaging is less useful initially because of the variable and often complicated anatomy.

4. Latin for sewer.

Reference

Jaramillo D, Lebowitz RL, Hendren WH: Cloacal malformation: radiologic findings and imaging recommendations, *Radiology* 177:441-448, 1990.

Cross-Reference

Genitourinary Radiology: THE REQUISITES, p 193.

Comment

Cloacal malformation occurs exclusively in females and is a congenital anomaly in which the urinary, genital, and intestinal tracts empty into a single orifice in the perineum, the cloaca. A cloaca exists in fish, birds, and amphibians, as well as the normal human embryo at 4 weeks' gestation. This congenital anomaly is believed to result from incomplete separation of the rectum and urogenital sinus by the urorectal septum. This anomaly is heterogeneous in that there are many variations in the connections between the bladder, vagina, and rectum. The rectum and vagina may empty into the ureter, the ureter and vagina may drain into the rectum, or the ureter and rectum may empty into the vagina.

Cloacal malformation is associated with a number of complications and anomalies. One large series reported uterine duplication in 55% of affected women, vaginal duplication in 46%, sacral agenesis in 40%, and bladder diverticula in 20%. The primary complications of this anomaly are renal failure resulting from obstruction, vesicoureteral reflux, or both and repeated urinary tract infections caused by contamination from the fecal stream.

The role of radiologic studies is to facilitate surgical correction of this disorder by precisely defining the complex anatomic relationships between the lower genital, urinary, and gastrointestinal tracts. Treatment of a cloacal malformation consists of diverting colostomy and correction of urinary reflux in the neonatal period, followed by definitive surgical repair to create separate openings for the urethra, vagina, and rectum.

Notes

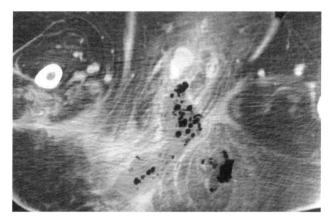 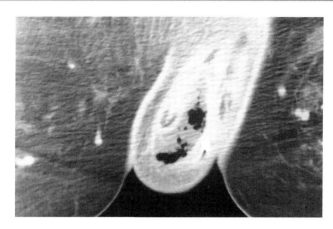

1. CT images of the scrotum and perineum are shown. True or False: The alpha toxin produced by clostridial bacteria, especially *Clostridium perfringens,* is the most common cause of this disease.

2. In women, where does this disease most often originate?

3. What are some of the findings of this disease on scrotal sonography?

4. True or False: This disease is a surgical emergency.

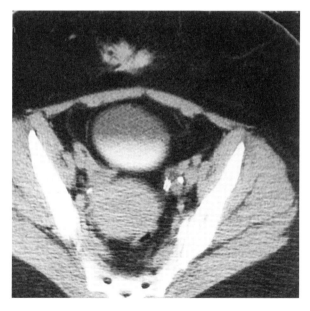 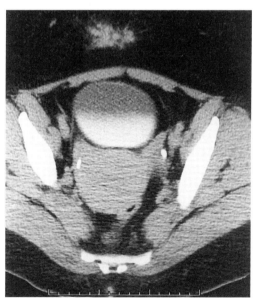

1. Two images from a CT examination performed to investigate severe, intermittent abdominal pain are shown. Where is the lesion located?

2. What is the radiologic differential diagnosis for the lesion?

3. On further questioning the patient describes cyclical pain that began after a cesarean section. Based on this information, should any other condition be added to the differential diagnosis?

4. Would MRI provide any new information? What might it show?

Fournier's Gangrene

1. False. Fournier's gangrene is usually a polymicrobial necrotizing fasciitis caused by gram-negative rods or streptococcal, staphylococcal, and anaerobic streptococcal organisms.

2. From abscesses of the vulva or Bartholin's gland.

3. Thickened scrotal wall containing gas and presence of peritesticular fluid; testes and epididymides often are unaffected.

4. Absolutely true.

Reference

Rajan DK, Scharer KA: Radiology of Fournier's gangrene, *Am J Roentgenol* 170:163-168, 1998.

Cross-Reference

Genitourinary Radiology: THE REQUISITES, pp 309-312.

Comment

Fournier's gangrene is a polymicrobial necrotizing fasciitis of the perineum. This disease is a surgical emergency because of the rapidity with which the fasciitis can spread to the anorectum and the lower genital, anterior abdominal, and pelvic retroperitoneal spaces. Surgical debridement within 24 hours of presentation reduces the mortality from 76% to 12%. Clinically the typical patient seeks treatment days after the onset of perineal pain, pruritus, and fever and appears toxic; the genitalia may be gangrenous. Crepitus is detected in 19% to 64% of patients at the time of diagnosis. The cause of Fournier's gangrene is usually an invasive infection from the perianal or colorectal area and may be preceded by regional trauma or surgery. An infectious obliterative endarteritis is responsible for the rapidly progressive necrotizing fasciitis. Diabetes is a risk factor.

The diagnosis usually is established clinically, and imaging is often unnecessary. Ultrasound and CT have been performed to confirm the clinical diagnosis and to reveal the full extent of disease. Sonography of the scrotum may demonstrate hyperechoic foci with posterior acoustical shadowing, typical of gas, in swollen scrotal and perineal soft tissues. CT may reveal an infected pelvic or abdominal fluid collection, perianal abscess, fistulous tract, incarcerated inguinal hernia, or other potential source for the necrotizing infection.

Notes

Scar Endometrioma

1. Subcutaneous fat in the anterior abdominal wall.

2. Hematoma, surgical scar, metastasis, or abscess.

3. Yes, endometriosis.

4. Possibly. It might show characteristic findings of hemorrhage.

Reference

Matthes G, Zabel DD, Nastala CL, Shestak KC: Endometrioma of the abdominal wall following combined abdominoplasty and hysterectomy: case report and review of the literature, *Ann Plast Surg* 40:672-675, 1998.

Cross-Reference

Genitourinary Radiology: THE REQUISITES, pp 258-264.

Comment

This unusual case of ectopic endometrial tissue in the subcutaneous fat occurred after cesarean section. The patient had severe, cyclical abdominal pain, and the correct diagnosis was made by the emergency room radiologist to the disbelief of the general surgeons.

Scar endometriosis reportedly occurs in up to 5% of patients who undergo cesarean section or hysterectomy. The pathogenesis is iatrogenic transplantation of endometrial tissue to the abdominal wall during surgery. Treatment is surgical excision. Biopsy should be avoided to prevent further seeding of the endometrial tissue along the biopsy tract. If the lesion is large, it may be reduced preoperatively by the administration of a gonadotropin-releasing hormone antagonist.

Notes

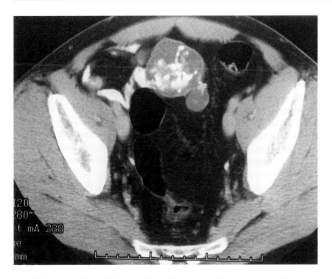 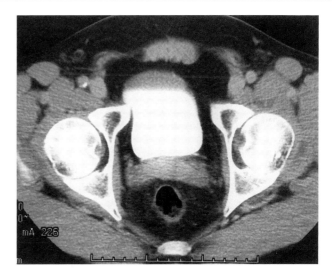

1. What is the differential diagnosis for this pelvic mass?

2. Is the retropubic space of Retzius extraperitoneal?

3. In what percentage of bladder transitional cell carcinomas is calcification identified?

4. True or False: The prognosis for patients with urachal carcinoma is better than that for those with nonurachal bladder malignancies.

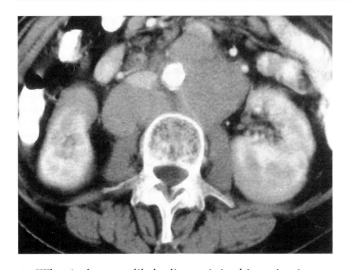 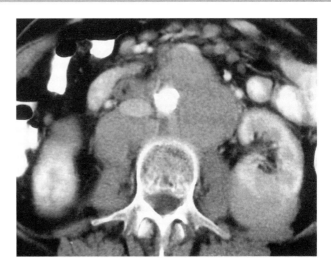

1. What is the most likely diagnosis in this patient?

2. What feature of the retroperitoneal mass makes the diagnosis of retroperitoneal fibrosis unlikely?

3. When bilateral solid renal masses are present, what are the major differential diagnoses?

4. Which type of lymphoma involves the kidneys?

CASE 181

Urachal Adenocarcinoma

1. Benign (e.g., hemangioma) or malignant bladder tumor, urachal adenocarcinoma, ovarian metastasis, and peritoneal metastasis from a gastrointestinal tumor.

2. Yes.

3. 1% to 7%.

4. False.

Reference

Korobkin M, Cambier L, Drake J: Computed tomography of urachal carcinoma, *J Comput Assist Tomogr* 12(6):981-987, 1988.

Cross-Reference

Genitourinary Radiology: THE REQUISITES, p 233.

Comment

Malignancy rarely arises from the urachus, the epithelium-lined fibrous cord (median umbilical ligament) connecting the bladder apex to the umbilicus. Urachal cancer accounts for less than 0.5% of all bladder cancers and arises in the extraperitoneal space from the juxtavesical segment of the urachus in 90% of patients. In general, any adenocarcinoma arising at or near the bladder dome should be considered to be of urachal origin. Two thirds of patients are men between the ages of 40 and 70 years. Of urachal cancers, 85% are mucinous adenocarcinomas, although squamous cell carcinoma, transitional cell carcinoma, and sarcoma also have been reported. The prognosis for urachal adenocarcinoma is much worse than that for bladder carcinoma because the tumor grows to a large size in a clinically occult space; the 5-year survival rate is only about 10%. Painless hematuria is the most common presenting symptom; gross or microscopic mucus is found in the urine in only 25% of patients.

The diagnosis is usually suggested on CT; conventional radiographs rarely reveal any abnormality, and excretory urography shows a deformity of the bladder apex in only about 10% of cases. On CT a urachal carcinoma appears as a soft tissue mass arising at or near the anterosuperior aspect of the bladder that may extend anterosuperiorly toward the umbilicus. These masses usually are large (6 to 10 cm in diameter), and calcification is recognized in 70% of cases on CT. Urachal carcinoma has a propensity to invade the abdominal wall, peritoneum, or small bowel.

Notes

CASE 182

Renal Lymphoma

1. Lymphoma.

2. Extensive soft tissue between the vertebra and the aorta and lateral ureteral deviation.

3. Metastases, including renal lymphoma, and renal cell carcinoma.

4. Non-Hodgkin's lymphoma.

Reference

Davidson AJ, Hartman DS, Davis CJ Jr, et al: Infiltrative renal lesions: CT-sonographic-pathologic correlation, *Am J Roentgenol* 150:1061-1064, 1988.

Cross-Reference

Genitourinary Radiology: THE REQUISITES, pp 115-116, 181.

Comment

This patient has massive retroperitoneal lymphadenopathy with enlarged lymph nodes surrounding both the inferior vena cava and the aorta. The aorta is pushed anteriorly away from the spine by the lymphadenopathy. There also are bilateral perirenal masses. These features strongly suggest lymphoma. Lymphoma involving the kidneys can present in several different patterns. There can be direct spread from the retroperitoneum along the lymphatics into the renal sinus and eventually the kidney. Multifocal infiltrative renal masses, diffuse infiltration of one or both of the kidneys, or a solitary renal mass mimicking primary renal neoplasm may occur. Unlike most other neoplasms, lymphoma also has a predilection for involvement of the perirenal space, as illustrated by this case. Perirenal soft tissue masses are uncommon; their presence suggests lymphoma. Alternative diagnoses include metastases from other tumors, such as melanoma, and, if the mass is solitary, a primary retroperitoneal sarcoma, such as malignant fibrous histiocytoma.

Renal involvement by lymphoma usually occurs with non-Hodgkin's lymphoma. Burkitt's lymphoma also has a predilection for extranodal disease, but it is uncommon in North America.

Notes

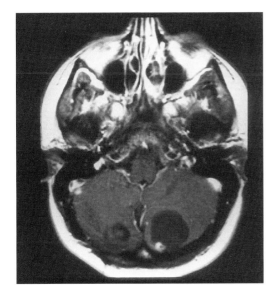 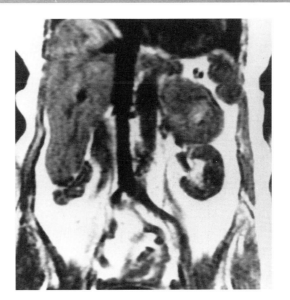

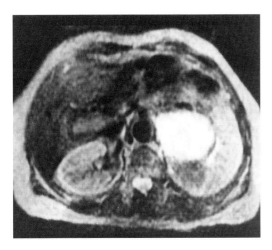

1. In patients with von Hippel-Lindau disease, what pancreatic lesion is most frequently associated with the development of pheochromocytoma?

2. In patients with von Hippel-Lindau disease, what percentage of pheochromocytomas are multiple or bilateral?

3. In patients with multiple endocrine neoplasia syndromes, what adrenomedullary pathologic condition may precede the development of a pheochromocytoma?

4. Name two other syndromes or diseases in which a pheochromocytoma may occur.

Pheochromocytoma in von Hippel-Lindau Disease

1. Islet cell tumor.

2. 50% to 80% (as opposed to approximately 10% of sporadic tumors).

3. Medullary hyperplasia of the adrenal gland.

4. Sturge-Weber syndrome, tuberous sclerosis, and Carney's syndrome (pulmonary chondromas and gastric stromal neoplasms [leiomyosarcoma]).

References

Choyke PL, Glenn GM, Walter MM, Patronas NJ, Linehan WM, Zbar B: von Hippel-Lindau disease: genetic, clinical, and imaging features, *Radiology* 194:629-642, 1995.

Melmon KL, Rosen SE: Lindau's disease, *Am J Med* 36:595-617, 1964.

Cross-Reference

Genitourinary Radiology: THE REQUISITES, pp 351-355.

Comment

Pheochromocytomas can be associated with a number of syndromes and diseases. Medullary carcinoma of the thyroid and pheochromocytoma are associated with both multiple endocrine neoplasia syndromes IIA (Sipple's syndrome) and IIB/III (ganglioneuromatosis and multiple mucosal neuromas). Approximately 10% of pheochromocytomas are inherited; the majority are inherited in an autosomal dominant pattern. About 1% of patients with neurofibromatosis develop pheochromocytomas.

The case presented is that of pheochromocytoma in a patient with von Hippel-Lindau disease. In 1926, Arvid Lindau, a Swedish ophthalmologist, observed that cerebellar and retinal hemangioblastomatosis is part of a heritable "angiomatous lesion of the central nervous system." The following diagnostic criteria for von Hippel-Lindau disease were proposed by Melmon and Rosen in 1964: (1) given a family history of retinal or cerebellar hemangioblastoma, only one hemangioblastoma (retinal, cerebellar, or spinal) or visceral lesion (renal tumor, pancreatic cyst or tumor, pheochromocytoma, or papillary cystadenoma of the epididymis) is necessary for the diagnosis, or (2) if there is no family history, at least two hemangioblastomas and a visceral manifestation are required.

Notes

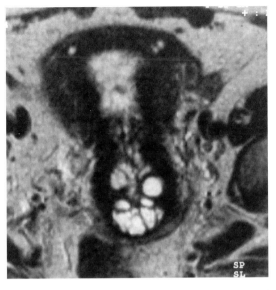 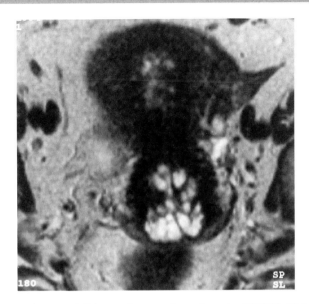

1. What is the differential diagnosis for the endocervical mass visible on these turbo spin-echo T2W MR images?
2. What clinical symptom is characteristic of this rare tumor?
3. This lesion may be associated with two other diseases. Name one of them.
4. True or False: This is a benign-appearing malignancy with an excellent prognosis.

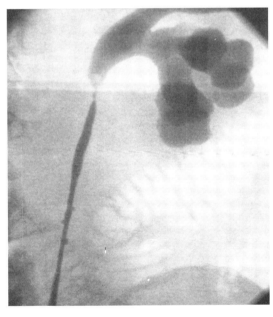 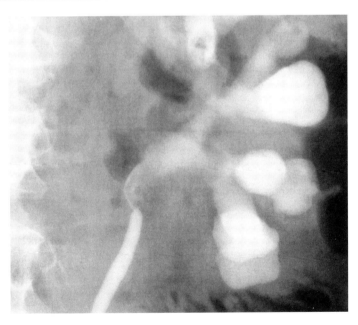

1. What is the diagnosis for the small outpouchings from the ureter?
2. Do these outpouchings represent a benign or malignant abnormality?
3. What is the significance of these outpouchings?
4. What is the most likely diagnosis for the filling defect in the upper pole calyx and the narrowing at the uretero-pelvic junction?

CASE 184

Adenoma Malignum

1. Cystic endometrial hyperplasia, deep nabothian cysts, and adenoma malignum.

2. Profuse, watery vaginal discharge.

3. Peutz-Jeghers syndrome or mucinous tumor of the ovary.

4. Unfortunately, false.

Reference

Doi T, Yamashita Y, Yasunaga T, et al: Adenoma malignum: MR imaging and pathologic study, *Radiology* 204:39-42, 1997.

Cross-Reference

Genitourinary Radiology: THE REQUISITES, pp 295-301.

Comment

Adenocarcinoma accounts for about 10% of all cases of cervical carcinoma; adenoma malignum or minimal deviated adenocarcinoma of the cervix makes up about 3% of all cervical adenocarcinomas. This malignancy may be associated with Peutz-Jeghers syndrome, and an association with mucinous tumor of the ovary also has been described. The most common presenting symptom is watery cervical discharge; vaginal bleeding is uncommon.

Macroscopically this neoplasm presents as a multicystic mass; cysts range from microscopic to several centimeters in diameter. Even solid and enhancing areas on MRI are composed of minute cysts with edematous cervical tissue. Although the gross appearance is deceptively benign, this tumor deeply invades the cervical stroma. The walls of these cysts are lined with a single layer of mucin-secreting columnar cells, which resemble normal cervical glands. For the pathologist the diagnosis of malignancy may be difficult because tumor cells usually are well differentiated. Despite this difficulty, the clinical course of adenoma malignum is characterized by early dissemination, poor response to treatment, and a dismal long-term prognosis.

The differential diagnosis of adenoma malignum includes cystic endometrial hyperplasia and deeply invasive nabothian cervical cysts. Contrast-enhancing solid tissue should not be associated with nabothian cysts, and stromal invasion is not present in cases of cystic endometrial hyperplasia.

Notes

CASE 185

Ureteral Pseudodiverticula

1. Ureteral pseudodiverticula.

2. Benign.

3. They indicate increased risk of synchronous or metachronous transitional cell carcinoma (TCC).

4. TCC.

Reference

Wasserman NF, Zhand G, Posalaky IP, Reddy PK: Ureteral pseudodiverticula: frequent association with uroepithelial malignancy, *Am J Roentgenol* 157:69-72, 1991.

Comment

Ureteral pseudodiverticula are uncommon but not rare. They represent intramural outpouchings from the ureteral lumen. In and of themselves, ureteral pseudodiverticula are completely benign and represent invagination of the urothelium into hyperplastic nests of cells in the ureteral wall. These pouches are visible on both retrograde pyelograms and intravenous urograms, although they are most commonly identified on retrograde studies because of the pressure of injection. The significance of these diverticula is their association with TCC. Up to one fourth of patients with ureteral pseudodiverticula have a coexisting TCC, as does this patient, or will develop a TCC within several years. The TCC can occur ipsilateral to the pseudodiverticula or within the bladder. It has been postulated that pseudodiverticula result from chronic ureteral inflammation, which also may predispose these patients to development of urothelial neoplasms. When ureteral pseudodiverticula are evident, careful evaluation of the entire urothelium should be performed to exclude coexisting TCC. If none is found, follow-up imaging is recommended semiannually.

Notes

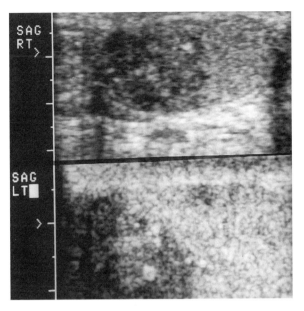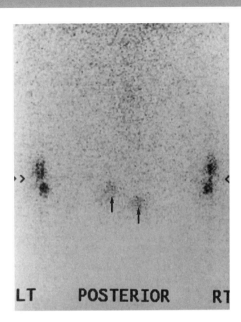

1. Images from scrotal sonography and adrenocortical scintigraphy are shown. Arrows indicate activity in the testes. What radiopharmaceutical is used in adrenocortical scintigraphy?

2. What is the most likely diagnosis for these testicular lesions?

3. Elevated levels of which hormone causes these lesions?

4. What is the most common disease associated with these testicular masses?

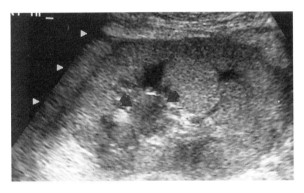

1. A sagittal sonogram of a transplanted kidney is shown. To what do the arrows point?

2. What is the differential diagnosis for this mass?

3. List several factors that can predispose an individual to fungal infections of the kidney.

4. How are fungal infections of the urinary tract treated?

Testicular Adrenal Rests Associated with Congenital Adrenal Hyperplasia

1. NP-59 (^{131}I-6β-iodomethyl-19-norcholesterol).

2. Adrenal rests.

3. Adrenocorticotrophic hormone (ACTH), or corticotropin.

4. Congenital adrenal hyperplasia (adrenogenital syndrome).

Reference

Avila NA, Premkumar A, Shawker TH, Jones JV, Laue L, Cutler GB Jr: Testicular adrenal rest tissue in congenital adrenal hyperplasia: findings at gray-scale and color Doppler US, *Radiology* 198:99-104, 1996.

Cross-Reference

Genitourinary Radiology: THE REQUISITES, pp 312-316.

Comment

Elevated serum levels of corticotropin may result in the growth of rests of adrenal tissue in the testes, celiac plexus region, broad ligaments, or fetal ovarian tissue. Adrenal rests most often occur in association with congenital adrenal hyperplasia (CAH) but also have been reported in patients with Addison's disease or Cushing's syndrome. CAH is caused by an autosomal recessive defect in the production of an adrenocortical enzyme, most often 21-hydroxylase. Elevated levels of ACTH cause rests, which are identical to hyperplastic adrenal cortex, to grow in adrenal tissue. In patients with CAH, adrenal rest tissue may hypertrophy when there is inadequate glucocorticoid replacement and may atrophy when high doses of glucocorticoid are administered. Most adrenal rests are detected in patients with CAH, but in as many as 18% of patients, adrenogenital syndrome is not discovered until testicular enlargement develops.

Adrenal rests are bilateral in 75% of cases and may be mistaken for testicular lymphoma, leukemia, or metastases. Unilateral rests may be difficult to distinguish from primary tumors of the testicle. On ultrasound, rests are often visible in the periphery of the testicle and do not distort the outer contour of the gonad. Testicular adrenal rests differ from other intratesticular mass lesions in that the echogenic line of the testicular mediastinum or parenchymal vessels on Doppler may course through an adrenal rest undisturbed. In most cases testicular adrenal rests are hypoechoic, but they may have a hyperechoic rim or a focus of calcification, as in the case presented. Large hypoechoic rests may be associated with marked attenuation on ultrasound. When the diagnosis is in doubt, the existence of functional adrenal tissue may be established by adrenocortical scintigraphy or testicular venous sampling.

Notes

Fungal Infection in a Transplanted Kidney

1. Mass in the renal collecting system.

2. Blood clot, fungus ball, neoplasm, and lymphoproliferative disease.

3. Immunosuppression, diabetes, neurogenic bladder, use of an indwelling catheter for long periods, and long-term antibiotic or steroid use.

4. Systemic antifungal agents, bladder irrigation with antifungal agents, and percutaneous extraction.

Reference

Kennedy CA, Panosian CB: Infectious complications of kidney transplantation. In Danovitch GM, editor: *Handbook of kidney transplantation,* Boston, 1992, Little, Brown and Co.

Cross-Reference

Genitourinary Radiology: THE REQUISITES, pp 182-189.

Comment

Immunosuppressive therapy has contributed to the long-term success of renal transplantation, but with it come many associated problems. Chief among these problems is a susceptibility to opportunistic infections. Urinary tract infection is the most common infection after organ transplantation, occurring in approximately 40% of renal allograft recipients. This incidence has been reduced to around 10% since the institution of prophylactic therapy with trimethoprim-sulfamethoxazole. Gram-negative organisms, such as *Escherichia coli* and *Klebsiella* species, are the most common causative agents (76%), followed by gram-positive bacteria (22%) and fungi (1%). The most common fungal pathogens are *Candida* and *Aspergillus* species. Predisposing factors for posttransplant urinary tract infection include extensive manipulation during surgery, placement of indwelling urinary catheters, anatomic abnormalities resulting in urostasis, and neurogenic bladder. Infection most commonly occurs in the first 6 months after transplantation. After this time, infection is usually related to impaired allograft function.

Renal parenchymal fungal infection usually occurs via hematogenous dissemination. In contrast, infection in the lower urinary tract usually occurs via an ascending route from the bladder. Fungus balls are found in the urinary bladder more often than in the upper collecting system. Detection of a fungus ball relies on signs and symptoms of obstruction coupled with funguria. Hydronephrosis may or may not be present. The fungus ball is an echogenic, weakly shadowing mass within the collecting system.

Notes

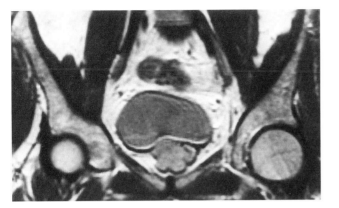
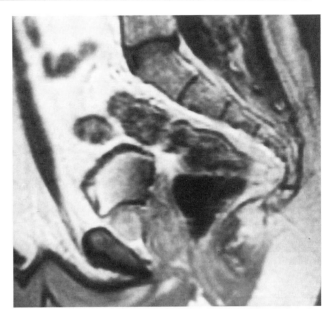

1. What is the pulse sequence shown on the sagittal image?

2. This patient complained of diaphoresis during and after micturition. What other clinical symptoms might be expected in this patient?

3. In what other sites may this tumor occur?

4. What precautions should be taken before the lesion is surgically removed?

Bladder Paraganglioma (Pheochromocytoma)

1. Proton density–weighted spin echo (the fat is bright, the urine in the bladder is bright, and the CSF is dark).

2. Headache, palpitations, and other symptoms related to catecholamine excess.

3. Adrenal glands (in 90% of patients), the paravertebral sympathetic plexus, and the organ of Zuckerkandl (paraganglion cells along the lower abdominal aorta from the inferior mesenteric artery to the iliac arteries).

4. Patient should be pretreated with α-adrenergic blockers, such as phenoxybenzamine, to prevent a hypertensive crisis.

References

Atiyeh BA, Baraket AJ, et al: Extra-adrenal pheochromocytoma, *J Nephrol* 10:25-29, 1997.

Whalen RK, Althausen AF, et al: Extra-adrenal pheochromocytoma, *J Urol* 147:1-10, 1992.

Cross-Reference

Genitourinary Radiology: THE REQUISITES, pp 205-206, 351-355, 364.

Comment

Extraadrenal pheochromocytoma arises from the paraganglion chromaffin cells of the sympathetic nervous system. These abnormalities occur most commonly in the paraadrenal area, followed by the region of aortic bifurcation (organ of Zuckerkandl). Other sites include the bladder, mediastinum, and heart. Extraadrenal pheochromocytomas are estimated to occur in 10% of adults and up to 40% of children. These lesions are larger, more likely to recur, and more likely to metastasize than their adrenal counterparts. The work-up for a suspected pheochromocytoma consists of measurement of urinary catecholamine levels and noncontrast CT of the abdomen and pelvis. Treatment is surgical excision. Radiation therapy and chemotherapy are ineffective. Follow up after resection should include annual measurement of urinary catecholamine levels and, if these levels are elevated, repeat cross-sectional imaging. MRI and adrenomedullary scintigraphy with metaiodobenzylguanidine I 131 are adjunctive examinations if CT is not diagnostic.

Notes

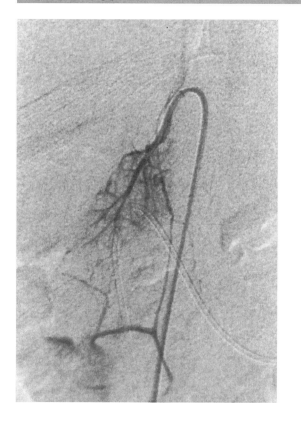
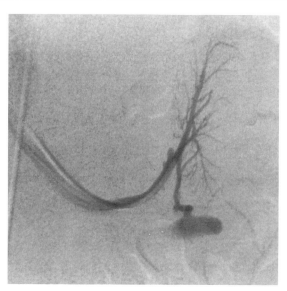

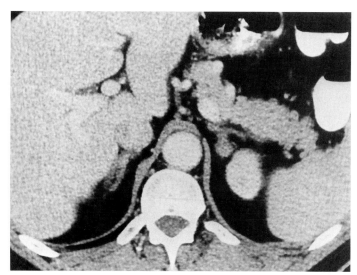

1. What are the causes of primary aldosteronism?
2. Why is it important to distinguish among the various causes?
3. When is CT alone diagnostic?
4. What is the most common complication of adrenal venography and venous sampling?

Primary Aldosteronism

1. Autonomous adrenocortical adenoma (80%), adrenal hyperplasia (20%), and adrenocortical carcinoma (<1%).

2. Unilateral adrenalectomy cures a hyperfunctional adenoma, whereas hyperplasia is managed medically.

3. When a unilateral hypodense adrenal mass that is smaller than 4 cm in diameter and a normal or atrophic contralateral adrenal gland are identified.

4. Adrenal venous extravasation occurs in about 4% of cases and often results in loss of function. It is an absolute contraindication to contralateral adrenal venography and venous sampling.

Reference

Doppman JL, Gill JR: Hyperaldosteronism: sampling the adrenal veins, *Radiology* 198:309-312, 1996.

Francis IR, et al: Integrated imaging of adrenal disease, *Radiology* 184:1-13, 1992.

Cross-Reference

Genitourinary Radiology: THE REQUISITES, pp 49, 366-367.

Comment

Only about 1% of patients with hypertension have primary aldosteronism. The radiologist's task is to distinguish among the causes so as to direct treatment. Thin-section noncontrast CT is the initial modality of choice. It is 98% sensitive for nodules that are larger than 1 cm in diameter. However, it is difficult to distinguish between a smaller adenoma and adrenal hyperplasia on CT. Therefore when CT demonstrates normal adrenal glands, bilateral hyperplasia, or a nodule with contralateral hyperplasia, adrenal function must be evaluated by ^{131}I-6β-iodomethyl-19-norcholesterol (NP-59) scintigraphy or adrenal venous sampling because a significant number of patients will have a small unilateral aldosteronoma.

Despite being nearly 100% accurate, selective adrenal venous sampling is performed infrequently because of a failure to sample the right adrenal vein in 30% of cases. However, subselective sampling is acceptable because measuring the aldosterone/cortisol (A/C) ratio in the venous blood can correct for dilution. An aldosteronoma resides in the gland with an A/C ratio that increases significantly after corticotropin stimulation and is at least 5 times greater than the contralateral A/C ratio. Suppressed aldosterone levels and a blunted response to corticotropin from the contralateral adrenal gland are the best predictors for the success of unilateral adrenalectomy.

Notes

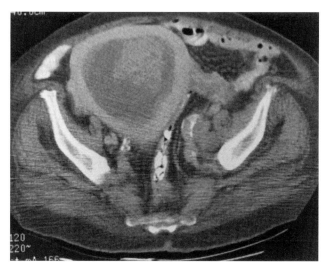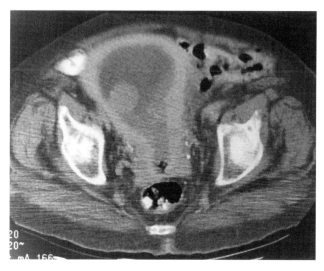

1. What is the most likely diagnosis in this 81-year-old woman?

2. True or False: Excessive estrogen is linked to most risk factors associated with endometrial carcinoma.

3. True or False: Leiomyosarcoma is the most common nonepithelial endometrial malignancy.

4. True or False: Prior pelvic radiation has been linked to endometrial sarcoma.

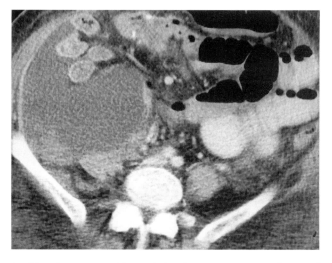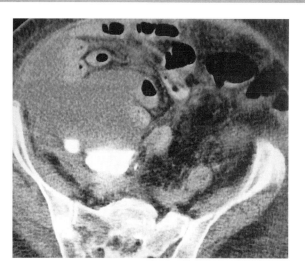

1. Two images, performed 5 minutes apart, are shown from an intravenous contrast enhanced CT examination in a patient with a history of recent gynecologic surgery. What is the most likely diagnosis, and what is the most common cause of this lesion?

2. What is the most appropriate imaging technique when this diagnosis is suspected?

3. What is the diagnostic significance of the radiodensity of the material in the fluid collection?

4. True or False: For this lesion, surgery performed early is the treatment of choice.

Malignant Mixed Müllerian Tumor of the Uterus

1. Endometrial carcinoma.

2. True.

3. False.

4. True.

Reference

Costa MJ, Khan R, Judd R: Carcinosarcoma (malignant mixed müllerian [mesodermal] tumor) of the uterus and ovary: correlation of clinical, pathologic, and immunohistochemical features in 29 cases, *Arch Pathol Lab Med* 115:583-590, 1991.

Cross-Reference

Genitourinary Radiology: THE REQUISITES, p 294.

Comment

Only about 3% of uterine cancers are sarcomas, but of these the malignant mixed müllerian tumor (MMMT or triple MT) is the most common. These tumors are considered biphasic neoplasms of the female genital tract because they are composed of both carcinomatous and sarcomatous elements (carcinosarcoma). Recall that the paramesonephric ducts are formed by mesenchyme of the urogenital ridge and are lined by coelomic epithelium. The epithelial component of the MMMT is typically an adenocarcinoma of the endometrioid type, and the most common mesenchymal components are fibrosarcoma and endometrial stromal sarcoma.

Because MMMT is uncommon and the clinical and radiologic presentations are not specific, a prebiopsy diagnosis of this tumor is a real home run. These tumors are associated with a clinical history of pelvic radiation treatment. In one study, 9.5% of patients had a history of radiotherapy and the median latent period between pelvic radiation and the diagnosis of MMMT was 16 years. MMMT is known for its very aggressive clinical course and poor prognosis. Even with stage I disease the 5-year survival rate is not greater than 35%; 85% of recurrences and metastases occur within the first 2 years of follow up. Prognostic factors are similar to those for endometrial carcinomas and include depth of myometrial invasion (when the tumor is confined to the uterus), stage of disease, presence of lymphatic or vascular space invasion, and size of the resected tumor. As many as half of all cases are in an advanced stage (stage III or IV) at the time of diagnosis.

Notes

Traumatic Injury of the Ureter

1. Ureteral disruption, which is most commonly iatrogenic in nature (i.e., caused by surgery). A less common cause is traumatic injury (blunt or penetrating).

2. CT after intravenous contrast administration (but without oral contrast enhancement); both early and delayed images should be performed.

3. Very dense contrast, as shown in this case, has been concentrated by the kidney and therefore is more radiodense than intravascular contrast.

4. False.

Reference

Kenney PJ, Panicek DM, Witanowski LS: Computed tomography of ureteral disruption, *J Comput Assist Tomogr* 11(3): 480-484, 1987.

Lask D, Abarbanel J, Luttwak Z, et al: Changing trends in the management of iatrogenic ureteral injuries, *J Urol* 154(5): 1693-1695, 1995.

Cross-Reference

Genitourinary Radiology: THE REQUISITES, pp 189-190.

Comment

Ureteral injury accounts for 3% to 5% of all traumatic injuries of the urinary tract. The majority of cases are the result of iatrogenic injury. Although gynecologic surgery leads the list, abdominal–perineal resection, cystectomy, vascular surgery, and spinal fusion all have been implicated. The ureter is well protected, and therefore traumatic injury is rare; penetrating trauma is much more likely than blunt trauma to cause injury.

Typical CT findings in ureteral disruption include normal renal enhancement, medial perirenal contrast extravasation, and nonopacification of the ipsilateral distal ureter. Extrarenal contrast has been concentrated by the kidney and is more radiodense than intravascular or oral contrast material. When there is a question of ureteral injury, early imaging, followed by delayed imaging (5 minutes after intravenous contrast administration), is suggested.

Antegrade pyelography can be performed to diagnose the ureteral tear and may be followed by interventions such as percutaneous nephrostomy or nephroureteral stent placement. One study of 44 patients with ureteral injury compared treatment with surgery to that with percutaneous nephrostomy alone. Those patients treated with percutaneous nephrostomy had significantly fewer secondary operations, had lower morbidity, and had spontaneous repair of the damaged ureter in the majority of cases.

Notes

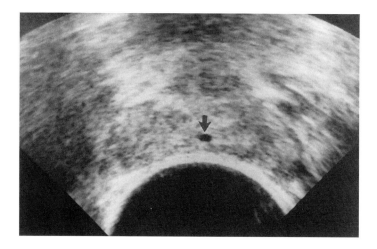

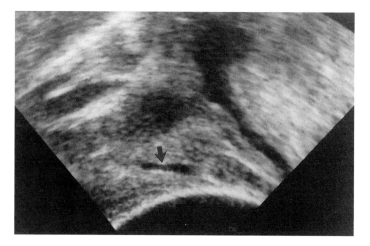

1. Transaxial and sagittal ultrasound images of the prostate in a patient with primary infertility are shown. Both seminal vesicles were hypoplastic. To what lesion does the arrow point?

2. What are some of the most common abnormalities that can be seen in infertile men on transrectal sonography?

3. What criteria can be used to diagnose seminal vesicle hypoplasia and atrophy?

4. In the infertile man what is the value of ultrasound-guided aspiration of a supraprostatic cyst?

Ejaculatory Duct Ectasia and Seminal Vesicle Hypoplasia

1. Ectatic ejaculatory duct.

2. Bilateral absence of the vas deferens; obstruction of the vas deferens, seminal vesicles, and ejaculatory ducts by prostatic calcification or fibrosis; and cysts of the seminal vesicles, vas deferens, ejaculatory ducts, or prostate.

3. Seminal vesicle size; hypoplastic seminal vesicles are defined as being smaller than 11 mm but larger than 7 mm, and atrophic seminal vesicles are smaller than 7 mm.

4. It may relieve obstruction of the vas deferens. Cystic fluid may contain viable sperm that can be used for in vitro fertilization.

Reference

Kuligowska E, Fenlon HM: Transrectal US in male infertility: spectrum of findings and role in patient care, *Radiology* 207:173-181, 1998.

Cross-Reference

Genitourinary Radiology: THE REQUISITES, pp 276, 304-305.

Comment

Medical imaging plays an important part in the evaluation of the infertile man. In particular, the distal genital tract can be investigated for congenital defects or obstruction with vasography, transrectal sonography (TRUS), or MRI. The patient in this case had bilateral vasal and seminal vesicle hypoplasia and a dilated ejaculatory duct on TRUS.

In the cited reference, Kuligowska and Fenlon evaluated 276 infertile men with azoospermia and low ejaculate volumes (<1.5 ml) using TRUS. The single largest group of abnormalities was congenital anomalies of the vas deferens—unilateral or bilateral absence or aplasia of the vas. There was a constant association between vasal agenesis with abnormalities of the seminal vesicles or ejaculatory ducts, including cyst formation or obstruction by fibrosis or calcification. This constellation of abnormalities is explained by the common origin of the distal male genital tract from the mesonephric (Wolffian) duct. Bilateral vasal agenesis also may be associated with renal anomalies (renal agenesis, cross-fused ectopia, or an ectopic pelvic kidney) in up to 43% of patients and may occur as part of the clinical spectrum of cystic fibrosis.

Some ductal anomalies confined to the distal two thirds of the ejaculatory ducts are surgically correctable. These anomalies include ejaculatory duct cysts, calculi, fibrosis, and calcification. Agenesis, obstruction, or occlusion of the ductal system proximal to this level is not correctable by surgery; in vitro fertilization with epididymal aspirates may be necessary in these cases.

Notes

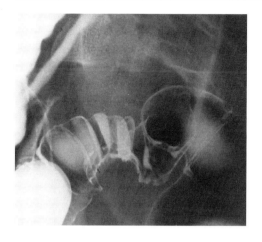
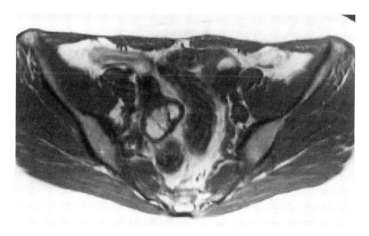
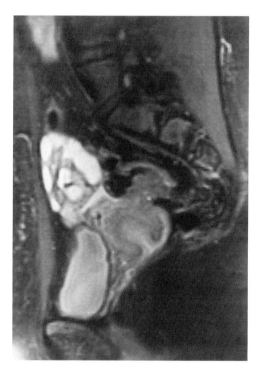

1. What is the differential diagnosis for the abnormal finding on the air-contrast barium enema?
2. What are the abnormal findings on MRI?
3. What primary malignancies are associated with colonic serosal metastases?
4. Could the diagnosis be made by colonoscopic biopsy in this case?

Endometriosis of the Sigmoid Colon

1. Polyp or other submucosal tumor.

2. The T1W and fat saturated T2W images show a right adnexal mass; the fat saturated T2W image shows a mass, similar in signal intensity to myometrium, involving the rectosigmoid colon.

3. Ovarian carcinoma and melanoma.

4. Probably not; mucosa looks intact.

Reference

Weed JC, Ray JE: Endometriosis of the bowel, *Obstet Gynecol* 69:727-730, 1987.

Cross-Reference

Genitourinary Radiology: THE REQUISITES, pp 258-260.

Comment

Endometriosis most commonly involves the ovaries, uterosacral ligaments, Douglas cul-de-sac, serosal surface of the uterus, and fallopian tubes. However, it has been estimated that 50% of patients with severe endometriosis have some degree of bowel involvement. Progressive endometriosis of the alimentary or lower urinary tract may produce fibrotic masses that can mimic a serosal or submucosal mass, or postoperative or postinflammatory adhesions.

Endometriosis of the alimentary tract most often affects the rectosigmoid colon, ileum, or appendix. Although multiple symptoms have been reported (diarrhea, constipation, rectal bleeding, abdominal distention, and partial or complete bowel obstruction), virtually all are cyclic, coinciding with menstrual function. Because the serosa is involved first, a stricture-forming lesion or an eccentric mural filling defect is most often visible on barium enema examination. In some cases endometriosis may encircle the bowel and mimic an "apple core" carcinoma. Deep penetration of endometriosis may even result in mucosal destruction, but this finding is unusual. Unlike rectosigmoid endometriosis, colon cancer is generally painless and causes intermittent rather than cyclic bleeding. Endometriosis of the bowel may require implant or bowel resection if medical treatments (i.e., medroxyprogesterone acetate, combined estrogen and progestin oral contraceptives, androgen derivatives, or gonadotropin-releasing hormone agonist) are unsuccessful.

Notes

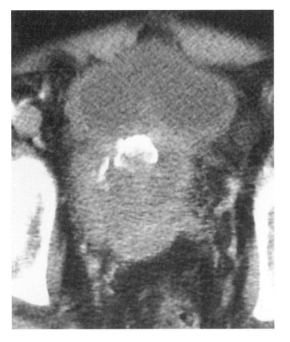 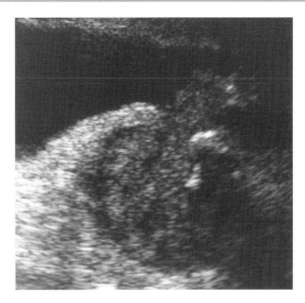

1. Explain the abnormal shape of the urinary bladder.
2. Worldwide, what is the most common cause of bladder wall calcification?
3. What is alkaline encrustation cystitis?
4. What is the most likely diagnosis in this case?

Carcinoma Arising in a Bladder Diverticulum

1. There is a large bladder diverticulum.

2. Bilharzial cystitis.

3. A form of chronic cystitis in which the inflamed or devitalized mucosa is covered by a layer of calcium phosphate, the precipitation of which is enhanced by alkaluria.

4. Carcinoma arising from a bladder diverticulum.

Reference

Dondalski M, White EM, Ghahremani GG, Patel SK: Carcinoma arising in urinary bladder diverticula: imaging findings in six patients, *Am J Roentgenol* 161:817-820, 1993.

Cross-Reference

Genitourinary Radiology: THE REQUISITES, pp 211-212.

Comment

In this case a transitional cell carcinoma (TCC) is growing from the dextrolateral wall of a bladder diverticulum, and the diverticular neck arises from the posterior wall of the urinary bladder. The ultrasound study shows that a papillary component of the TCC has grown through the neck of the diverticulum and into the lumen of the bladder.

Stasis of urine or long-standing infection may incite inflammatory changes in the mucosa of bladder diverticula, and neoplasm develops in 2% to 7%. In 80% of cases the histologic tumor type is TCC, but squamous cell carcinoma, adenocarcinoma, and mixed carcinoma have been reported. Carcinoma arising within bladder diverticula has a poorer prognosis than cancers of the native bladder because of early transmural spread. In the case presented note the thickened dextrolateral wall of the diverticulum and the lacy strands of tumor in the perivesical fat that indicate transmural spread (stage C or T_{3b}).

Cystography and cross-sectional imaging are more reliable than excretory urography and cystoscopy for the evaluation of complications of bladder diverticula. Although bladder diverticula are often demonstrated on urography, masses that arise within diverticula may be overlooked. Cystoscopy is a reliable method for diagnosing most mucosal bladder tumors, but those arising in diverticula may be inaccessible to the cystoscope, particularly if the diverticular neck is narrow. A diverticular bladder neoplasm may appear as an intraluminal filling defect, mass, or focus of mucosal irregularity. Incomplete contrast opacification of a diverticulum, failure of a previously identified diverticulum to fill, and ipsilateral ureteral obstruction are additional signs.

Notes

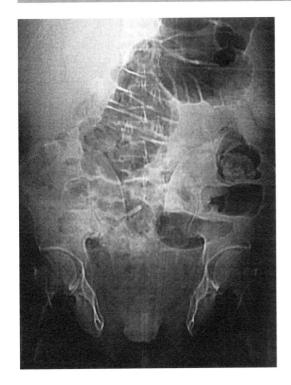
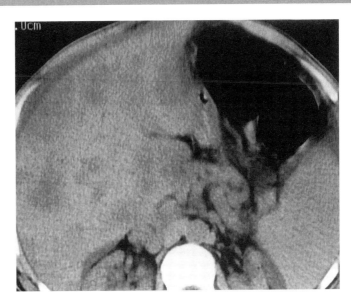
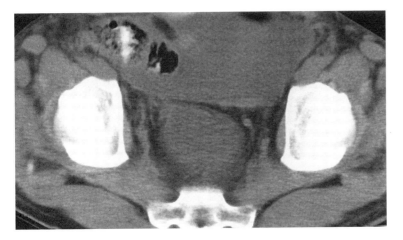

1. What is the major finding on the digital radiograph?
2. What conditions are associated with this finding?
3. What surgical procedure is performed on these patients?
4. What complications are associated with this surgery?

Metastatic Rectal Carcinoma After Urinary Diversion

1. Wide diastasis of the symphysis pubis.

2. Primary conditions are bladder exstrophy, epispadias, and cleidocranial dysplasia; a secondary consideration for pubic diastasis is traumatic injury.

3. Ureteral diversion.

4. Patients are at increased risk for bladder carcinoma and rectal carcinoma if ureteral diversion is performed to an undiverted segment of colon.

Reference

deRiese W, Warmbold H: Adenocarcinoma in exstrophy of the bladder: a case report and review of the literature, *Int Urol Nephrol* 18(2):159-162, 1986.

Cross-Reference

Genitourinary Radiology: THE REQUISITES, p 193.

Comment

Bladder exstrophy is an extremely rare condition, with an estimated incidence of 1 in 50,000 births. There is a 3:1 male predominance. The condition is caused by a defect in closure of the lower anterior abdominal wall and the anterior bladder. The anomaly is always associated with diastasis of the symphysis pubis and epispadias. Complications resulting from untreated disease include urinary tract infection and an increased risk of bladder carcinoma, particularly adenocarcinoma. Treatment is surgical and includes closure of the anterior abdominal wall defect and creation of a urinary diversion to an ileal conduit or isolated loop of colon. The epispadias (malformation where the urethra opens on the dorsum of the penis) can be repaired surgically, and these patients have normal fertility.

Initially the ureters were diverted to nonisolated colon. However, these sigmoid diversions were associated with an increased risk for colon carcinoma, presumably caused by the chemical irritation resulting from mixing urine with fecal material in the rectum. This patient had a urinary diversion to a loop of nondiverted sigmoid colon 28 years earlier but had no medical follow up. He had abdominal pain and on CT was found to have advanced rectal carcinoma with hepatic metastases.

Notes

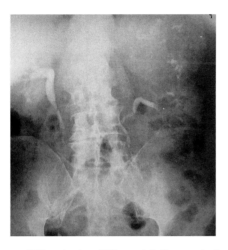 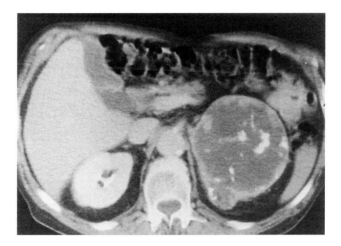

1. What is the differential diagnosis for this large left suprarenal mass?
2. To make a management recommendation, is knowledge about adrenal hyperfunction necessary?
3. If a surgeon is asked to biopsy this mass, does he or she need to know about adrenal hyperfunction?
4. What are phleboliths?

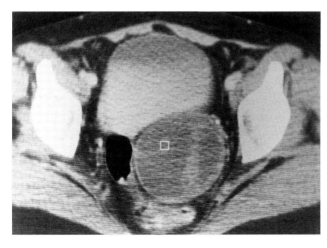 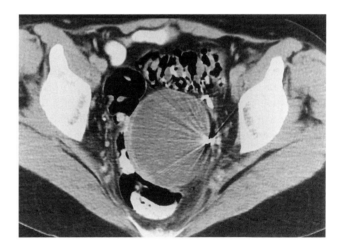

1. What are the four most common histologic types of ovarian cancer?
2. The CT image on the left was obtained 15 years before the image on the right. Does this time course suggest a particular type of ovarian tumor?
3. Hormone production is a characteristic of which pathologic type of ovarian neoplasm?
4. Name several clinical presentations of hormone-producing ovarian tumors.

Adrenal Hemangioma

1. Chronic adrenal hemorrhage, pheochromocytoma, metastasis, adrenocortical carcinoma, and mesenchymal tumor.

2. Yes.

3. Yes.

4. *Dorland's Medical Dictionary* defines a phlebolith as a calculus or concretion in a vein; a vein stone.

Reference

Sabanegh E Jr, Harris MJ, Grider D: Cavernous adrenal hemangioma, *Urology* 42:327-330, 1993.

Cross-Reference

Genitourinary Radiology: THE REQUISITES, pp 361-364.

Comment

Hemangiomas can occur in almost any organ; there have been roughly 30 reported cases of these benign, mesenchymal tumors arising from the adrenal gland. Because they are usually non-hyperfunctional, hemangiomas are usually large (more than 10 cm in diameter) at the time of incidental discovery. Calcifications have been reported in two thirds of cases and can appear as dystrophic clumps or crescents, can be more characteristic phleboliths, or can be both; the facetious question about phleboliths was intended to be a clue. When large, hemangiomas can be complicated by areas of fibrosis, necrosis, thrombosis, or hemorrhage. Peripheral, nodular enhancement can be evident on CT and may be an important clue to the diagnosis.

Given its size and heterogeneous appearance on urography and enhanced CT, this tumor was removed. The intent of the second and third questions was to caution the radiologist about the risks of biopsy or surgery on an unsuspected pheochromocytoma.

Notes

Ovarian Stromal Tumor (Granulosa Cell Tumor)

1. Epithelial, germ cell, stromal sex cord, and metastatic disease.

2. Yes. A benign, solid neoplasm, such as a stromal tumor or a benign germ cell tumor.

3. Stromal.

4. Menstrual abnormalities, sexual precocity, vaginal bleeding (estrogen production), and virilization or hirsutism (androgen production).

References

Hines JF, Khalifa MA, Moore JL, et al: Recurrent granulosa cell tumor of the ovary 37 years after initial diagnosis: a case report and review of the literature, *Gynecol Oncol* 60(3):484-488, 1996.

MacSweeney JE, King DM: Computed tomography, diagnosis, staging and follow-up of pure granulosa cell tumor of the ovary, *Clin Radiol* 49(4):241-245, 1994.

Cross-Reference

Genitourinary Radiology: THE REQUISITES, pp 278-281.

Comment

Ovarian neoplasm has four main histologic types with various subtypes. Epithelial ovarian neoplasms are the most common, accounting for 65% of ovarian malignancies. Approximately 65% of epithelial neoplasms are benign.

The two least common tumors of the ovary are sex cord stromal tumors and metastatic disease to the ovary. Each accounts for approximately 5% of ovarian neoplasms. Sex cord stromal tumors have three subtypes—fibroma-thecoma, granulosa cell tumor, and Sertoli-Leydig tumor (listed in descending order of frequency). The fibroma-thecoma is a benign fibrous tumor that may be associated with ascites and a right effusion, or Meigs syndrome. Granulosa cell tumors originate from the ovarian stroma and can secrete estrogen; 66% occur in postmenopausal women, may lead to endometrial hyperplasia or endometrial carcinoma, and can present with postmenopausal bleeding. In younger patients the estrogen production may cause precocious puberty. This case is typical of granulosa cell tumors in that the tumor responds to surgical therapy but can recur up to 20 years after the original resection. Patients with this tumor have a good prognosis; the 10-year survival rate is greater than 85%.

Notes

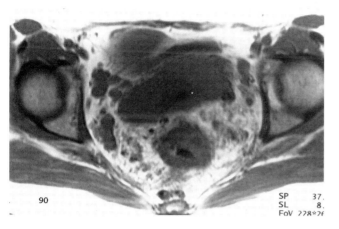 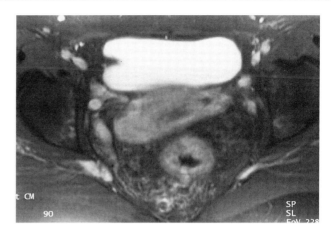

1. Describe the findings on the MR image to the left.
2. Describe the findings on the MR image to the right. Is this a T1W image?
3. What parts of the uterus normally enhance on MRI?
4. What is the differential diagnosis of the lesion shown in this case?

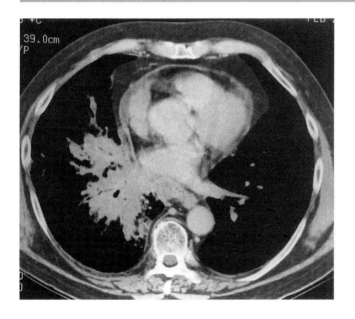 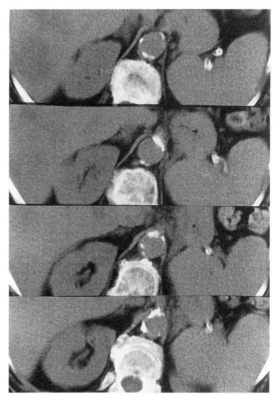

1. CT scans of the chest and abdomen in a patient with Cushing's syndrome are shown. What is the potential cause of the endocrinopathy?
2. What other tumors can cause ectopic corticotropin syndrome?
3. What is the most common cause of ectopic corticotropin-releasing hormone syndrome?
4. What are the causes of corticotropin-independent Cushing's syndrome?

CASE 198

Cavernous Hemangioma of the Rectum

1. Transaxial spin-echo T1W image shows multiple, small, round and ovoid masses around the rectum and uterus.

2. On this enhanced transaxial spin-echo T1W image with fat saturation, abnormal enhancement of these masses is evident.

3. Junctional zone of the uterus does not enhance as much as the endometrium or outer myometrium.

4. Vascular malformation or tumor and acute radiation proctitis.

Reference

Tan TCF, Wang JY, Cheung YC, Wan WYL: Diffuse cavernous hemangioma of the rectum complicated by invasion of pelvic structures: report of two cases, *Dis Colon Rectum* 41:1062-1066, 1998.

Cross-Reference

Genitourinary Radiology: THE REQUISITES, pp 33-37.

Comment

This 43-year-old woman had a history of recurrent rectal bleeding and had already undergone several unsuccessful hemorrhoidectomies. The MR images show multiple vessels in the perirectal fat that appear to radiate outward from the rectum, and the uterus is encompassed by this tangle of vessels.

The invasive growth pattern of diffuse cavernous hemangioma of the rectum distinguishes it from other vascular lesions of the intestines, including capillary hemangioma, circumscribed cavernous hemangioma, multiple phlebectasia, and angiomatosis. The typical clinical history consists of multiple episodes of progressive, painless, and often massive rectal bleeding. In contrast to circumscribed cavernous hemangioma, which typically presents as a focal polypoid mass, diffuse cavernous hemangioma of the rectum begins in the rectal wall but infiltrates the pelvic retroperitoneum in a manner similar to pelvic lipomatosis. As in this case, the uterus may be invaded, and infiltration of the bladder also has been reported. Mass effect from the tumor may obstruct the ureter or iliac veins, and fistulas may form when the tumor erodes through the rectal wall into contiguous organs.

The diagnosis can be suggested from a battery of imaging tests. Multiple pelvic phleboliths are visible on conventional radiographs in about half of all cases. Narrowing of the rectum on barium enema may mimic an infiltrating carcinoma. CT and MRI demonstrate the engorged rectum, multiple enhancing serpentine vessels radiating from the rectum, and abnormal enhancement of infiltrated pelvic organs. Definitive therapy for this tumor usually requires surgery because transcatheter vascular ablation only temporarily controls rectal hemorrhage.

Notes

CASE 199

Cushing's Syndrome: Ectopic Corticotropin Syndrome

1. Small cell carcinoma of the lung.

2. Carcinoid tumors of the bronchus, thymus, or pancreas; medullary carcinomas of the thyroid or pheochromocytoma; or other neuroendocrine tumors.

3. Bronchial carcinoid tumor.

4. Adrenocortical tumors and nodular adrenal hyperplasia.

Reference

Orth DN: Cushing's syndrome, *N Engl J Med* 332(12):791-803, 1995.

Cross-Reference

Genitourinary Radiology: THE REQUISITES, pp 364-366.

Comment

The causes of Cushing's syndrome may be corticotropin dependent (i.e., inappropriately high levels of plasma corticotropin) or corticotropin independent (i.e., abnormal adrenocortical tissue produces excessive cortisol). By a five to one ratio, the most common cause of corticotropin-dependent Cushing's syndrome is Cushing's disease (excessive secretion of corticotropin by pituitary corticotroph tumors, usually microadenomas). Acute ectopic corticotropin syndrome is associated with small cell carcinoma of the lung in 75% of cases and results in hypertension, edema, hypokalemia, and glucose intolerance. The chronic ectopic corticotropin syndrome is clinically indistinguishable from Cushing's disease and is caused by various neuroendocrine tumors listed above. These same tumors also can cause Cushing's syndrome by the excessive production of corticotropin-releasing hormone (CRH). CRH is normally synthesized in the hypothalamus and is the most potent regulator of corticotropin secretion by the anterior pituitary.

Excluding exogenous corticosteroid administration, overproduction of cortisol or cortisol precursors is the main cause of corticotropin-independent Cushing's syndrome. Adrenal adenomas tend to synthesize cortisol exclusively, so that precursor production is relatively low and virilization is rare. In contrast, adrenocortical carcinomas are relatively inefficient at producing cortisol, androgenic precursors also are secreted in excess, and virilization is common.

Notes

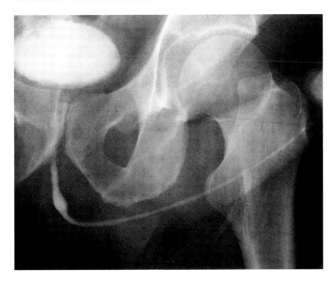

1. What type of study was performed?
2. What is the abnormal finding?
3. What is the differential diagnosis?
4. True or False: One cause of this lesion has been linked to urethral sarcoma.

Balanitis Xerotica Obliterans

1. Cystourethrogram.

2. Diffuse narrowing of the penile urethra.

3. Postinfectious urethritis, long-term urethral catheterization, chemical urethritis (rare), and balanitis xerotica obliterans (BXO) (rare).

4. False (squamous cell carcinoma of the penis).

Reference
Staff WG: Urethral involvement in balanitis xerotica obliterans, *Br J Urol* 47:234-237, 1970.

Cross-Reference
Genitourinary Radiology: THE REQUISITES, pp 235-237.

Comment
Don't worry about making the correct diagnosis of BXO in this case; it is truly the "spotted zebra" of urethral inflammatory diseases. BXO is a localized variant of lichen sclerosis et atrophicus, a skin disease of unknown etiology that causes white, thickened plaques on the glans, penis, prepuce, and urethral meatus. It may result in phimosis or meatal stenosis. Uncommonly the fossa navicularis and the anterior urethra may be involved, and in these cases urethrography may reveal smooth narrowing of the anterior urethra of varying lengths.

The significance of BXO is that it is a premalignant lesion. Penile squamous cell carcinoma may be discovered long after BXO has been treated with topical steroid cream or, if this treatment is not successful, local excision. An interesting aside is that phimosis is found in as many as 75% of patients with squamous cell penile carcinoma and is the most common coexisting abnormality in patients with this malady. It is believed that the closed preputial cavity promotes the development of penile cancer by a carcinogen in smegma (the debris of desquamated cells on the inner surface of the prepuce).

The more common (and therefore more likely) diagnosis for this appearance is a postinfectious urethritis. Postinfectious (either gonococcal or nongonococcal urethritis) strictures may be multiple and may involve several centimeters of the urethra. Rarely the entire anterior urethra may narrow as a result of long-standing inflammation and fibrosis.

Notes